An Introduction to Population-Level Prevention of Non-Communicable Diseases

An Introduction to Population-Level Prevention of Non-Communicable Diseases

Edited by

Mike Rayner
British Heart Foundation Centre on Population Approaches for Non-Communicable Diseases Prevention, Nuffield Department of Population Health, University of Oxford, UK

Kremlin Wickramasinghe
British Heart Foundation Centre on Population Approaches for Non-Communicable Diseases Prevention, Nuffield Department of Population Health, University of Oxford, UK

Julianne Williams
British Heart Foundation Centre on Population Approaches for Non-Communicable Diseases Prevention, Nuffield Department of Population Health, University of Oxford, UK

Karen McColl
Freelance consultant/writer

Shanthi Mendis
Geneva Learning Foundation, Geneva, Switzerland

OXFORD
UNIVERSITY PRESS

OXFORD
UNIVERSITY PRESS

Great Clarendon Street, Oxford, OX2 6DP,
United Kingdom

Oxford University Press is a department of the University of Oxford. It furthers the University's objective of excellence in research, scholarship, and education by publishing worldwide. Oxford is a registered trade mark of Oxford University Press in the UK and in certain other countries

First Edition published in 2017

Impression: 1

Published in the United States of America by Oxford University Press
198 Madison Avenue, New York, NY 10016, United States of America

British Library Cataloguing in Publication Data
Data available

Library of Congress Control Number: 2017930524

ISBN 978–0–19–879118–8

Printed in Great Britain by Ashford Colour Press Ltd, Gosport, Hampshire

Foreword

Non-communicable diseases (NCDs), including heart disease, stroke, cancer, diabetes, and chronic lung disease, are collectively responsible for more than two-thirds of all deaths worldwide. Primarily four risk factors are responsible for the burden of NCDs: tobacco use, physical inactivity, the harmful use of alcohol, and unhealthy diets.

Almost three-quarters of all deaths from NCDs before the age of 70 occur in low- and middle-income countries. For a long time there was a strong belief that NCDs are associated with affluent lifestyles. But current statistics clearly show that not just developed countries, but low- and middle-income countries face a growing burden of NCDs and that it is in some of the poorest populations around the world where NCDs have the greatest impact.

In 2011 a high-level meeting of the United Nations recognized the growing burden of NCDs as a threat to global development and called for actions from heads of state to tackle the issue. The inclusion of a goal to reduce premature mortality from NCDs by one-third in the Sustainable Development Goals agreed in 2015 was a turning point in scaling up the global response. The World Health Organization (WHO) recommends a series of actions to tackle NCDs and they can be categorized as the following: improved governance, tackling risk factors more effectively, strengthening health systems, and better monitoring and evaluation. Health systems in all but a few countries are more focused on treatment of individuals with disease than prevention. Population-level prevention approaches such as national-level policies to raise taxes on tobacco or restrict the marketing of unhealthy food and drinks to children are likely to be extremely cost-effective, but many countries lack the capacity to implement such actions.

Since 2012 the WHO Collaborating Centre on Population Approaches for Non-Communicable Disease Prevention at the Nuffield Department for Population Health, University of Oxford has organized a regular short course on population approaches to NCD prevention. With the participation of other experts, including representatives of WHO, the course aims to build capacity for population-level action to tackle NCDs. However, given the large number of trained professionals needed to tackle this global issue, a face-to-face training programme is not able to reach everyone who requires the knowledge and skills necessary for effective action.

An Introduction to Population-Level Prevention of Non-Communicable Diseases is mainly based on material presented at the course, and it provides an exciting opportunity for this to be shared with a greater global audience. This book brings together evidence about different aspects of the problem of NCDs and their solution for academics, policy-makers, and other practitioners. It is structured around the key steps of the policy cycle and encourages evidence-based policy-making and evaluation at a population level.

While providing the general principles and scientific basis to population-level prevention for NCDs, it also provides case studies from countries around the world seeking to implement such prevention in practice.

I hope this book will play a significant role in our global response to the prevention of NCDs in coming years and decades. I congratulate the authors on this publication and wish every success for the dissemination and future updates.

Dr Oleg Chestnov
Assistant Director-General—Noncommunicable Diseases
and Mental Health World Health Organization

Acknowledgements

We would like to thank all the participants and resource persons who have presented at the short course on Prevention Strategies for Non-Communicable Diseases run by the University of Oxford. This book is based on presentations made during short courses held between 2012 and 2015. Presenters during these courses included the following: Steve Allender, Virginia Arnold, Prachi Bhatnagar, Francesco Branca, Adam Briggs, Simon Capewell, Sudeep Chand, Michel Coleman, Gill Cowburn, Aiden Doherty, Kaia Engesveen, Charlie Foster, Gauden Galea, Simon Gillespie, Celina Gorre, Corinna Hawkes, Shabbar Jaffar, Prasad Katulanda, Mike Kelly, Paul Kelly, Mike Knapton, Alexandra Krettek, David Matthews, Karina McHardy, Klim McPherson, Shanthi Mendis, Bente Mikkelsen, Colin Mitchell, Modi Mwatsama, Oliver Mytton, Melanie Nichols, Brian Oldenburg, Richard Peto, Emma Plugge, Johanna Ralston, Mike Rayner, Srinath Reddy, Aaron Reeves, Justin Richards, Harry Rutter, Peter Scarborough, David Stuckler, William Summerskill, Nick Townsend, Temo Waqanivalu, Kremlin Wickramasinghe, Denis Xavier, and Xuefeng Zhong.

This book contains a number of case studies. The following individuals contributed to these cases studies or provided other additional material for the book: Luke Allen, Simone Bösch, Hannah Brinsden, Linda Cobiac, Dylan Collins, Alessandro de Maio, Randa Hamadeh, Erin Hoare, Nousin Hussain, Kiran Jobanputra, Sandeep Kishore, Alexandra Krettek, Tim Lang, Nijole Gostautaite Midttun, Modi Mwatsama, Jessica Pullar, Nabil Sulaiman, Anne-Marie Thow, Daniel Vujcich, Temo Waqanivalu, and Rouham Yamout.

We also appreciate the help of Sahar Bhatti, Oluwatosin Ogunmoyero, Anja Mizdrak, and Lizzie Wilkins, who documented presentations and discussions from the short course. We would also like to thank all our colleagues at the British Heart Foundation Centre on Population Approaches for Non-Communicable Disease Prevention, Nuffield Department of Population Health, University of Oxford and the Department for Continuing Education, University of Oxford for their support throughout this publication. Finally, we are so grateful for the team at the Oxford University Press, who worked very hard to publish this book on a tight timeline. Thank you to James Cox, Geraldine Jeffers, Catherine Barnes, and Nicola Wilson for their tireless help as we prepared the manuscript for publication.

Contents

Abbreviations

ANGELO	analysis grid for elements linked to obesity
ATLAS	Active Teen Leaders Avoiding Screen Time
BMI	body mass index
BMJ	British Medical Journal
BRFSS	Behavioural Risk Factor Surveillance Study
BSE	bovine spongiform encephalopathy
CASH	Consensus Action on Salt and Health
CDC	Centers for Disease Control and Prevention
CER	cost-effectiveness ratio
CFIR	Consolidated Framework for Implementation Research
CHD	coronary heart disease
CHP	community health programme
COPD	chronic obstructive pulmonary disease
CPG	Coronary Prevention Group
CVD	cardiovascular disease
DALY	disability-adjusted life years
DfID	Department for International Development
DHS	Demograghic and Health Survey
DNAP	District Nutrition Action Plan
FCTC	Framework Convention on Tobacco Control
FFQ	Food Frequency Questionnaire
FSA	Food Standards Agency
GBD	Global Burden of Disease
GDA	guideline daily amount
GSHS	Global School-Based Health Survey
HARDIC	Heart-Health Associated Research and Dissemination in the Community
HDSS	Health Demographic Surveillance System
INFORMAS	International Network for Obesity Research, Monitoring and Action Support
INPARD	Integrating Nutrition Promotion and Rural Development
ISH	Internal Society of Hypertension
IMF	International Monetary Fund
LMIC	low- and middle-income countries
LY	life year
MAFF	Ministry of Agriculture, Fisheries and Food
MOPH	Ministry of Public Health
MSAP	multisectoral action plan
MSF	*Médecins sans Frontières*
NCD	non-communicable disease

NGO	Non-governmental organization
NICE	National Institute for Health and Care Excellence
NNCDC	National NCD Committee
NSDF	National Strategic Development Framework
OECD	Organisation for Economic Cooperation and Development
PAR	population attributable risk
PBAC	Pharmaceutical Benefits Advisory Committee
PHARMAC	Pharmaceutical Management Agency
QALY	quality-adjusted life year
RCT	randomized controlled trial
SDG	sustainable development goal
SES	socioeconomic status
SPAGHL	Samoan Parliamentary Advocacy Group on Healthy Lifestyles
SSB	sugar-sweetened beverages
UN	United Nations
UNDP	United Nations Development Programme
WHA	World Health Assembly
WHO	World Health Organization
WHO PEN	WHO Package of Essential NCD Interventions for Primary Health Care in Low-Resource Settings
WTO	World Trade Organization
YLD	years lived with disability
YLL	years of life lost
YP-CDN	Young Professionals-Chronic Disease Network

Part I

Introduction

Chapter 1

Introduction

1.1 Aims of the book

This book is intended to capture the material covered in an accredited six-day short course on Prevention Strategies for Non-communicable Diseases which takes place in Oxford. This course is organized by the British Heart Foundation Centre on Population Approaches for Non-communicable Disease Prevention of the Nuffield Department of Population Health at the University of Oxford and the Department of Continuing Education at the University Oxford. This document also encompasses material discussed during a workshop on Non-communicable Disease Prevention: Policy Development and Implementation Issues in Low- and Middle-Income Countries, organized jointly by the World Health Organization and the University of Oxford, which has drawn the first two courses to an end. Speakers for both the course and the workshop are selected to share their expertise and engage in debates on some of the most contentious and challenging issues facing non-communicable disease (NCD) prevention today. To complement the content of the short courses and workshops, some additional contributors have provided material on issues not previously covered. In addition, many case studies are included to illustrate NCD prevention in practice.

This document reflects the breadth of the material covered and also highlights some key discussion points. It is expected that this document will provide useful information for individuals and organizations interested in NCDs and their prevention, in particular public health practitioners, policy-makers, post-graduate students, and early career level professionals working in the field of NCDs. There is a need for training courses and materials to help equip such interested parties to design, implement, and evaluate strategies for NCD control; this document has been designed with this need in mind, particularly in the context of low- and middle-income countries (LMICs).

1.2 How the book is structured

This document is structured to reflect the strategy- or policy-making cycle shown in Figure 1.1.

Part II covers problem definition, the first stage of the policy cycle. Problem definition involves establishing the nature and the extent of the problem of NCDs in a particular

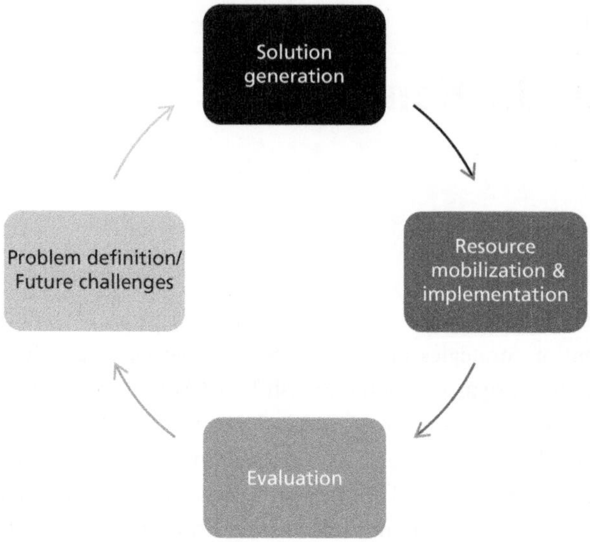

Figure 1.1 The strategy/policy-making cycle.

situation. It also involves consideration of the causes of the problem (such as NCD risk factors) and the wider determinants of health. Chapter 2 sets out an initial understanding of what NCDs are and the burden they present to low-, middle-, and high-income countries. It goes on to explore the risk factors and determinants of NCDs throughout the life course (Chapter 3) and the sociopolitical landscape, including the competing interests that can render NCD prevention more challenging (Chapter 4). The section then sets out how the global response to NCDs is shifting from apathy to action (Chapter 5) and the important role of public health advocacy in tackling NCDs (Chapter 6). Finally, the section takes a more operational look at how to define the problem in a particular context, through use of screening and/or surveillance (Chapter 7).

The second stage of the policy-making cycle is solution generation, which involves assessing the evidence for the potential costs and benefits of a particular intervention, considering potential barriers to, and facilitators of, different solutions and prioritizing possible actions, and finally, developing a plan. Solution generation is explored in Part III (Chapters 8–10). Chapters 8 and 9 examine the types of evidence required for population-level approaches to NCD prevention. More specifically, addressing approaches to evaluating effectiveness and cost effectiveness and modelling different interventions. Chapter 10 outlines the steps involved in building a prevention strategy and introduces some tools for priority setting.

Part IV addresses the important issue of resource mobilization and implementation (sometimes referred to as 'capacity building'). Chapter 11 provides some pointers for implementation, including the critical importance of strengthening health systems (Chapter 12), how to consider tackling inequalities, the key role of disadvantaged groups as stakeholders in the process, and the fundamental need to reach beyond the health sector and develop multisectoral solutions to the challenges of NCDs (Chapter 13).

It is vital that progress towards goals and targets is monitored and that programmes and interventions are evaluated. Part V addresses evaluation and monitoring, which is the fourth stage of the policy cycle. Evaluations may assess whether the interventions for preventing NCDs, once implemented, met their aims and objectives or to generate evidence which may be generalized to other situations. Chapter 14 outlines different types of evaluation and identifies some of the core issues to consider when evaluating a programme. It also sets out the issues in formulating an evaluation plan, and the choice of reliable and valid measures, as well as highlighting some of the challenges in relation to reporting and monitoring progress towards goals. Finally, Chapter 15 emphasizes policy-making as a cyclical process in which the various steps must be revisited in order to ask new questions about the problem and the solutions before proceeding to a new round of implementation.

1.3 **Key concepts**

The three concepts of prevention, treatment (or control), and care are not competing and should instead be seen as complementary in the fight against NCDs. Prevention, treatment, and care are all important responses to the global NCD problem. It is notable, for example, that two of the nine voluntary targets in Global NCD Action Plan relate to treatment. The main focus of this book, however, is on population approaches to prevention.

1.4 **Prevention**

While the primary focus of this document is on prevention, it is important to recognize that it is neither feasible nor desirable to devote all resources to prevention. In effect, this would mean ignoring the millions of people already affected by NCDs who would then go on to develop complications or have their conditions deteriorate. There are considerable areas of overlap and prevention, cure, and care can be seen to exist on a continuum of activities that are needed to successfully tackle any disease (see Figure 1.2).

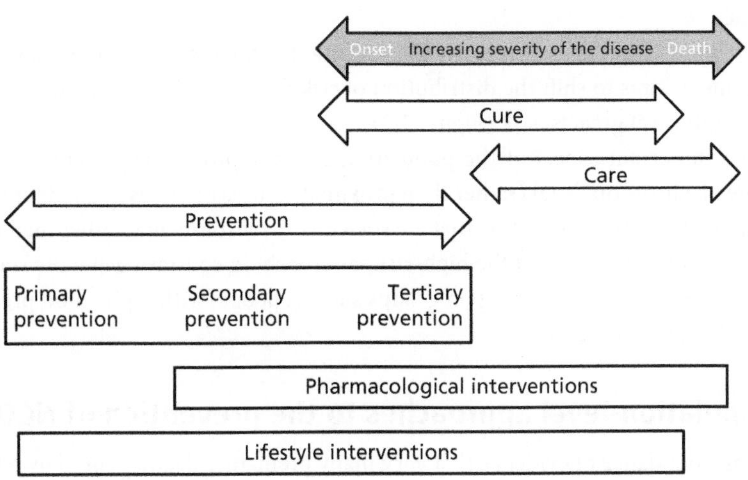

Figure 1.2 Continuum of care, cure, and prevention.

As shown in the figure, there are different levels of prevention:

- **Primary prevention** applies before the onset of a disease and aims to prevent it from occurring;
- **Secondary prevention** is used before the onset of a disease with individuals at high risk of developing that disease with the aim of detecting those individuals as early as possible;
- **Tertiary prevention** applies when the person already has established disease and aims to prevent or limit the condition from worsening, to slow down its progression, or to prevent complications.

Some authors would add 'primordial prevention' to this list, referring to a form of prevention—prior to primary prevention—that aims to establish and maintain the conditions for promoting health.

All forms of prevention, whether primary, secondary, or tertiary, can involve pharmacological interventions—aimed at reducing intermediate risk factors such as raised blood pressure or raised blood cholesterol levels—as well as interventions aimed at behavioural risk factors. This document focuses on prevention via behaviour change but this is not to say that pharmacological interventions do not also have an important role to play in the prevention of NCDs.

1.5 Population-level approaches to prevention

Public health can be defined as 'the science and art of preventing disease and promoting health through the organized efforts of society, organizations, communities, families and individuals'.[1] Crucially, public health programmes aim to improve the health, not only of individuals but also of groups (families, communities, the whole population of a country). WHO's global action plan recognizes that it is not possible to tackle NCDs by only aiming interventions at individuals, and embraces both the population and individual approaches.

A population-based approach to NCD prevention, which is the predominant focus of this document, aims to shift the distribution of risk factors in the population as a whole, rather than those at greatest risk (Figure 1.3).

Another important aspect of the population-based approach to prevention is that it puts more of a focus on distal (rather than proximal) causes of disease—in other words, it places more importance on factors that are societal or environmental rather than individual. The individual (also called the high-risk) approach, in contrast, generally starts with intermediate risk factors, focusing on groups such as people with high blood pressure or high blood cholesterol levels.

1.6 Population-level approaches to the prevention of NCDs

There is an abundance of evidence that very many premature deaths caused by NCDs are avoidable and that prevention can work.

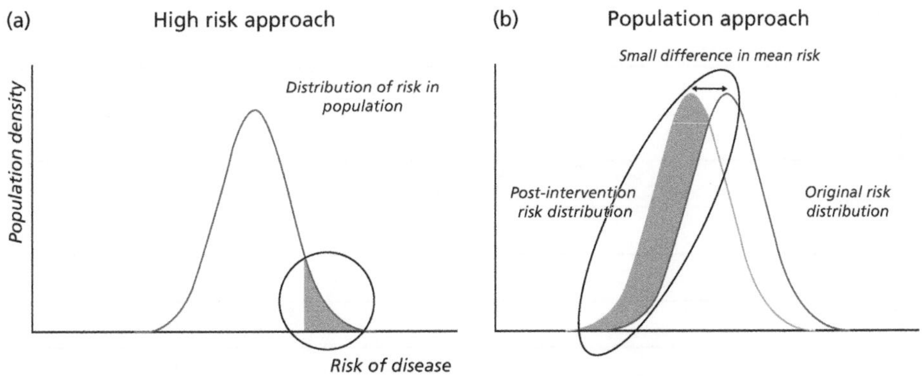

Figure 1.3 Relative gains of a population approach versus a high-risk approach. These figures, adapted from Geoffrey Rose's seminal work *The Strategy of Preventive Medicine*, illustrate the benefits of a population-based approach. The curve on the left illustrates how risk is distributed in a normal population—with much larger numbers with an intermediate level of risk and smaller numbers at high or low risk. A prevention approach which targets high-risk individuals (a) would have the effect of cutting off the tail of the curve with reduced risk shown as the shaded area. A population-based approach, which aims to bring about small changes in the population as a whole, would shift the whole disease curve to the left (b). The health gains, again shown by the shaded area, are therefore much larger, reducing the risk in many more people.

Adapted with permission from Rose G. *Rose's strategy of preventive medicine*. Revised edition with commentary from Kay-Tee Khaw and Michael Marmot. Oxford: Oxford University Press, Copyright © 2008 Oxford University Press.

Factors that point to the substantial avoidability of premature deaths from NCDs include the following:

- Geographic variation—every disease common in one place is much less common elsewhere;
- Differences between population disease rates are not chiefly genetic;
- Trends—the big changes in disease over time reflect changes in particular causes; and
- Several major causes have been identified, so it is likely that there will be others identified in the future.

There is strong evidence that prevention works in reducing death and disease. Figure 1.4 illustrates the tremendous gains made in reducing death rates from coronary heart disease in several high-income countries in the latter half of the twentieth century. These health gains show that NCD deaths are preventable. Modelling work to analyse the factors contributing to these falling death rates estimates that about 50% of the drop in mortality can be attributed to prevention though reduced exposure to behavioural risk factors[2,3] (see the section in Chapter 8 on impact modelling), and about 50% to improvements in treatment and prevention through pharmacological interventions and surgery.

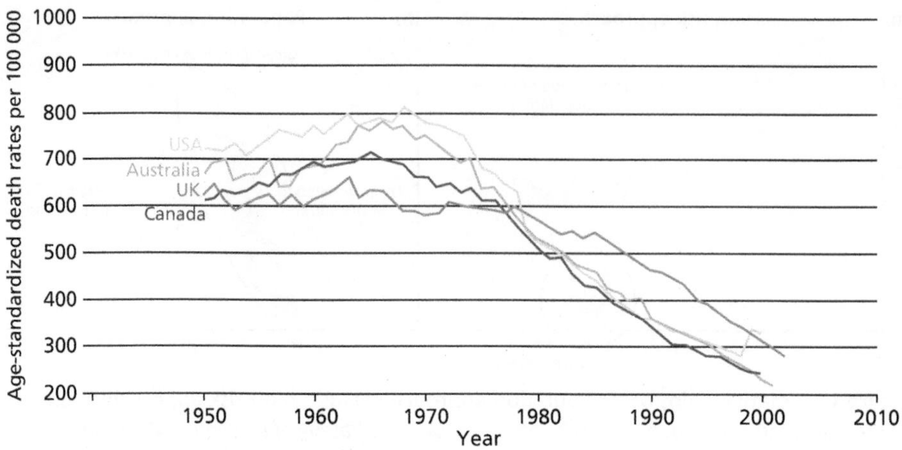

Figure 1.4 NCD deaths are preventable: falling heart disease death rates in four high-income countries, 1950–2002.

Reproduced from WHO. *Preventing chronic diseases: a vital investment.* Geneva: World Health Organization, http://www.who.int/chp/chronic_disease_report/contents/part1.pdf?ua=1, accessed 02 Feb. 2014, Copyright © 2005 World Health Organization.

Examination of the specific example of smoking, this time in the UK alone, also shows that prevention is effective. Figure 1.5 shows how the population risk of dying from smoking in the United Kingdom has changed between 1960 and 2010.

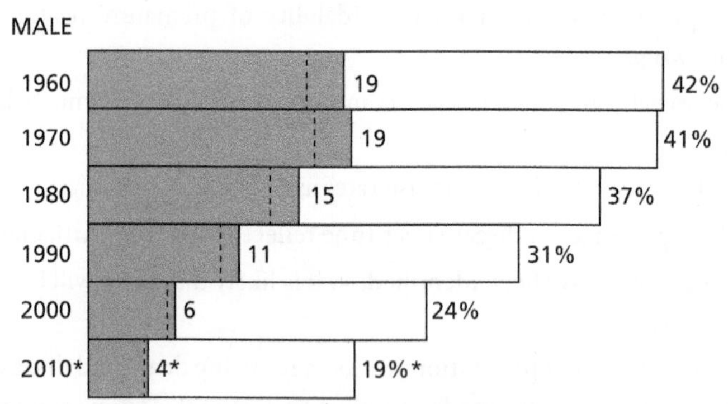

Figure 1.5 Smoking deaths in the UK, 1960–2010. Population risk of a 35 year old dying at ages 35–69 from smoking (shaded) or from any cause (shaded and white). Note: Most of those killed by smoking would otherwise have survived beyond age 70, but a minority (shaded area to right of dotted line) would have died by 70 anyway.

Reproduced with permission from Peto R. Harveian Oration 2012: Halving premature death. *Clinical Medicine*, Volume 14, Issue 6, pp. 643–57, Copyright © 2014 Royal College of Physicians.

Acknowledgements

This chapter is based on presentations by Professor Mike Rayner, Professor Simon Capewell, Professor Brian Oldenburg, and Professor Richard Peto.

References

1. **Winslow CA.** (1920). The untilled fields of public health. *Science* **51**(1306):23–33.
2. **Bajekal M, Scholes S, Love H, Hawkins N, O'Flaherty M, Raine R**, et al. (2012). Analysing recent socioeconomic trends in coronary heart disease mortality in England, 2000-2007: A population modeling study. *PLoS Med* **9**(6): e1001237.
3. **Smolina K, Wright FL, Rayner M, Goldacre MJ.** (2012). Determinants of the decline in mortality from acute myocardial infarction in England between 2002 and 2010: linked national database study. *BMJ* **344**:d8509. Available from: http://www.bmj.com/content/344/bmj.d8059

Further reading

Rose G. Rose's strategy of preventive medicine. Revised edition with commentary from Kay-Tee Khaw and Michael Marmot. Oxford: Oxford University Press, 2008.

Part II

Problem definition

Chapter 2

Understanding NCDs

2.1 What are NCDs?

This chapter explains what is meant by the term non-communicable diseases (NCDs) in the context of this document and outlines the burden presented by NCDs in low-, middle-, and high-income countries.

The term non-communicable disease can refer to any condition which is not transmissible between people. In this book the term focuses on the four most prominent NCDs: cardiovascular disease (heart disease and stroke), diabetes, cancers, and chronic respiratory diseases.

It is important to note that the full NCD burden also includes death and illness caused by accidents and a range of other diseases. The approach taken here of focusing on cardiovascular diseases, cancers, chronic respiratory diseases, and diabetes mirrors that of WHO and the wider United Nations (UN) system (see Box 2.1).

2.2 Cardiovascular disease, cancer, diabetes, chronic obstructive pulmonary disease

Cardiovascular diseases—principally, heart disease and stroke—are the most common cause of death worldwide, responsible for over 17 million deaths in 2012. Of these, 4.73 million deaths were in the western Pacific region, 4.58 million in Europe, 3.62 million in South East Asia, 1.94 million in the Americas, 1.25 million in Africa, and 1.19 million in the eastern Mediterranean. Cardiovascular diseases account for nearly half of all NCD deaths.

Cancer is another leading cause of death and ill health, and the growing cancer burden is a major cause for concern. On a worldwide basis, there were an estimated 14.1 million cancer cases in 2012 and this is expected to reach 24 million by 2025. In the same year 8.2 million deaths were attributable to cancer.[1] Globally, lung cancer was the most common, responsible for 13% of new cases diagnosed in 2012, followed by breast cancer (1.7 million new cases in women) and colorectal cancer (nearly 1.4 million new cases).[2] Specifically in men, the most common cancers were lung, prostate, and colorectal cancers, accounting together for nearly 4% of all cancers (excluding non-melanoma skin cancer).[2] For women, breast cancer was most

Box 2.1 Scope of the 2011 political declaration of the high-level meeting of the General Assembly on the Prevention and Control of Non-communicable Diseases

The UN political declaration on NCDs which emerged from the high-level meeting in September 2011 sets out the scope of UN action on NCDs and the subsequent global action plan as highlighted by this selection of quotes (emphasis added):

Note with profound concern that, according to the World Health Organization, in 2008, an estimated 36 million of the 57 million global deaths were due to non-communicable diseases, ***principally cardiovascular diseases, cancers, chronic respiratory diseases, and diabetes****, including about 9 million deaths before the age of 60, and that nearly 80 per cent of those deaths occurred in developing countries.*

Note further that ***there is a range of other non-communicable diseases and conditions****, for which the risk factors and the need for preventive measures, screening, treatment, and care are linked with the four most prominent non-communicable diseases.*

Recognize that ***mental and neurological disorders****, including Alzheimer's disease, are an important cause of morbidity and contribute to the global non-communicable disease burden, for which there is a need to provide equitable access to effective programmes and health-care interventions.*

Recognize that ***renal, oral, and eye diseases*** *pose a major health burden for many countries and that these diseases share common risk factors and can benefit from common responses to non-communicable diseases.*

Recognize that the most prominent non-communicable diseases are linked to common risk factors, namely ***tobacco use, harmful use of alcohol, an unhealthy diet, and lack of physical activity****.*

Recognize that the ***conditions in which people live and their lifestyles*** *influence their health and quality of life and that poverty, uneven distribution of wealth, lack of education, rapid urbanization, population ageing, and the economic social, gender, political, behavioural, and environmental determinants of health are among the contributing factors to the rising incidence and prevalence of non-communicable diseases.*

Note with grave concern the vicious cycle whereby ***non-communicable diseases and their risk factors worsen poverty, while poverty contributes to rising rates of non-communicable diseases****, posing a threat to public health and economic and social development.*

common (more than 25% of new cases) and this was followed by colorectal and lung cancers, on a worldwide basis.[2]

In 2015, 415 million people worldwide were living with diabetes—equivalent to one in 11 adults—and this total is projected to reach 642 million by 2040. It is also estimated that one in two adults with diabetes is undiagnosed. Nearly 1.5 million deaths were attributed to diabetes in 2015. On the basis of 2010 data, an estimated 46.8 million disability-adjusted life years (DALYs) were lost to diabetes. People with diabetes are at higher risk of developing other serious diseases—persistently high blood sugar levels can affect the heart, circulatory system, eyes, kidneys, nerves, and teeth. In many countries diabetes is a leading cause of cardiovascular disease, blindness, kidney failure, and lower limb amputation. Damage to the nerves can lead to problems with digestion, erectile dysfunction, and peripheral neuropathy (pain and loss of feeling), particularly in the feet. Women with diabetes are also at higher risk of complications during pregnancy and their children are at risk of adverse health outcomes in later life.

Chronic obstructive pulmonary disease (COPD) is a life-threatening lung condition that interferes with normal breathing (due to a persistent blockage of airflow from the lungs). It is an umbrella term used to describe progressive lung diseases, such as chronic bronchitis and emphysema (these terms are no longer used). The condition is characterized by increasing breathlessness and other symptoms include abnormal sputum, a chronic cough, wheezing, and tightness in the chest. COPD was the third largest cause of death globally in 2012, when more than 3.1 million people died of the condition, representing 6% of all deaths. Of these deaths, more than 90% occur in low- and middle-income countries. In the 2013 Global Burden of Disease study, COPD was the fifth biggest cause of loss of DALYs.[3]

2.3 **Other NCDs**

The full NCD burden also includes death and illness caused by non-communicable conditions other than the four main diseases described in section 2.2. They include accidents (globally, road injury was the ninth biggest cause of death in 2012 and falls were ranked 22nd as a cause of DALYs in 2013) and a range of other diseases. These include mental and neurological disorders and renal, oral, and eye diseases.

The death and disability caused by these conditions should not be underestimated or ignored. Mental and behavioural disorders were responsible for over 257,000 deaths in 2012[1] and depressive disorders were the 11th largest cause of DALYs lost worldwide in 2013.[3] Neurological conditions—such as Alzheimer's disease and other dementias, Parkinson's disease, epilepsy, and multiple sclerosis—accounted for 1.4 million deaths in 2012. Eye and ear diseases (sense organ diseases) were the 13th largest cause of disability and death (DALYs) in 2013.[1] Oral conditions were responsible for 1.57 million deaths in 2012, including over 1.1 million due to dental caries. Digestive diseases accounted, in 2012, for 2.26 million deaths, including over a million due to cirrhosis of the liver.

Musculoskeletal disorders are a major source of disability, with low back and neck pain the fourth leading cause of DALYs in 2013.

For this group of NCDs, many of the risk factors—and the need for prevention, screening, treatment, and care—are linked. Conditions such as dementia and dental caries, for example, have dietary risk factors in common with cardiovascular disease. Cirrhosis of the liver, to take another example, is linked to alcohol use, also a risk factor for certain cancers.

All of these conditions, therefore, can benefit from efforts to tackle the four major NCDs and action on their major risk factors and determinants.

2.4 **The burden of NCDs**

Globally, NCDs are responsible for death and disability on a massive scale. NCDs are the single biggest cause of death in the world—of 56 million deaths in the world in 2012, 38 million (68%) were due to all NCDs.[4]

The burden of NCD mortality has risen rapidly in recent decades. The proportion of deaths attributed to all NCDs rose from 57% in 1990 to 65% in 2008.[5] The proportion of

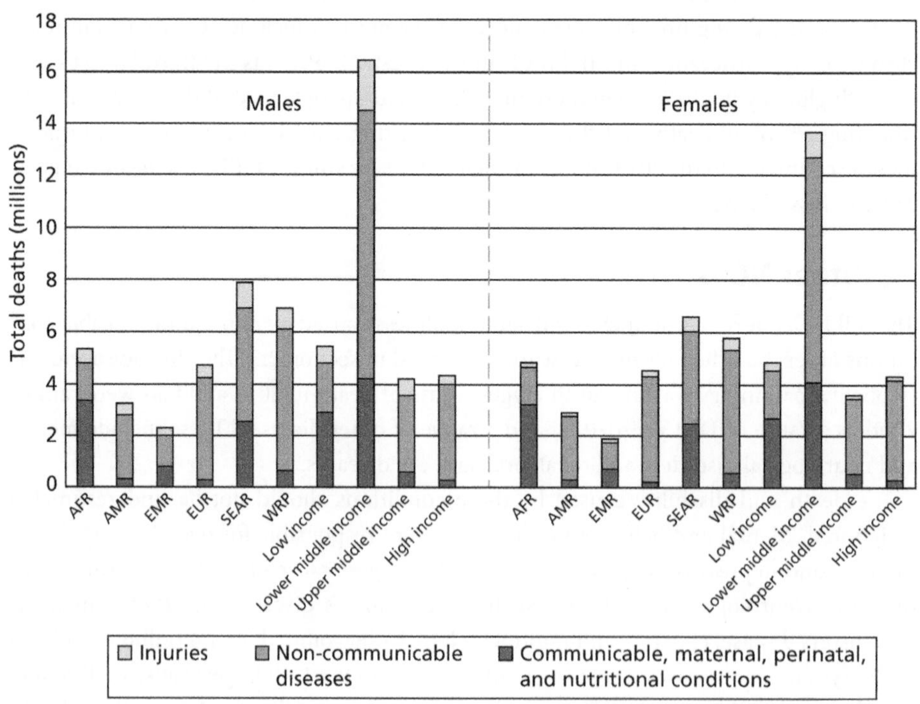

Figure 2.1 Total deaths by cause, by WHO region, by World Bank income group, and by sex, 2008.

Reproduced with permission from World Health Organization. *Global status report on non-communicable diseases 2010*. Geneva: World Health Organization, Copyright © 2011 WHO, http://www.who.int/nmh/publications/ncd_report_full_en.pdf, accessed 01 Aug. 2016.

global deaths caused by communicable, maternal, and neonatal causes, along with nutritional deficiencies, dropped from 34% to 25% over the same period, and, by 2008, was exceeded by NCD deaths in every region except Africa (Figure 2.1).[5]

WHO projections estimate that deaths from all NCDs would increase to 44 million deaths annually (an increase of 15%) globally between 2010 and 2020.[6] Figure 2.2 shows projections for different causes of death for 2015 and 2030, illustrating that the proportion of deaths caused by all NCDs is projected to rise in high-, middle-, and low-income countries (see Chapter 4 for discussion of NCDs in low- and middle-income countries).

Not only are NCDs responsible for millions of deaths, they cause ill health and disability on a massive scale. Estimates of morbidity are challenging (Box 2.2), but the 2013 global burden of disease analysis estimates that 1.43 billion DALYs are due to all NCDs, accounting for over half (58%) of the 2.45 billion DALYs which make up the total global burden of premature death, disease, and injury.[7]

The human suffering caused by this burden of disease also translates to economic loss. Globally, it has been estimated that the cumulative cost of lost output due to the four

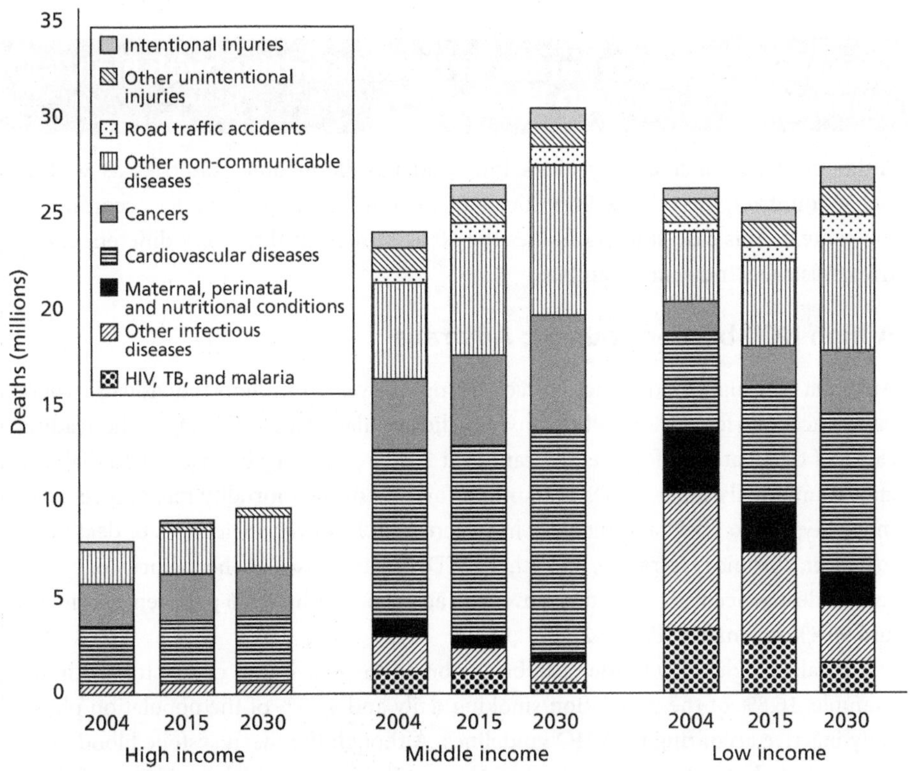

Figure 2.2 Projected global numbers of deaths by cause for high-, middle-, and low-income countries.

Reproduced with permission from World Health Organization. *The Global Burden of Disease: 2004 Update*. Geneva: World Health Organization, Copyright © 2008 WHO, http://www.who.int/healthinfo/global_burden_disease/2004_report_update/en/, accessed 01 Aug. 2016.

Box 2.2 Estimating NCD morbidity

Estimates of morbidity are considerably more difficult to obtain than estimates of mortality since reliable data on disease incidence and prevalence are more problematic than mortality data. A major initiative to address these issues and provide comparable data on the overall burden of death, premature death, disability disease, and injury by different causes is the Global Burden of Disease (GBD) study. The GBD study calculates the burden in terms of disability-adjusted life years by cause. DALYs are a summary metric of population health obtained by adding years of life lost and years lived with disability.[5]

major NCDs combined will lead to a loss of US$30 trillion dollars between 2011 and 2030.[8] When mental health conditions are added the figure rises to US$47 trillion—when divided by the 20-year period this loss is equivalent to about 5% of global GDP at 2010 levels.

Case study: The NCD burden in three countries, with high, moderate, and low NCD burdens

Although NCDs increasingly affect low- and middle-income countries as well as richer countries, the relative importance of the burden of NCDs varies according to the context. This case study examines the NCD burden in three very different countries: Australia, India, and Zambia.

A high NCD burden country: Australia

Australia is a high-income nation, consisting of over 23 million individuals, where NCDs account for 90% of all deaths. Cardiovascular disease (CVD) is the leading cause of death at 35% followed by cancer at 29%, respiratory disease at 6%, diabetes at 3%, and finally other NCDs accounting for 17% of the mortality rate.[9] Since 2000, mortality due to CVD and diabetes has decreased; however, incidences of death due to cancer, chronic respiratory, and other NCDs has increased.[10] The majority of NCD-related deaths occur in individuals over the age of 60, with 86.6% prevalence in males and 90.8% in females (Figure 2.3).

Australia's high NCD burden can be attributed to behavioural risk factors with, for example, 16.8% of the population smoking daily and 40.3% of the population physically inactive according to WHO guidelines. Although the mean systolic blood pressure and cholesterol is on the decline, there still remains a high incidence of these metabolic risk factors, with 36.4% prevalence of raised blood pressure and 57.4% of raised cholesterol. Body mass index is also rising, with 63.2% of the population overweight and 26.8% obese (Figure 2.4).[9]

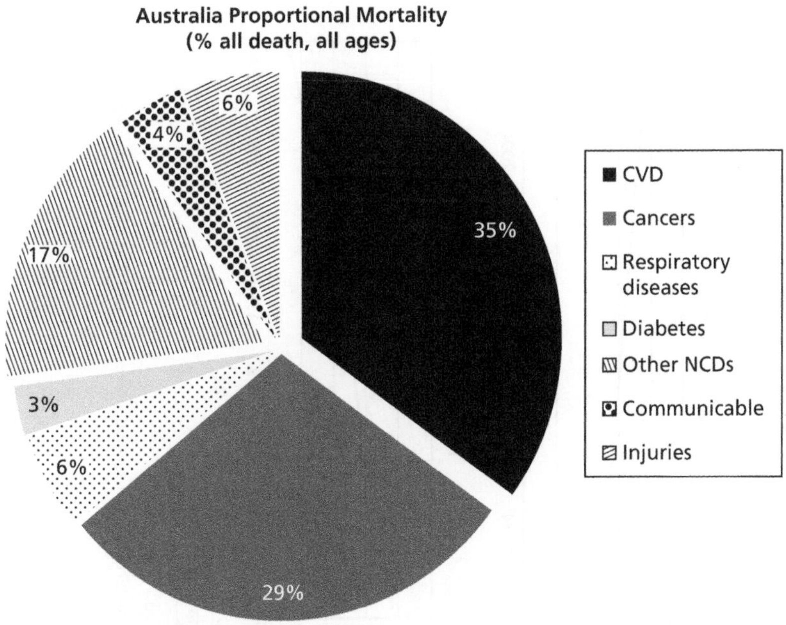

Figure 2.3 Causes of death in Australia, 2011.

Reproduced with permission from **WHO**. *NCD Country Profiles: Australia*, http://www.who.int/nmh/countries/aus_en.pdf?ua=1, accessed 01 Jul. 2016, Copyright © 2011 World Health Organization.

Australia has funding available for NCD treatment and control, prevention and health promotion, surveillance, monitoring, and evaluation. As a country, it has an operational integrated or topic-specific programme for cancer, alcohol, unhealthy diet/overweight/obesity, physical activity, and tobacco but lacks policy pertaining to cardiovascular diseases, chronic respiratory disease, and diabetes. Currently, it has an operational multisectoral national strategy integrating major NCDs and their shared risk factors. It has established national indicators to complement a set of national targets that fully encompass all three areas of nine voluntary targets including morbidity and metabolic and behavioural risk factors. However, these targets are not time-bound commitments.[11] Australia has a robust health surveillance system that generates reliable cause-specific mortality data on a routine basis, and has implemented a comprehensive health examination survey every five years. To address risk factors, Australia has taken measures to reduce tobacco demand and harmful consumption of alcohol, increase availability of healthy foods, and decrease physical inactivity. Tobacco-demand reductions have included indoor smoke-free policies, restricted advertising, health warnings, excise taxes and legislation for plain tobacco packaging.[12] Australia has not implemented any pricing policies on alcohol nor does it regulate marketing of food and beverages to children.[10]

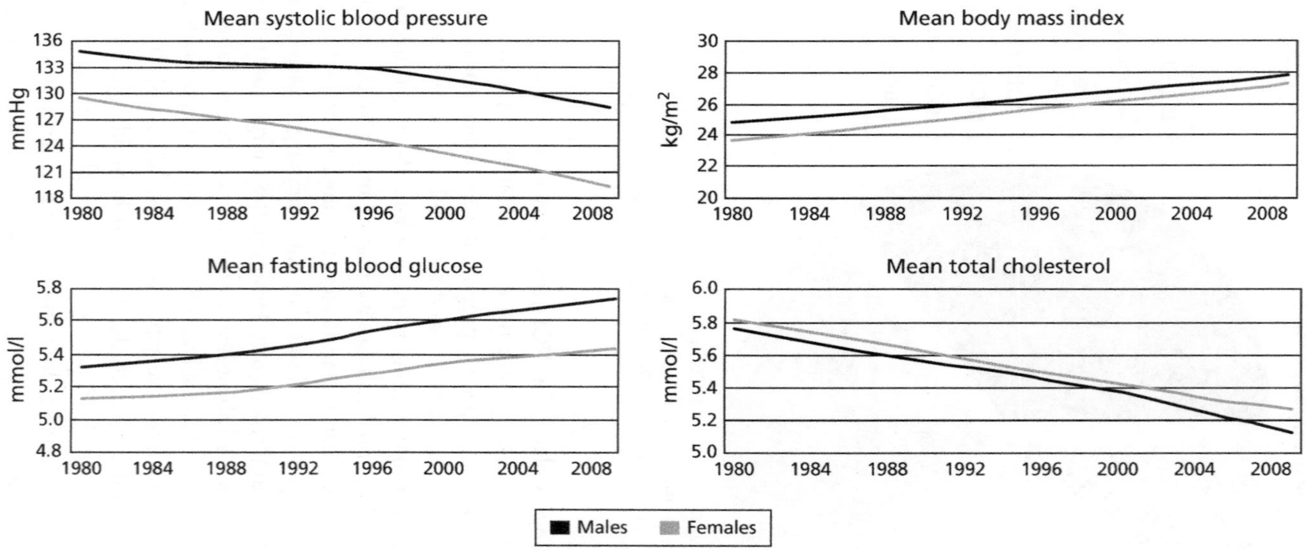

Figure 2.4 Trends in metabolic risk factors in Australia between 1990 and 2006.

Reproduced with permission from **WHO**. *NCD Country Profiles: Australia*, http://www.who.int/nmh/countries/aus_en.pdf?ua=1, accessed 01 Jul. 2016, Copyright © 2011 World Health Organization.

A moderate NCD burden country—India

India is an emerging economy, with a population of over 1.2 billion individuals, where NCDs account for 53% of all deaths (Figure 2.5). Though on the decline, India also continues to be plagued with a communicable disease burden, accounting for 37% of total deaths. CVD accounts for the greatest portion of the NCD burden with 24% of total deaths, followed by respiratory disease at 11%, cancer at 6%, and diabetes at 2%.[13] Since 2000, incidences of death due to all four of these major NCDs have risen.[14] A significant portion of NCD-related death occurs in individuals under the age of 60 with 38% in males and 32% in females.

India's rising NCD burden is associated with many harmful behavioural factors including physical inactivity, with a prevalence of 17.3% in females and 10.8% in males. Daily incidence of tobacco smoking has a high prevalence in males at 25.1%, as compared to 2.0% in females. Though the mean total cholesterol is declining, all other metabolic risk factors are on the rise in India as 32.5% of the population has raised blood pressure and 27.2% has raised cholesterol. The mean body index is steadily increasing, with 11% of the population overweight (Figure 2.6).

Like Australia, India has funding available for the different aspects of NCD prevention, treatment, and control. There is an operational integrated policy for CVD, cancer, diabetes, alcohol, unhealthy diet/overweight/obesity, physical inactivity, and tobacco.

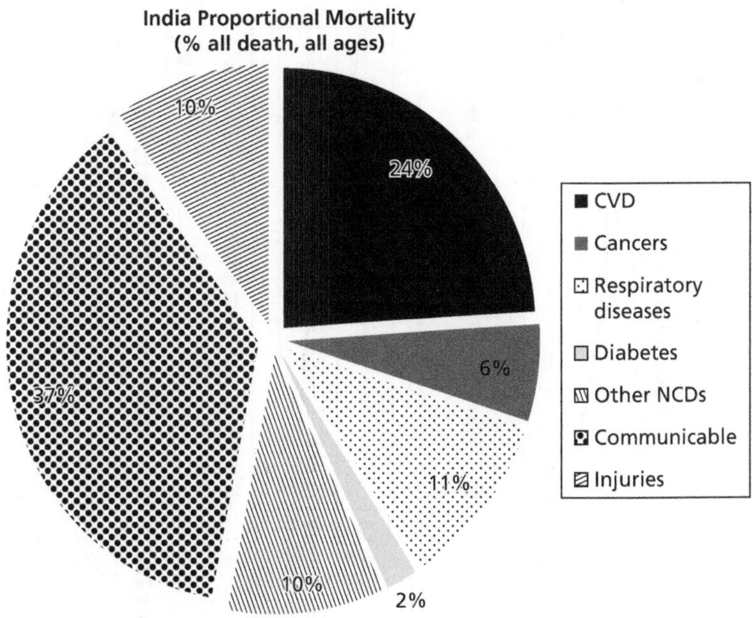

Figure 2.5 Causes of death in India, 2011.

Reproduced with permission from **WHO**. *NCD Country Profiles: India*, http://www.who.int/nmh/countries/ind_en.pdf?ua=1, accessed 01 Jul. 2016, Copyright © 2011 World Health Organization.

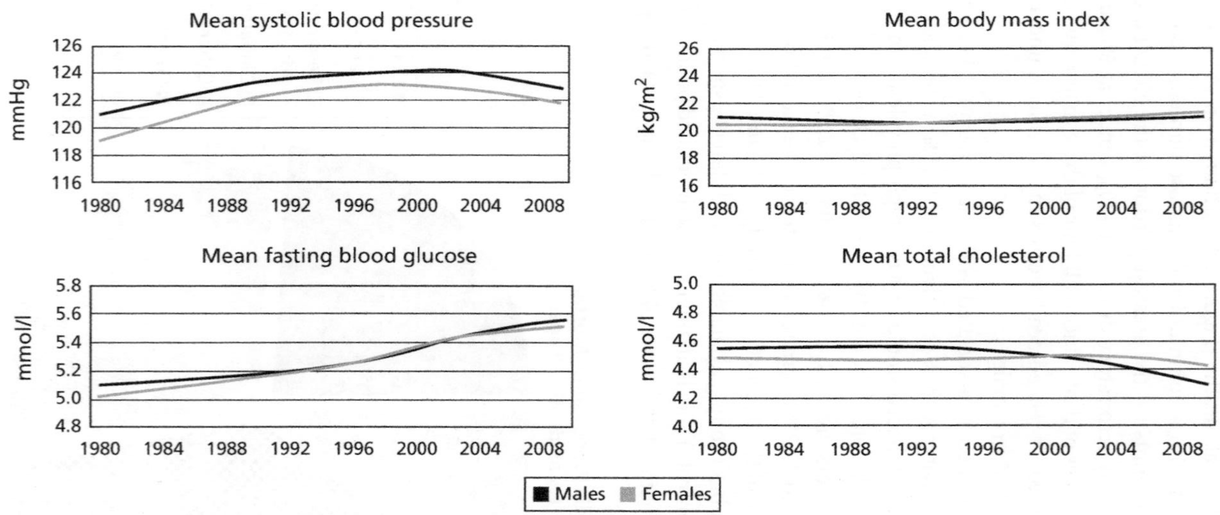

Figure 2.6 Trends in metabolic risk factors in India between 1990 and 2006.

Reproduced with permission from **WHO**. *NCD Country Profiles: India*, http://www.who.int/nmh/countries/ind_en.pdf?ua=1, accessed 01 Jul. 2016, Copyright © 2011 World Health Organization.

However, there is a lack of policy action for chronic respiratory diseases. India has developed a set of time-bound national targets and indicators to reduce the NCD burden based on WHO guidance that encompass all nine voluntary targets.[10] The country has additionally added a tenth target, related to chronic respiratory disease, which aims to reduce household use of solid fuel by 50% by 2025.

India is also developing a national multisectoral action plan that outlines actions by various sectors in addition to the health sector.[15] India lacks a sound health surveillance system for generating reliable cause-specific mortality data on a routine basis and for conducting a periodic comprehensive health examination survey. The country has initiated measures to manage risk factors and has implemented several key policies. They have imposed smoke-free policies, banned advertising, legislated pictorial health warnings on packages, but have not yet imposed taxation on tobacco products. Public awareness has been raised on diet and physical activity but further measures need to be taken for the reduction in the harmful use of alcohol and unhealthy diets.[10]

Country with a low NCD burden—Zambia

Zambia is a low-income country, with a population of 14.1 million, where NCDs account for 23% of all deaths (Figure 2.7).[16] Though it has significantly decreased since 2000,[17] the country still faces a considerable communicable disease burden, accounting

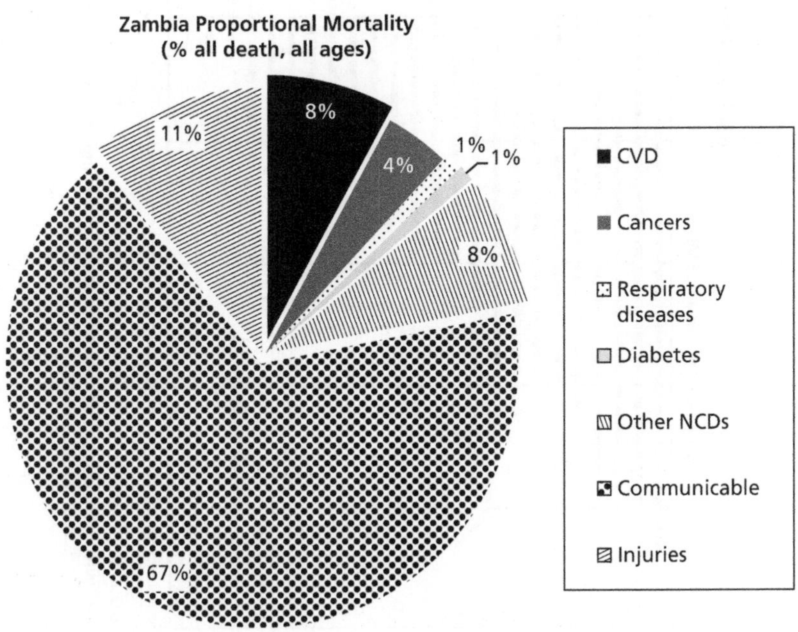

Figure 2.7 Causes of death in Zambia, 2014.

Reproduced with permission from **WHO**. *NCD Country Profiles: Zambia*, http://www.who.int/nmh/countries/zmb_en.pdf?ua=1, accessed 01 Jul. 2016, Copyright © 2011 World Health Organization.

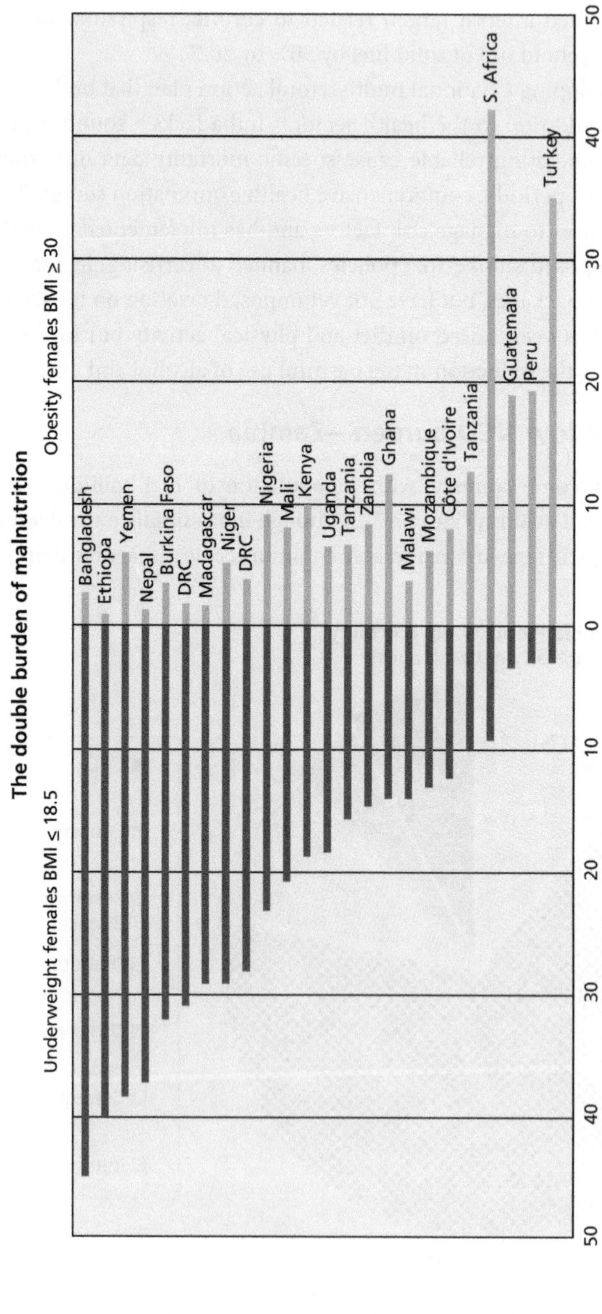

Figure 2.8 Double burden of malnutrition in females.

Source: data from **WHO**, *WHO Global Database on Body Mass Index*, http://apps.who.int/bmi/index.jsp, accessed 01 Jul. 2016, Copyright © 2006 World Health Organization.

for 67% of all deaths. The majority of NCD-related deaths can be attributed to CVD, at 8%, followed by cancer at 4%, and diabetes and chronic respiratory diseases both at 1%. For individuals aged 30–70, the probability of dying from the four main NCDs remains low at 18%.[13] Although at a population level deaths due to cancer and chronic respiratory disease have not changed since 2000, mortality due to CVD and diabetes has increased.[14]

Prevalence of risk factors such as smoking and alcohol consumption is relatively low. Incidence of raised blood pressure, however, remains high at 32.8% and there is 3.6% obesity.[13] Furthermore, Zambia now faces the double burden of malnutrition where 15% of females are underweight and 8% are overweight (Figure 2.8).

Even with limited infrastructure and funding, Zambia has set time-bound national targets and indicators and has an operational NCD department within the Ministry of Health, establishing guidelines for the management of major NCDs through primary care approaches. The country has an operational policy to reduce the harmful use of alcohol, physical inactivity, burden of tobacco, and unhealthy diet. However, there has been little progress in implementing measures to reduce these behavioural risks and the country is lacking a multisectoral national policy or any plan to integrate several NCDs and shared risk factors. Zambia has developed a comprehensive routine health examination but a more robust NCD surveillance system needs to be developed to generate reliable cause-specific mortality data on a routine basis.[10] Due to the low NCD burden, compared to India and Australia, Zambia has limited information on NCD reduction initiatives, behavioural and metabolic risk, and their subsequent trends.

Comparisons of age-standardized mortality

When comparing proportional mortality among Australia, India, and Zambia, it is evident that NCDs account for the greatest number of deaths in Australia, followed by India and Zambia. However, the age-standardized mortality rates for NCDs contradict the perceived NCD burden and changes the landscape for the global burden of NCDs (Table 2.1). This discrepancy can be attributed to the comparatively young populations in low- to middle-income countries. Due to relatively high birth and death rates, the

Table 2.1 Age-standardized mortality by cause in Australia, India and Zambia, 2012

	Age-standardized mortality rate by cause (per 100,000 population)				
Countries	**Cancer**	**CVD**	**Diabetes**	**Chronic respiratory diseases**	**All NCDs**
Australia	111	92.4	9.5	22.2	302.9
India	71.9	306.3	26.3	154.8	682.3
Zambia	105	271.7	39.3	23.8	587.4

Source: data from World Health Organization. 'Global Health Observatory data repository: Mortality and global health estimates', http://apps.who.int/gho/data/node.main.686?lang=en, accessed 01 Aug. 2016, Copyright © 2016 WHO.

populations of India and Zambia have a median age of 27 and 17, respectively, while Australia's median age is 38.[18] Thus, India and Zambia's proportional mortality figures are dominated by younger age groups who are less likely to be affected by NCDs. Following age standardization, however, it is evident that NCDs are of concern for both low- and middle-income countries, as well as high-income nations.

2.5 Differences in the burden within countries: health inequities and inequalities

Health inequities and inequalities[19] should be considered when describing the NCD burden. As well as the major differences in patterns of NCDs between regions and countries, shown in Figure 2.1 and Figure 2.2, there are often significant differences between groups within populations (see Box 2.3).

Box 2.3 Health inequities and health inequalities

Health inequities are *avoidable* inequalities in health between groups of people within countries and between countries. These inequities arise from inequalities within and between societies. Social and economic conditions and their effects on people's lives determine their risk of illness and the actions taken to prevent them becoming ill or treat illness when it occurs.[20]The term socioeconomic should be interpreted very widely, to include, for example, gender and ethnicity as well as social differences based on occupation, education, and/or income levels.

Case study: Socioeconomic status and cardiovascular health

Cardiovascular disease remains a leading public health problem that contributes 30% to the annual global mortality and 10% to the global disease burden. The conventional risk factors of CVD are tobacco use, raised blood pressure, raised blood cholesterol, and diabetes mellitus. Many other factors increase the risk of CVD including low socioeconomic status (SES), income distribution, education and literacy, housing and living conditions, and employment and employment security. Evidence on social determinants and inequities related to CVD indicates an inverse relationship between SES and CVD incidence and mortality. An individual's SES influences behavioural risk factors, the development of CVD, and outcomes of CVD.

Quality of life differs greatly between countries, but health and illness follow a social gradient. The poorest health is not confined to those who are worst off; at all levels of income, the lower the socioeconomic position, the worse the health. Health inequities between and within countries are caused by the unequal distribution of power, income, goods, and services, globally and nationally. This greatly influences the visible circumstance of individuals' lives, including their access to health care and education; their conditions of work and leisure; their homes, communities, towns, or cities; and their chances of leading a flourishing life.

This unequal distribution of health-damaging experiences is the result of a combination of poor social policies and programmes, unfair economic arrangements, and bad politics. Together, the structural determinants and conditions of daily life constitute the social determinants of health and cause much of the health inequity between and within countries. Protecting the cardiovascular health of those in lower socioeconomic strata through population-based prevention strategies is a priority.[21] The needs of those at high risk of CVD should be addressed, with a special focus on disadvantaged sectors. Reduction of CVDs in disadvantaged groups is necessary to achieve substantial decreases in the total NCD burden, making them mutually reinforcing priorities.

Michael Marmot and Sharon Friel's[21] work on social determinants of health suggests three key principles of action: improve the conditions of daily life; tackle the inequitable distribution of power and money; and measure and understand the problem by expanding the knowledge base. This acknowledgement of health inequity and social determinants of health is the key step essential for action. National governments and international organizations should set up national global health-equity surveillance systems for routine monitoring of health inequity and the social determinants of health. Further, addressing this health inequity and inequitable conditions of daily living requires addressing inequities in the way society is organized. This falls at the core of strengthening governance with a capable and adequately financed public sector and private sector that are held accountable for their actions.

Finally, ameliorating daily living conditions includes improving the well-being of girls and women, putting major emphasis on early child development and education, improving living and working conditions, and creating social protection policy supportive of health communities.

Coronary heart disease and cerebrovascular disease make the largest contribution to the global CVD burden. They develop slowly through life due to atherosclerosis of blood vessels caused by lifelong exposure to behavioural risk factors influenced by SES. The Global Burden of Disease Study 2010 confirmed that strokes disproportionately affect low- and middle-income countries, though incidences are continuing to rise in high-income countries. Even in wealthier nations high-quality evidence shows that low socioeconomic status is generally associated with an increased risk of stroke.[22] This disproportionality can be attributed to the global inequalities that exist in risk factors and health care. Major NCD risk factors are increasingly concentrated in low- and middle-income populations—the very same population that has limited access to primary care and NCD treatments.[23]

There are significant equity gaps in the implementation of cost-effective interventions and provisions of quality care for CVD. These discrepancies are particularly emphasized in low-income countries where health systems are not geared for providing chronic care and the per capita expenditure is inadequate, yet coronary heart disease is among the ten leading causes contributing to the disease burden. These gaps can only be addressed if there is a modest increase in public spending coupled with efficient use of resources and investment. This should be designed to benefit persons of low socioeconomic position as people of higher socioeconomic status have been found more likely to receive treatment and have been reported to be prescribed medications for secondary prevention.

The variation that is seen in coronary heart disease incidence across the social gradient is due to numerous risk factors. Those of low socioeconomic position have a poorer risk factor profile. Differential stress among socioeconomic tiers has been shown to play a part in the causation and prognosis of heart disease in patients. Comorbidity could also be a potential explanation for higher case fatality and worse prognosis of patients in low social categories. Often, diabetes and hypertension go undetected, leading to the eventual development of CVD. Occupational status and income have been shown to have an effect on mortality through their impact on lifestyle-related risk factors both before and after a stroke. The adverse impact on cardiovascular health of both globalization and urbanization is greater for poorer countries and for the poor within countries. Most existing data suggest that low childhood SES negatively impacts levels of adult cardiovascular risk factors.

Interventions should be targeted to decrease social stratification, reduce exposure to risk factors, lessen vulnerability, reduce unequal consequences, and reduce differential outcomes. There are complex links between CVD and cardiovascular risk factors to poverty, literacy, employment, and other social determinants, which provide entry-points to address CVD inequities. Two complementary approaches are required: first, strategies for primary and secondary prevention must pay special attention to disadvantaged groups; and, second, policy and structural interventions must address root social causes. It is only then that disadvantaged segments of the population will be able to utilize opportunities to make choices that protect and promote cardiovascular health.

From a public health perspective, it is a challenge to advocate for behavioural changes to reduce CVD risks if basic obstacles remain. For people to understand messages and advertisements promoting and advocating lifestyle changes, they need at least to have primary education; it is only then that they will internalize the info and act upon it. Measures such as housing and poverty alleviation may also be important for addressing the social gradient of CVD—there is evidence that a personal lack of control over one's life and environment increases the risk of morbidity from coronary heart disease. Social determinants have a substantial impact on the uptake of interventions, from affecting affordability and accessibility to differences in health knowledge, beliefs, and behaviour. Inequities are further punctuated by health-care systems that do not provide essential non-communicable disease services through a primary health-care approach. Lack of health-care support, for example for people with hypertension and diabetes, may expose them to catastrophic health-care costs due to acute cardiac events or stroke.

In order to successfully implement CVD interventions, social determinant-conscious efforts are needed across CVD and NCD programmes. Dedicated human and financial resources need to be identified within CVD and NCD programmes to deal with social determinants across promotion, prevention, and management areas of work in an integrated fashion. To address CVD inequities, social protection needs to be extended to all people throughout the course of their lives. The social gradient of CVD may be attributed to multiple interacting factors, including cardiovascular risk, social determinants, comorbid conditions, general health status, health-seeking behaviours, use of specialized cardiac and stroke services, access to health-care services, and clinical practice patterns.

This case study is largely adapted from WHO's *Equity, Social Determinants and Public Health Programmes*, Chapter 3 and WHO's Country statistics. Accessed July 2016. http://www.who.int/gho/countries/en/.[24]

Acknowledgements

This chapter draws on presentations by Prachi Bhatnagar and Dr Aaron Reeves, with case study material prepared by Nousin Hussain.

References

1. **World Health Organization.** Global Health Estimates 2014 Summary Tables.
2. **Ferlay J, Soerjomataram I, Ervik M, Dikshit R, Eser S, Mathers C,** et al. *GLOBOCAN 2012 v1.1, Cancer Incidence and Mortality Worldwide: IARC CancerBase no. 11* [Internet]. Lyon, France: International Agency for Research on Cancer, 2014. Available from: http://globocan.iarc.fr.
3. **Global Burden of Disease Study 2013 Collaborators.** Global, regional, and national incidence, prevalence, and years lived with disability for 301 acute and chronic diseases and injuries in 188 countries, 1990-2013: a systematic analysis for the Global Burden of Disease Study 2013. *Lancet* 2015; **386**(9995):743–800.
4. **World Health Organization.** *Global Status Report on Non-communicable Diseases, 2014.* Geneva: WHO, 2015.
5. **Murray CJ, Vos T, Lozano R, Maghavi M, Flaxman AD, Michaud C,** et al. Disability-adjusted life years (DALYs) for 291 diseases and injuries in 21 regions, 1990-2010: a systematic analysis for the Global Burden of Disease Study 2010. *Lancet* 2012; **380**:2197–223.
6. **World Health Organization.** *Global Status Report on Non-communicable Diseases, 2010.* Geneva: WHO, 2011.
7. **GBD 2013 DALYs and HALE Collaborators.** Global, regional, and national disability-adjusted life years (DALYs) for 306 diseases and injuries and healthy life expectancy (HALE) for 188 countries, 1990–2013: quantifying the epidemiological transition. *Lancet* 2015; **386**(10009):2145–91.

8. **Bloom DE, Cafiero ET, Jané-Llopis E, Abrahams-Gessel S, Bloom LR, Fathima S**, et al. *The Global Economic Burden of Noncommunicable Diseases*. Geneva: World Economic Forum, 2011.

9. **World Health Organization.** *Australia. Noncommunicable Diseases (NCD) Country Profiles, 2014*. Available at: http://www.who.int/nmh/countries/aus_en.pdf?ua=1

10. **World Health Organization.** *Australia: WHO statistical profile, 2014*. Available at: http://www.who.int/gho/countries/aus.pdf?ua=1

11. **World Health Organization.** *Noncommunicable Diseases Progress Monitor 2015*. Geneva: WHO, 2015. Available at: http://www.who.int/nmh/publications/ncd-progress-monitor-2015/en/

12. **Department of Health,** Australian Government. Introduction of tobacco plain packaging in Australia. Available at: http://www.health.gov.au/internet/main/publishing.nsf/Content/tobacco-plain

13. **World Health Organization.** *India. NCD Country Profiles, 2011*. Available at: http://www.who.int/nmh/countries/ind_en.pdf?ua=1

14. **World Health Organization.** *India: WHO statistical profile, 2015*. Available at: http://www.who.int/gho/countries/ind.pdf?ua=1

15. **World Health Organization.** India: first to adapt the Global Monitoring Framework on noncommunicable diseases (NCDs). Available at: http://www.who.int/features/2015/ncd-india/en/

16. **World Health Organization.** *Zambia. Noncommunicable Diseases (NCD) Country Profiles, 2014*. Available at: http://www.who.int/nmh/countries/zmb_en.pdf?ua=1

17. **World Health Organization.** *Zambia: WHO statistical profile, 2015*. Available at: http://www.who.int/gho/countries/zmb.pdf?ua=1

18. **World by Map.** Median age: the age for all countries of the world that divides a population into two equal-sized groups. Available at: http://world.bymap.org/MedianAge.html

19. For definition of terms see http://www.who.int/social_determinants/thecommission/finalreport/key_concepts/en/

20. **World Health Organization.** Social determinants of health: key concepts. Available at: http://www.who.int/social_determinants/thecommission/finalreport/key_concepts/en/

21. **Marmot M, Friel S, Bell R, Houweling TA,** and **Taylor, S.** Closing the gap in a generation: Health equity through action on the social determinants of health. *Lancet* 2008; 372(9650), 1661–9. Available at: http://www.sciencedirect.com/science/article/pii/S0140673608616906

22. **Marshall IJ, Wang Y, Crichton S, McKevitt C, Rudd AG,** and **Wolfe CDA.** The effects of socioeconomic stroke risk and outcomes. *Lancet Neurology* 2015; 14(12):1206–18. Available at: http://www.thelancet.com/pdfs/journals/laneur/PIIS1474-4422(15)00200-8.pdf

23. **Di Cesare M, Khang Y-H, Asaria P, Blakely T, Cowan MJ, Farzadfar F**, et al. Inequalities in non-communicable diseases and effective responses. *Lancet* 2013; 381(9866):585–97. Available at: http://www.sciencedirect.com/science/article/pii/S0140673612618510

24. **Blas E,** and **Kurup AS.** *Equity, Social Determinants, and Public Health Programmes*. Geneva: World Health Organization, 2010.

Chapter 3

NCDs: Risk factors and determinants

3.1 Introduction

There are a variety of risk factors and broader determinants involved in the development of non-communicable diseases (NCDs). The World Health Organization (WHO) has developed a simplified model to illustrate this (Figure 3.1). Note that the WHO has recently concluded that alcohol intake is also a major common modifiable risk factor.

3.2 Causal webs help us to understand NCDs

With this wide array of determinants, from societal to individual, and the interactions between them it is clear that the aetiology of non-communicable diseases is complex. Causal webs have been developed to document and illustrate the factors involved in NCD development and the relationships between these factors. These models can help with understanding the issues and, crucially, the opportunities for intervention.

Some causal webs seek to simplify the picture by highlighting key factors. Figure 3.2 illustrates a relatively simple causal web for the development of cancer and cardiovascular disease.

Causal webs can combine the biological, social, psychosocial, socioeconomic, and environmental factors. Figure 3.3 illustrates the complex inter-relationships between a number of different pathways—biological, social, sociobiological, and biosocial—that may influence lung function and/or respiratory disease.

Figure 3.2 and Figure 3.3 are relatively crude, in order to represent in a relatively simplified way the aetiology of multifactorial conditions. Other causal webs, however, are extremely complicated by design, seeking to illustrate the complexity of NCD aetiology. For example, the obesity system map developed for the UK's Foresight report illustrates a highly intricate plethora of factors, a multitude of interactions, and feedback loops. An interactive version is available online.[1]

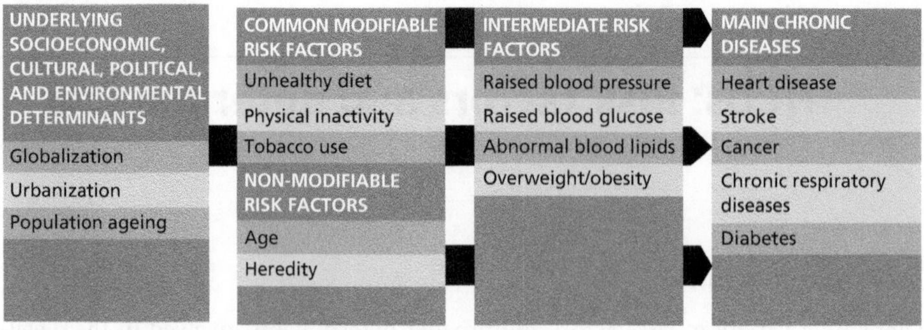

Figure 3.1 WHO model of the causes of chronic diseases.

Note: Alcohol is also a common modifiable risk factor.

3.3 Key behavioural risk factors: smoking, alcohol, diet, and physical activity

The four major NCDs share a small number of common, behavioural risk factors. Four are particularly important: tobacco use, physical inactivity, unhealthy diet, and the harmful use of alcohol. These behaviours lead, in turn, to four metabolic or physiological changes, or intermediate risk factors (raised blood pressure, overweight/obesity, hyperglycaemia, and hyperlipidaemia).

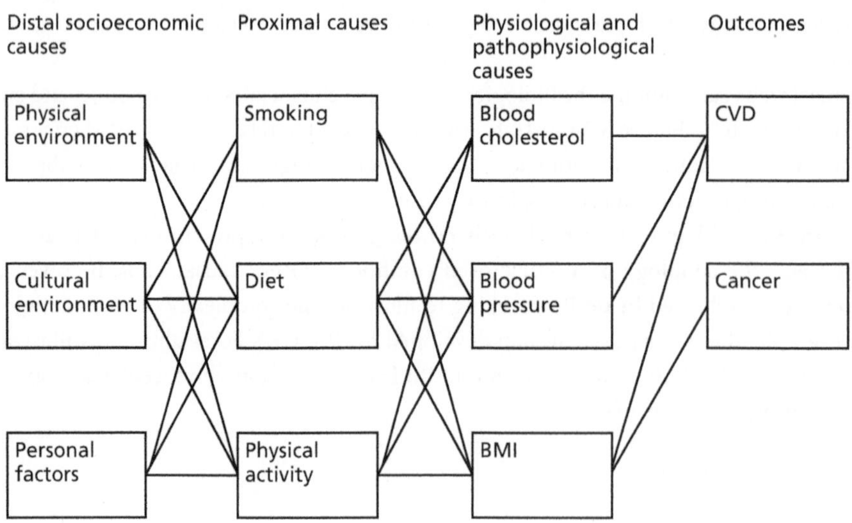

Figure 3.2 Causal web for cancer and cardiovascular disease

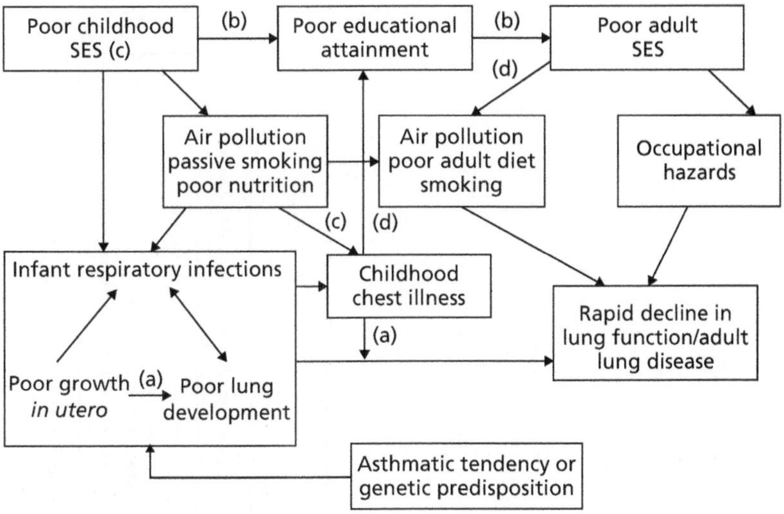

Figure 3.3 Lung function and respiratory disease: biological and psychosocial exposures across the life course. Path (a) shows the mainly biological pathway whereby impaired foetal development is associated with later harm from infection and greater susceptibility to impaired lung function and/or chronic obstructive pulmonary disorder (COPD) in later life. Path (b) shows the social pathway, whereby low socioeconomic status (SES) influences which adverse factors children are exposed to and is associated with lower SES status and smoking in adulthood. Path (c) is a sociobiological pathway in which poor childhood SES status increases the risk of infection—and, through other factors, the ability of the immune system to stave off infection—with potential impact on lung function in childhood and adulthood. Path (d) is a biosocial pathway, in which repeated childhood infections result in poorer educational attainment and, therefore, lower SES status in later life.

Figure reproduced with permission and text adapted from Ben-Shlomo Y and Kuh D. A life course approach to chronic disease epidemiology: conceptual models, empirical challenges and interdisciplinary perspectives. International Journal of Epidemiology, Volume 31, Issue 2, pp. 285–93, Copyright © 2002 International Journal of Epidemiology.

The Global Burden of Disease Study ranked 79 risk factors or clusters of risks according to their contribution to disability-adjusted life years (DALYs) worldwide. The vast majority of the top risk factors (Figure 3.4) are linked to NCDs. Some links—such as the link between childhood underweight and NCDs—may be less obvious, but there is evidence of a link between malnutrition and development of NCDs later in life or in future generations.[2]

The leading risk factors had changed substantially between 2000 and 2013. The leading cause of attributable DALYs in 2000 was child and maternal malnutrition, but this dropped to fourth. Several risks related to NCDs became more prominent, with the top three leading risks being high blood pressure, smoking, and high body mass index (Figure 3.5). More than half of the top 25 risks are clearly associated with the four major NCDs.

The authors of another major study, the InterHeart study, estimated that about 90% of coronary heart disease risk can be explained by nine risk factors: smoking,

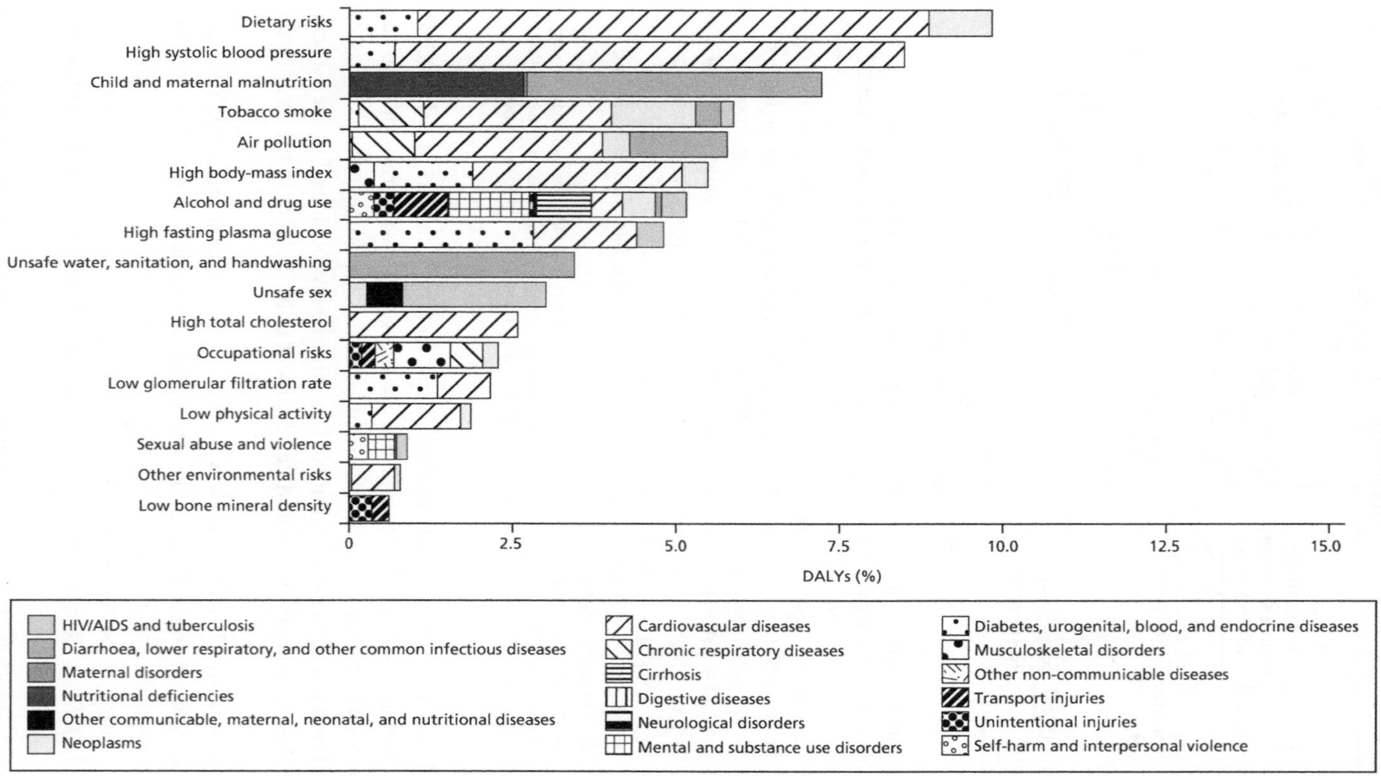

Figure 3.4 Burden of disease attributable to leading risk factors in 2013 (burden of disease expressed as a percentage of global disability-adjusted life years in both sexes combined).

Reprinted from *The Lancet*, Volume 386, GBD 2013 Risk Factors Collaborators, Global, regional, and national comparative risk assessment of 79 behavioural, environmental and occupational, and metabolic risks or clusters of risks in 188 countries, 1990-2013: a systematic analysis for the Global Burden of Disease Study 2013, pp. 2287–323, Copyright © 2015, with permission from Elsevier.

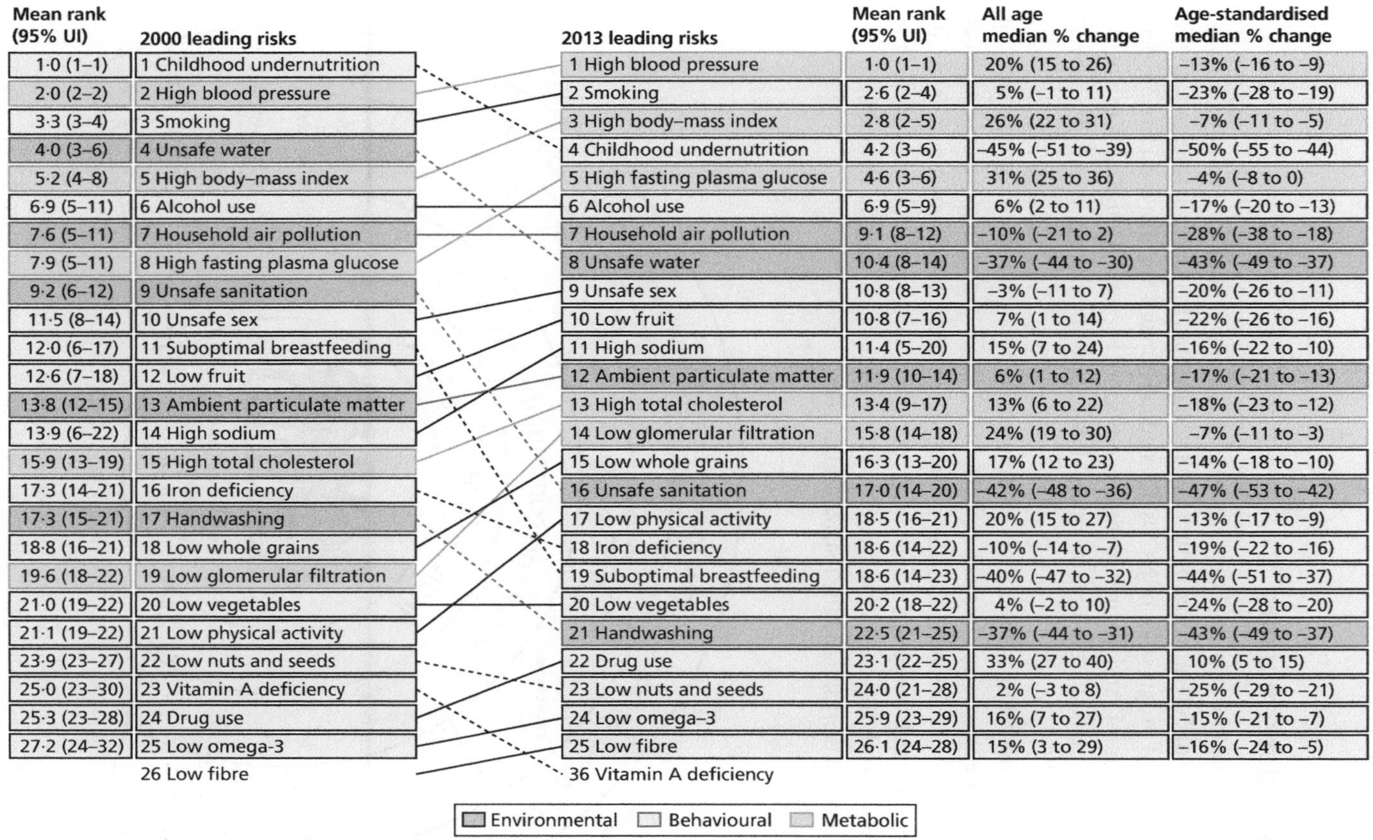

Mean rank (95% UI)
2000 leading risks
2013 leading risks
Mean rank (95% UI)
All age median % change
Age-standardised median % change
1·0 (1–1) 1 Childhood undernutrition
2·0 (2–2) 2 High blood pressure
3·3 (3–4) 3 Smoking
4·0 (3–6) 4 Unsafe water
5·2 (4–8) 5 High body–mass index
6·9 (5–11) 6 Alcohol use
7·6 (5–11) 7 Household air pollution
7·9 (5–11) 8 High fasting plasma glucose
9·2 (6–12) 9 Unsafe sanitation
11·5 (8–14) 10 Unsafe sex
12·0 (6–17) 11 Suboptimal breastfeeding
12·6 (7–18) 12 Low fruit
13·8 (12–15) 13 Ambient particulate matter
13·9 (6–22) 14 High sodium
15·9 (13–19) 15 High total cholesterol
17·3 (14–21) 16 Iron deficiency
17·3 (15–21) 17 Handwashing
18·8 (16–21) 18 Low whole grains
19·6 (18–22) 19 Low glomerular filtration
21·0 (19–22) 20 Low vegetables
21·1 (19–22) 21 Low physical activity
23·9 (23–27) 22 Low nuts and seeds
25·0 (23–30) 23 Vitamin A deficiency
25·3 (23–28) 24 Drug use
27·2 (24–32) 25 Low omega-3
26 Low fibre
1 High blood pressure 1·0 (1–1) 20% (15 to 26) –13% (–16 to –9)
2 Smoking 2·6 (2–4) 5% (–1 to 11) –23% (–28 to –19)
3 High body–mass index 2·8 (2–5) 26% (22 to 31) –7% (–11 to –5)
4 Childhood undernutrition 4·2 (3–6) –45% (–51 to –39) –50% (–55 to –44)
5 High fasting plasma glucose 4·6 (3–6) 31% (25 to 36) –4% (–8 to 0)
6 Alcohol use 6·9 (5–9) 6% (2 to 11) –17% (–20 to –13)
7 Household air pollution 9·1 (8–12) –10% (–21 to 2) –28% (–38 to –18)
8 Unsafe water 10·4 (8–14) –37% (–44 to –30) –43% (–49 to –37)
9 Unsafe sex 10·8 (8–13) –3% (–11 to 7) –20% (–26 to –11)
10 Low fruit 10·8 (7–16) 7% (1 to 14) –22% (–26 to –16)
11 High sodium 11·4 (5–20) 15% (7 to 24) –16% (–22 to –10)
12 Ambient particulate matter 11·9 (10–14) 6% (1 to 12) –17% (–21 to –13)
13 High total cholesterol 13·4 (9–17) 13% (6 to 22) –18% (–23 to –12)
14 Low glomerular filtration 15·8 (14–18) 24% (19 to 30) –7% (–11 to –3)
15 Low whole grains 16·3 (13–20) 17% (12 to 23) –14% (–18 to –10)
16 Unsafe sanitation 17·0 (14–20) –42% (–48 to –36) –47% (–53 to –42)
17 Low physical activity 18·5 (16–21) 20% (15 to 27) –13% (–17 to –9)
18 Iron deficiency 18·6 (14–22) –10% (–14 to –7) –19% (–22 to –16)
19 Suboptimal breastfeeding 18·6 (14–23) –40% (–47 to –32) –44% (–51 to –37)
20 Low vegetables 20·2 (18–22) 4% (–2 to 10) –24% (–28 to –20)
21 Handwashing 22·5 (21–25) –37% (–44 to –31) –43% (–49 to –37)
22 Drug use 23·1 (22–25) 33% (27 to 40) 10% (5 to 15)
23 Low nuts and seeds 24·0 (21–28) 2% (–3 to 8) –25% (–29 to –21)
24 Low omega–3 25·9 (23–29) 16% (7 to 27) –15% (–21 to –7)
25 Low fibre 26·1 (24–28) 15% (3 to 29) –16% (–24 to –5)
36 Vitamin A deficiency
Environmental
Behavioural
Metabolic

Figure 3.5 Leading global risk factors for disability adjusted life years in both sexes combined in 2000 and 2013.

Reprinted from *The Lancet*, Volume 386, GBD 2013 Risk Factors Collaborators, Global, regional, and national comparative risk assessment of 79 behavioural, environmental and occupational, and metabolic risks or clusters of risks in 188 countries, 1990-2013: a systematic analysis for the Global Burden of Disease Study 2013, pp. 2287–323, Copyright © 2015, with permission from Elsevier.

diabetes, hypertension, abdominal obesity, psychosocial factors, fruit and vegetables, exercise, alcohol, and the ratio of ApoB to ApoA1 (fat-transporting proteins) in the blood.[3]

3.4 **Other determinants**

In addition to the four principal behavioural risk factors identified in section 3.3, there are a wide range of determinants of those behaviours that, in other ways, impact on the development and progression of NCDs These determinants include a variety of socioeconomic, cultural, and environmental conditions. Figure 3.6 illustrates this wide array of determinants, according to a model developed by Dahlgren and Whitehead in 1991.

The 2008 Commission on the Social Determinants of Health made the case for tackling the 'causes of the causes' of disease, in other words the 'fundamental global and national structures of social hierarchy and the socially determined conditions these create in environments which people grow, live, work and age'.[4] A conceptual framework for the Commission's work (Figure 3.7) suggests that interventions can aim to change both the circumstances of daily life and their structural drivers.

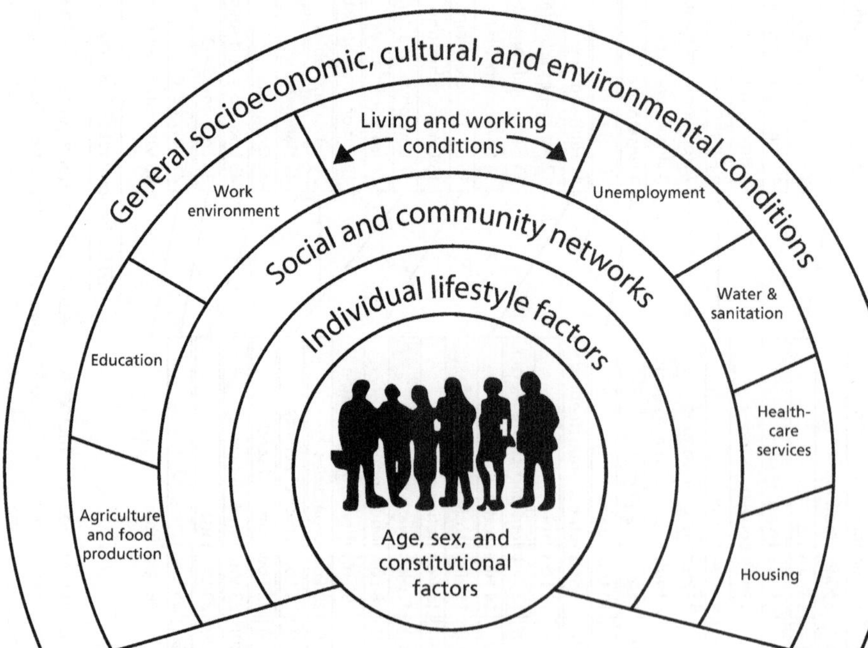

Figure 3.6 Model of broad range of determinants of health.

Reproduced with permission from Dahlgren G and Whitehead M. *Policies and strategies to promote social equity in health: Background document to WHO—Strategy paper for Europe*. Copenhagen: World Health Organization Regional Office for Europe, Copyright © 1992 World Health Organization.

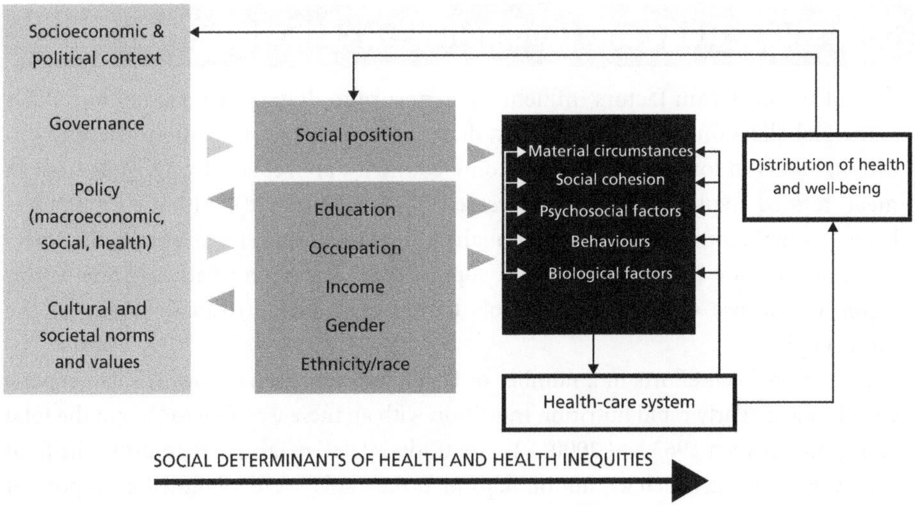

Figure 3.7 Conceptual framework of social determinants of health.
Reproduced with permission from Commission on Social Determinants of Health (WHO). *Closing the gap in a generation: Health equity through action on the social determinants of health*, http://www.who.int/social_determinants/final_report/csdh_finalreport_2008.pdf, accessed 10 Aug. 2016, Geneva: WHO, Copyright © 2008 World Health Organization.

The Commission set out three principles of action, closely reflected in three overarching recommendations:

- Improve the conditions of daily living—the circumstances in which people are born, grow, live, work, and age.
- Tackle the inequitable distribution of power, money, and resources—the structural drivers of those conditions of daily life—globally, nationally, and locally.
- Measure the problem, evaluate action, expand the knowledge base, develop a workforce that is trained in the social determinants of health, and raise public awareness about the social determinants of health.

It has also been widely argued that actions need to go further still. Stuckler and colleagues called for understanding of the 'causes of the causes of the causes', i.e. upstream factors such as trade liberalization and market integration, privatization and deregulation, and rapid economic growth.[5]

For any particular disease, a variety of environmental factors interact with an individual's genes to influence the development of that disease. Growing understanding of genetic propensity to develop diseases might, in future, help to prevent, diagnose, or treat conditions. There is also growing evidence of the importance of epigenetics, whereby environmental factors *in utero* or in very early childhood influence the expression of genes. It is important to remember, however, that genes interact with environmental factors, and a holistic approach, which considers the environment as well as genetics, to tackling NCDs remains vital (see Section 3.5 A life-course approach to NCDs).

Case study: Trade and food policy—a case study from Tonga

One of the upstream factors influencing exposure to dietary risk factors for NCDs is the globalization of the food supply, driving the nutrition transition whereby traditional diets in low- and middle-income countries are replaced with diets high in meat, refined staples, and other processed foods (Figure 3.8). Although much has been written about the impact of globalization—including, for example, the liberalization of trade rules—on the food supply, there has been relatively little exploration of the use of trade policy tools to improve the nutritional quality of the food supply.

There have been efforts in a number of Pacific island countries—which had experienced a particularly rapid nutrition transition with an increase of up to 80% in the total fat supply between 1963 and 2000[6]—to use trade-related measures to improve the food supply. Fatty meats, such as mutton flaps or turkey tails, were identified as important contributors to the population fat consumption—by 2004 Tongans, for example, were consuming, on average, around 600 g of mutton flaps per week, representing about 18% of all meat consumption on the island.[7]

In response to this situation, the Tongan Ministry of Health developed a proposal for an import quota to restrict the volume of imports of any product with a fat content of more than 40%, which could be readily identifiable through import coding, and which made a significant contribution to Tongans' fat and saturated fat intakes. At the time of the proposal the only product to meet these criteria was mutton flaps. The proposal was justified on the basis of calculations that replacing 50% of mutton flaps with the same quantity of fish would reduce average energy intake by around 100 kcal/person/week.

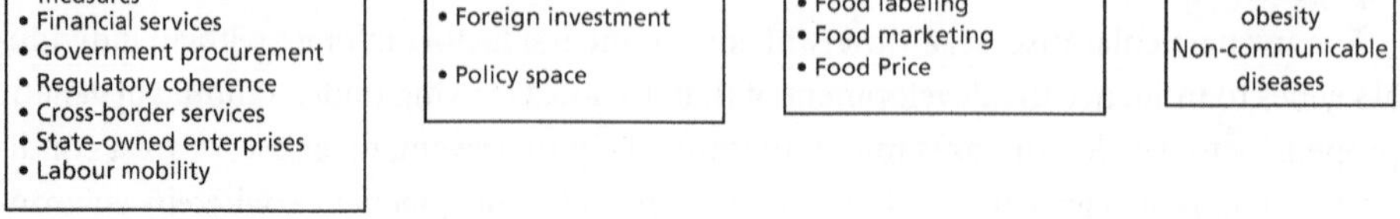

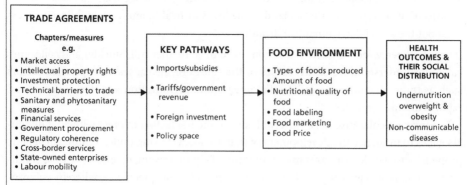

Figure 3.8 Conceptual framework of the relationships among trade agreements, food environments, and diet-related health.

Reproduced from Friel S, Gleeson D, Thow A-M, Labonte R, Stuckler D, Kay A, et al. A new generation of trade policy: potential risks to diet-related health from the trans pacific partnership agreement. *Globalization and Health*, Volume 9, Article 46, Copyright © 2013 Friel et al.

The draft Fatty Meat Import Quota Act, however, was never submitted to the cabinet—despite an earlier indication that the cabinet offered in-principle support—and was never implemented. Suggested reasons for this include concerns about the possible impact on Tonga's negotiations to join the World Trade Organization, and policy-makers' worries about the broader implications of restricting the supply of products exported by two of the country's significant aid donors (namely, Australia and New Zealand). In addition, some stakeholders did not consider the import quota to be the right instrument to use, since it did not provide any alternative product for consumption and was not the preferred option under World Trade Organization commitments to tariffication of quantitative restrictions.

An analysis by Thow and colleagues[7] examined the Tongan experience, and contrasted this with the experience of Fiji and Samoa, where bans of similar products were implemented. These measures successfully reduced the amount of the targeted fatty meat in the food supply and raised consumer awareness about the health effects of such fatty meats. The researchers were able to identify, therefore, factors that enabled policy uptake and barriers which hindered policy progress.

One of the important factors identified was ownership of the initiative by multiple stakeholders from the early stages of the policy cycle. In Fiji and Samoa the proposals were put forward by other political leaders (the Ministry of Commerce, the Prime Minister) with the Ministry of Health. In Tonga, the proposal was developed within the Ministry of Health and was promoted in cabinet by the Minister for Health.

There was another factor that may have eased the passage of the measures in Fiji and Samoa—the widespread public perception that these products are considered to be unacceptable for human consumption in the countries of origin and were being 'dumped'. This created an open 'policy window' for a health-promoting measure.

The instrument chosen is also important—in Tonga's case the mechanism chosen was a quota. This was at a time when the World Trade Organization (WTO) was explicitly phasing out quotas. Although the policy-makers would have been able to argue, under WTO rules, that the measure was justified on health grounds, there was a lack of clarity about the extent to which implementation of this measure was compatible with Tonga's accession to the WTO. In Fiji and Samoa, the policy process was simpler because the measures were implemented under legislative mechanisms.

The evidence suggests that it is possible to use trade policy tools to improve diets, but such approaches need to be used strategically. One promising example comes from Ghana, where the government implemented an innovative food standards policy to limit the amount of fatty meat in the food supply. For more details about their particular strategy, along with a broader discussion about how trade and investment agreements may constrain governments' policy options to prevent non-communicable diseases, please see the Further Reading section at the end of this chapter. A number of critical elements are needed to enable implementation of trade policy tools: effective advocacy, active involvement of those responsible for implementation of the policy from the outset, and taking advantage of any aspects of the cultural context that might create open windows for health-related measures. A number of potential barriers also emerge—limited scope of the measure, poor engagement from other (non-health) sectors, use of an inappropriate policy instrument and a lack of a clear mechanism for enforcement.

3.5 A life-course approach to NCDs

NCD prevention efforts have long recognized that health and well-being in later life are affected by what happens early in life and that there are critical points across the lifespan—including childhood, adolescence, and during pregnancy—where it may be possible to influence health-related behaviours.

The understanding of such a life-course approach to health is, however, changing in light of emerging evidence—from a variety of disciplines including genetics, epidemiology, psychology, neuroscience, economics, environmental, political, and social sciences—about the developmental origins of health and disease. Health outcomes are affected by a complex array of protective and risk factors, including genetic, epigenetic, and intrauterine factors, environmental exposures, nurturing family and social relationships, behavioural choices, social norms, and opportunities.

Increasingly, evidence suggests that the interplay between genetic and environmental factors is more complex than previously recognized and this helps to explain *how* social and environmental factors can influence biological processes. Exposure to various stressors during the period of early development (preconception, gestation, infancy, and early childhood), for example, is particularly important. In response to such exposures—such as poor maternal nutrition, foetal exposure to environmental toxins, or prolonged stress—individuals can adapt by, for example, altering the way genes are expressed or changing how the very young brain develops. Chronic stress in early life, for example, can decrease the levels of a genetic mechanism known as methylation and this, in turn, is associated with increased risk of common NCDs. Similarly, exposure to smoking or child maltreatment can shorten telomeres, the areas at the end of chromosomes that repair damage to DNA. Accelerated telomere shortening is linked to various health problems, including cardiovascular disease, diabetes, and cognitive decline.

This means that a life-course approach to NCD prevention involves much more than taking action at different points throughout the life course to encourage adoption of healthy behaviours or prevent recourse to risky behaviours. Rather, it implies taking action on the risk factors or protective factors that influence early development to maximize the peak of health. This should be followed by action on environmental factors during adulthood to maintain the peak for as long as possible and to slow the rate of loss (Figure 3.9).

Furthermore, research is providing new insights into how such interplay between biological mechanisms and social or environmental factors can have an impact on health

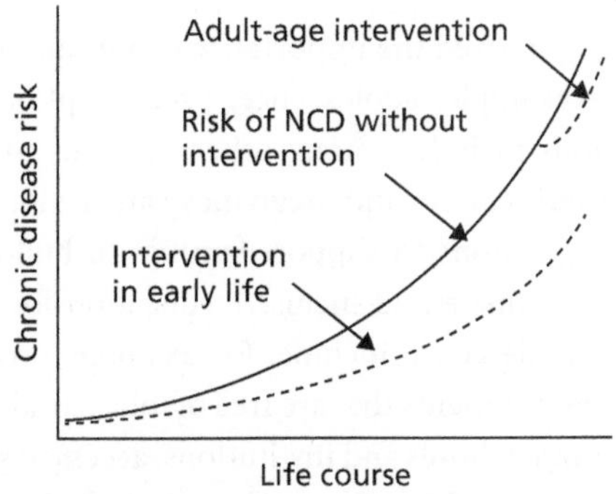

Figure 3.9 A life-course approach to NCD prevention.
Reproduced from Godfrey KM, Gluckman PD, and Hanson MA. Developmental origins of metabolic disease: life course and intergenerational perspectives. *Trends in Endocrinology and Metabolism*, Volume 21, Issue 4, pp. 199–205, Copyright © 2010 Elsevier Ltd.

inequities. This growing understanding of how health advantages and disadvantages accumulate over a person's lifetime—and the impact on health inequalities—translates into a wealth of opportunities to take timely action at different stages of life. Adoption of a life-course approach to health and well-being has, therefore, been advocated as part of efforts to close the health gap between the most disadvantaged and the least disadvantaged (Box 3.1).

Box 3.1 Minsk Declaration on a life-course approach

In the WHO European Region, the life-course approach was discussed at a Ministerial Conference in Minsk in October 2015. The resulting document, the Minsk Declaration[8] declared that 'adoption of the life-course approach across the whole of government would improve health and well-being, promote social justice, and contribute to sustainable development and inclusive growth and wealth in all our countries'.

The declaration focused on three types of action—namely, actions that are taken early, actions appropriate to transitions in life, and collective solutions. The declaration committed countries to considering national actions on a number of priorities in these three areas.

Priorities for early action target health during pregnancy and in infancy and early childhood. These include, among others, policies to minimize childhood exposure to poverty and health inequalities, policies to prevent intrauterine and early childhood exposure to poor nutrition, infection or environmental hazards, actions to minimize adverse childhood experiences such as injuries, violence, and neglect, interventions to maximize cognitive stimulation, learning, nurturing interaction with caregivers and access to quality health, social and child protection services, and actions to promote inclusive schools, kindergartens, and other educational opportunities.

The declaration also emphasized the importance of appropriate actions during life's transitions, such as, for example, adolescence, preconception and pregnancy, and retirement. Priority actions include, among others, actions to promote quality preconception information and services and pregnancy care, actions to promote, support, and protect breastfeeding, actions to support families to build parenting capacities, and policies to promote adequate and inclusive education for all. Other approaches which focus on healthy adolescence include, for example, promotion of knowledge and life skills, access to environments that are free of tobacco, alcohol, and recreational drugs, access to violence-free schools and institutions, access to supportive community networks, and access to basic qualifications and work skills. Universal health coverage for youth-friendly services was also highlighted, including provision of quality services and information for sexual and reproductive health and mental health. Priorities for healthy ageing include actions that facilitate social engagement, establishment of social protection systems, targeting supportive interventions for higher risk older people and investment in the prevention and management of conditions which limit a person's activity.

Priorities for 'acting together' emphasize the need for collective solutions that involve the whole of society, including government, academia, civil society, the private sector, and the media. In September 2016 WHO's governing body in Europe, the Regional Committee, adopted a Resolution based on the Minsk Declaration, urging Member States and the Regional Office to make greater user of the life-course approach.

Case study: Preventing substance use in adolescents in Iceland

Unhealthy behaviours, such as smoking, drinking, or drug use, often start in adolescence and can continue into adult life. Interventions targeted at adolescents, therefore, could potentially have a lifelong impact on unhealthy behaviours. For over a decade Iceland has pursued a multilevel approach, based in schools but involving the wider community, to preventing substance use in adolescents.

Annual cross-sectional surveys in all secondary schools in the country provide data on trends in substance use and insight into the role and influence of personal and social factors. The surveys have shown that a cohort which reports above-average substance use at the age of 13 will maintain that high use through to the age of 15. A cohort of 13 year olds that has lower than average substance use, in contrast, will continue to have relatively lower use for the next two years. On this basis, an approach was selected in the early 2000s to target younger adolescents, during their formative school years and before they have started to experiment with substance use.

Iceland's approach has been to try to reduce known risk factors and to strengthen a number of protective factors, such as participation in supervised youth activities or sport, parental support, responsible supervision, and monitoring. It also focused on close networks where parents know their children's friends and the friends' parents.

Key components of the intervention include the following:

- Communicating to parents about the importance of emotional support, reasonable monitoring, and spending more time with their adolescent children.
- Increasing the opportunities for young people to participate in organized recreational extracurricular activities and sport, and encouraging young people to take part.
- Working with local schools to strengthen the support network between schools parents and other relevant agencies. This network carries out various activities, including poster campaigns, weekend night parental walks, or 'patrols', to unobtrusively monitor young people's behaviour, and funding for adolescent membership of facilities offering youth and sports activities.

The evidence that this approach is working is promising, since Iceland has seen a 60% decline in adolescent substance use (in both experimentation and use of alcohol, tobacco, and cannabis) (Figure 3.10). Sigfusdottir and colleagues argue that this decline is 'due to the decade-long partnership between researchers, public health policymakers and practitioners that has sought to reduce substance abuse by reducing

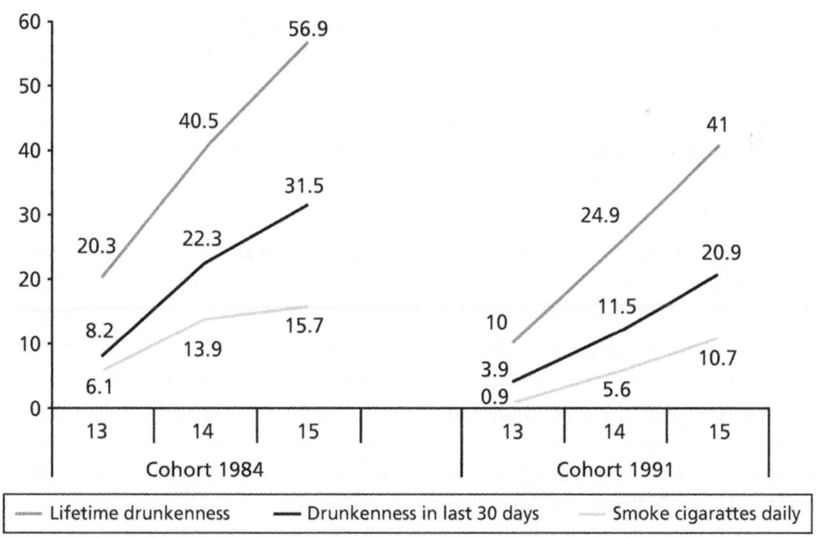

Figure 3.10 Trends in prevalence rates of substance abuse for two birth cohorts in Iceland seven years apart.

Reproduced with permission from Sigfusdottir ID, Kristjansson AL, Gudmundsdottir ML, and Allegrante JP. Substance use prevention through school and community-based health promotion: a transdisciplinary approach from Iceland. *Global Health Promotion*, Volume 18, Issue 3, pp. 23–26, Copyright © 2011 International Union for Health Promotion and Education.

known risk factors and strengthening a broad range of community-level protective factors'.

The authors conclude that primary prevention efforts that are organized around this type of multilevel intervention are likely to be more successful than single-focus efforts.

Adapted with permission from Sigfusdottir ID, Kristjansson AL, Gudmundsdottir ML, and Allegrante JP. Substance use prevention through school and community-based health promotion: a transdisciplinary approach from Iceland. *Global Health Promotion*, Volume 18, Issue 3, pp. 23–26, Copyright © 2011 International Union for Health Promotion and Education.

Acknowledgements

This chapter is largely drawn from a presentation by Professor Mike Rayner, information from the WHO Regional Office for Europe on the life-course approach, and the case study sources cited. Dr Anne-Marie Thow provided materials and feedback for the case study and reading on trade and food policy.

References

1. **Shiftn.** Obesity System Influence Diagram. Available at: http://www.shiftn.com/obesity/Full-Map.html.
2. **Victora CG, Adair L, Fall C,** et al., for the Maternal and Child Undernutrition Study Group. Maternal and child undernutrition: consequences for adult health and human capital. *Lancet* 2008; 371(9609):340–57.
3. **Yusuf S, Hawken S, Ounpuu S, Dans T, Avezum A, Lanas F** et al. Effect of potentially modifiable risk factors associated with myocardial infarction in 52 countries (the INTERHEART study): case-control study. *Lancet* 2004; **364**: 937–52.
4. **Commission on Social Determinants of Health.** *Closing the Gap in a Generation: Health Equity through Action on the Social Determinants of Health.* Geneva: WHO; 2008.
5. **Stuckler D, Basu S, McKee M.** Public health in Europe: Power, politics and where next? *Public Health Reviews* 2010; **32**:213–42.
6. **Friel S, Gleeson D, Thow A-M, Labonte R, Stuckler D, Kay A,** et al. A new generation of trade policy: potential risks to diet-related health from the trans pacific partnership agreement. *Globalization and Health. Globalization and Health* 2013; **9**:46.
7. **Thow A, Swinburn B, Colagiuri S, Diligolevu M, Quested C, Vivili P,** et al. Trade and food policy: Case studies from three Pacific Island countries. *Food Policy* 2010; **35**(6):556–64.
8. **World Health Organization.** *The Minsk Declaration: The Life-Course Approach in the Context of Health 2020.* Geneva: WHO, 2015. Available at: http://www.euro.who.int/en/media-centre/events/events/2015/10/WHO-European-Ministerial-Conference-on-the-Life-course-Approach-in-the-Context-of-Health-2020/documentation/the-minsk-declaration.

Further reading

On the methodology of quantifying health risks and causal webs:

Murray CJL, Ezzati M, Lopez AD, Rodgers A, Vander Hoorn S. Comparative quantification of health risks: Conceptual framework and methodological issues. *Population Health Metrics* 2003; **1**:1.

On the Global Burden of Disease and risk factors:

GBD 2013 Collaborators. Global, regional, and national comparative risk assessment of 79 behavioural, environmental and occupational, and metabolic risks or clusters of risks in 188 countries, 1990-2013: a systematic analysis for the Global Burden of Disease Study 2013. *Lancet* 2015; **386**(10010):2287–323.

On inequalities in health and underlying determinants:

Commission on Social Determinants of Health. *Closing the Gap in a Generation—Health Equity through Action on the Social Determinants of Health.* Geneva: WHO; 2008.

Stuckler D, Basu S, McKee M. Public health in Europe: Power, politics and where next? *Public Health Reviews* 2010; **32**:213–42.

On understanding the global picture on NCDs:

World Health Organization. *Global Status Report on Non-communicable Diseases, 2014.* Geneva: WHO; 2015.

On trade and food standards policies to prevent NCDs:

Thow A M, et al. Will the next generation of preferential trade and investment agreements undermine prevention of noncommunicable diseases? A prospective policy analysis of the Trans Pacific Partnership Agreement. *Health Policy* 2015; **119**(1):88–96.

Thow A M, et al. Development, implementation and outcome of standards to restrict fatty meat in the food supply and prevent NCDs: learning from an innovative trade/food policy in Ghana. *BMC Public Health* 2014; **14**(1):1.

Chapter 4

The sociopolitical landscape of NCDs, Part I

4.1 Introduction

In recent decades the world has witnessed rapid unprecedented transitions. Demographic shifts have placed new pressures on ageing populations whilst a double burden of infectious diseases and non-communicable diseases (NCDs) has developed in others. Additionally, globalization and urbanization have created new challenges, bringing profound dietary changes and more sedentary lifestyles for growing urban populations. Globalization is a powerful force exerting significant impacts on how both environmental structures and individual-level decisions, such as food availability and preferences, are made.

This chapter introduces the dramatic changes to the global landscape, which have created fertile ground for the rise in NCDs worldwide. It also highlights the process of health transition, which describes how patterns of disease and risk factors change with economic development and globalized markets. The chapter goes on to demonstrate why NCDs are an important issue for international development, to highlight the many competing voices and vested interests which also seek to influence policy, and to set out how the global response to NCDs have evolved.

4.2 Global health transitions and changes in NCD risk factors

The changes in disease patterns that affect low- and middle-income countries (LMICs) over time—as they transform into increasingly industrialized and urbanized societies—have been described as a process of health transition.

In fact, there are a number of different transitions that can shape public health. Rayner and Lang characterized nine such transitions: demographic, epidemiologic, rural to urban, nutritional, economic, energy, biological/ecological, cultural, and democratic.[1] These different transitions combine to have a major impact on the health of a population. The demographic transition, fuelled by falling birth rates and longer life expectancies, creates ageing populations. The rapid changes towards a high-fat, high-sugar 'western' diet brought about by the nutritional transition are exacerbated by the dramatic reductions in non-leisure physical activity brought about by urbanization (the rural–urban transition).

A model of health transition has been developed, and evolved in the decades since it was first proposed, to help explain the different stages in the process of transition.

Figure 4.1 shows the model and illustrates where different regions currently lie on the transition continuum.

Stage I Age of pestilence and famine	Stage II Age of receding pandemics	Stage III Age of 'man-made' degenerative diseases	Stage IV Age of delayed degenerative diseases	Stage V Age of social upheaval and health regression	Stage VI Era of environmental degradation
Dominant diseases are infections and nutritional deficiencies. Average life expectancy is extremely low (35). Any cardiovascular deaths are usually related to infectious or nutritional conditions (e.g. cardiomyopathies or rheumatic heart disease).	NCDs start to emerge, mainly in the form of high blood pressure and haemorrhagic stroke. Average life expectancy increases to around 50.	Coronary heart disease and both forms of stroke generally account for at least half of deaths. Changes in type of stroke depend on the changes in fat intakes and smoking prevalence, which favour thrombotic stroke.	Coronary heart disease and stroke still dominate, but deaths occur much later in life. Average life expectancy is over 70.	A period of upheaval can reverse the health gains, as occurred in central and eastern Europe during the 1990s.	This is a postulated period of environmental degradation which could dramatically alter the situation.

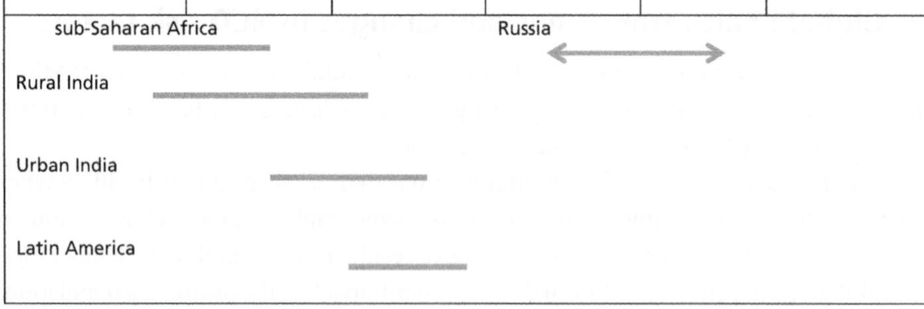

Figure 4.1 Stages of health transition

Source: data from **Omran AR**. The epidemiologic transition: A theory of the epidemiology of population change. *Milbank Memorial Fund Quarterly*, Volume 49, Issue 4, pp. 509–38, Copyright © 1971 Milbank Memorial Fund; **Olshansky ST** and **Ault AB**. The fourth stage of the epidemiologic transition: The age of delayed degenerative diseases. *The Milbank Quarterly*, Volume 64, Issue 3, pp. 355–91, Copyright © 1986 Milbank Memorial Fund; Yusuf S, Reddy S, Ounpuu S, and Anand S. Global burden of cardiovascular diseases, part I: General considerations, the epidemiological transition, risk factors, and impact of urbanization. *Circulation*, Volume 104, pp, 2746–53, Copyright © 2001 American Heart Association; Reddy KS, Nishtar S, and Thakker P. Public health in South Asia. In: Beaglehole R and Bonita R (eds.), *Global Public Health: A New Era*. Oxford: Oxford University Press, Copyright © 2009 Oxford University Press, pp. 209–24.

In the past, these changes tended to occur over a relatively long period of time. It took about a century for the USA, for example, to move from stage I to stage IV. In the recent context of globalization, however, some countries are now seeing these changes happen over a much shorter timeframe (see Box 4.1).

The health transition model is useful because it provides an evolving perspective that enables policy-makers to think beyond the immediate problems of the current health situation in their countries. It should help them to anticipate the epidemic and to provide a proactive, preventive response. The model focuses on the proportion of deaths from different causes, however, rather than age-standardized death rates. This means that there is a risk that policy-makers in the earlier stages of the transition fail to appreciate the scale of the NCD problem they are already facing (see Chapter 2 case study on Australia, India, and Zambia for an example). The reality is that many LMICs are now facing a double burden of disease.

The health transition generally has a dramatic impact on the differences in NCD and risk factor prevalence between various socioeconomic groups. At the earliest stages of the

Box 4.1 Rapid health transition in Mexico

Mexico is one country which experienced a highly compressed health transition between 1950 and 2010. The changes in causes of death which occurred over about a century in the USA took place over a much shorter period in Mexico (see Figure 4.2). Over this period, the country experienced a massive increase in total deaths with a large absolute and proportionate increase in NCDs, as well as a large absolute decrease in infectious disease.

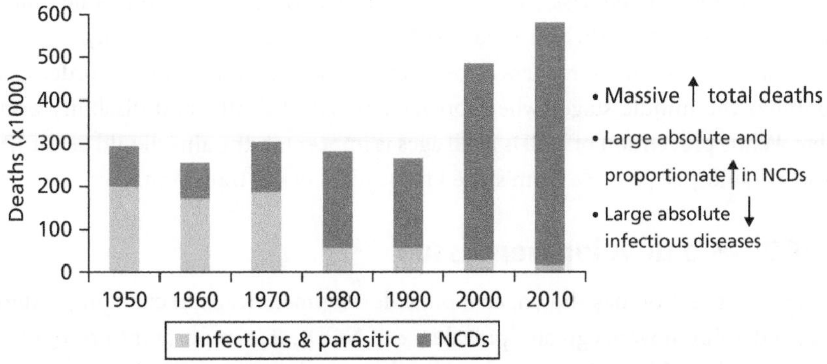

Figure 4.2 Rapid epidemiological transition from infectious and non-communicable diseases, Mexico, 1950–2010.

Source: data from **Fernald LC and Neufeld LM**. Overweight with concurrent stunting in very young children from rural Mexico: prevalence and associated factors. *European Journal of Clinical Nutrition*, Volume 61, pp. 623–32, Copyright © 2007 Macmillan Publishers Limited, part of Springer Nature.

Figure 4.3 illustrates the dramatic increase in overweight and obesity in the country.

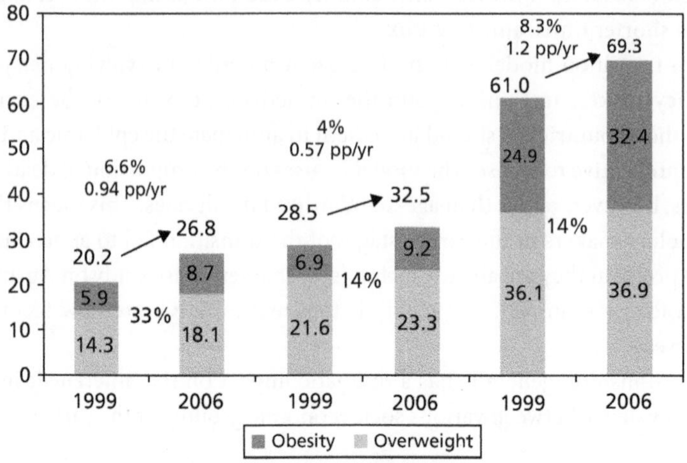

Figure 4.3 Trends in overweight and obesity in Mexico.

Source: data from **Fernald LC** and **Neufeld LM**. Overweight with concurrent stunting in very young children from rural Mexico: prevalence and associated factors. *European Journal of Clinical Nutrition*, Volume 61, pp. 623–32, Copyright © 2007 Macmillan Publishers Limited, part of Springer Nature.

transition, the poorest groups tend to be least affected by NCDs. As the socioeconomic and health transitions advance within each country, the social gradient for NCD events and NCD risk factors progressively reverses until the poor become most vulnerable. The social gradient for different risk factors will not necessarily reverse at the same time—the gradient reverses much earlier for tobacco use, for example, than for obesity.[2]

A key challenge for policy-makers is to anticipate the health transition in order to avoid or minimize the middle stages where preventable NCD deaths and disability occur in mid-life. While prevention of NCDs at all ages is important, the aim should be for LMICs to move as rapidly as possible from stage I to stage IV of the transition.

4.3 **NCDs as a development issue**

As the previous section has shown, economic development leads to changing patterns of disease, and a shift towards greater prevalence of NCDs. It is important to recognize that a growing burden of chronic disease can also have important implications for economic and social development. See age-standardized mortality rates for selected countries in Table 2.1.

As highlighted by the omission of any NCD-related goal from the millennium development goals which drove international development between 2000 and 2015,[3] NCDs have, until recently, been largely ignored as an important issue for development. Discussions on the post-2015 development agenda and the sustainable development goals recognized from the outset that a broader vision is needed and that NCDs had to be included. (See Chapter 5 for more on NCDs and the sustainable development goals.)

4.3.1 NCDs in LMICs

NCDs used to be thought by many as diseases of affluence that only affected richer countries. There has been growing realization in recent years, however, that NCDs already present a real and growing problem for poorer countries. Furthermore, as described in section 4.2 in relation to the health transition, many communities—and even families—have to bear the burden of NCDs alongside the already heavy burden of infectious disease and malnutrition. This double burden of disease places immense strain on communities, health systems, and economies.

Figure 4.4 shows that, while the proportion of deaths from NCDs is highest in high-income countries, the absolute number of deaths is actually higher in lower-middle income countries. In the poorest countries of sub-Saharan Africa the proportion of deaths attributed to NCDs is lower, but the absolute numbers of NCD-related deaths are high.

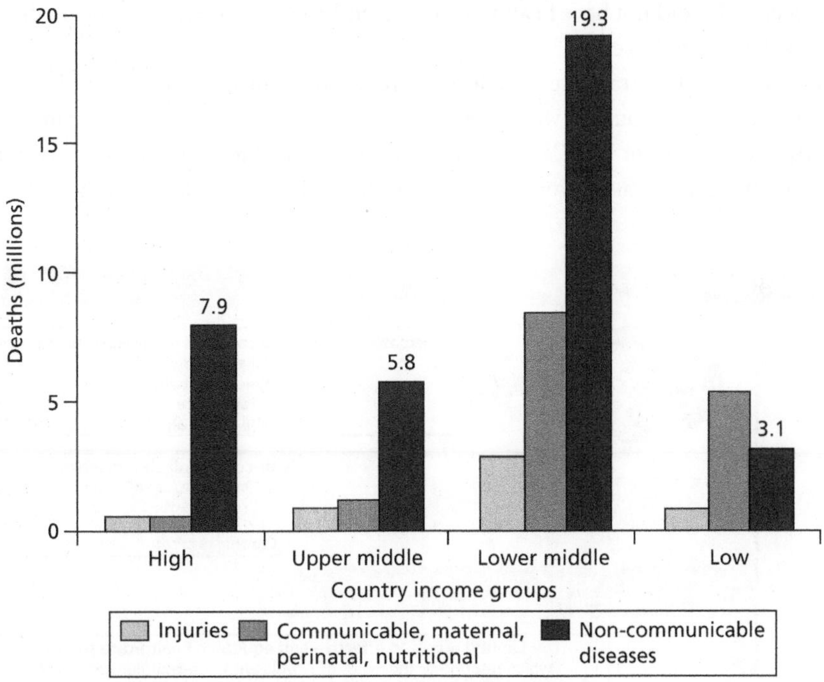

Figure 4.4 Causes of death by World Bank income groups, 2008.

Reprinted from *The Lancet*, Volume 378, Issue 9789, Beaglehole R, Bonita R, Alleyne G, Horton R, Li L, Lincoln P, et al. UN high-level meeting on non-communicable diseases: addressing four questions, pp. 449–55, Copyright © 2011, with permission from Elsevier Ltd.

The proportion of deaths caused by all NCDs is projected to rise in high-, middle-, and low-income countries by 2030 (see section 2.4). In every single region, a rise in the proportion of deaths from NCDs is predicted, with the biggest rise in sub-Saharan Africa for all ages, and in the age group 15–59 years.

When comparing populations it is also important to look at death rates standardized for age, to get a clear picture of the situation and how it will evolve with ageing populations. Age-standardized mortality rates for cardiovascular disease are highest in Africa, the Eastern Mediterranean, and South East Asia regions (see Table 2.1).

4.3.2 Economic impact of NCDs on societies

In addition to the pain and suffering which NCDs cause individuals and families, NCDs place a heavy economic burden on countries. People who die in middle age or are too unwell to work are not economically productive. This loss of income, often accompanied by high health-care costs, pushes many families into a cycle of poverty. In one study in China, 71% of 4,739 stroke survivors experienced catastrophic out-of-pocket expenditure which pushed 37% of patients and their families below the poverty line.[4] In a study of patients in Kerala in India, 40% of CVD patients lost their sources of income secondary to their illness, 82% did not have health insurance, and 13% could not continue medication due to factors related to costs.[5]

For economies, this translates to a loss of productivity through premature deaths and prolonged disability, coupled with escalating health-care costs. These costs can be particularly hard to bear for LMICs. NCDs have been estimated to cost developing countries between 0.02 and 6.77% of gross domestic product.[6] This is greater than the economic

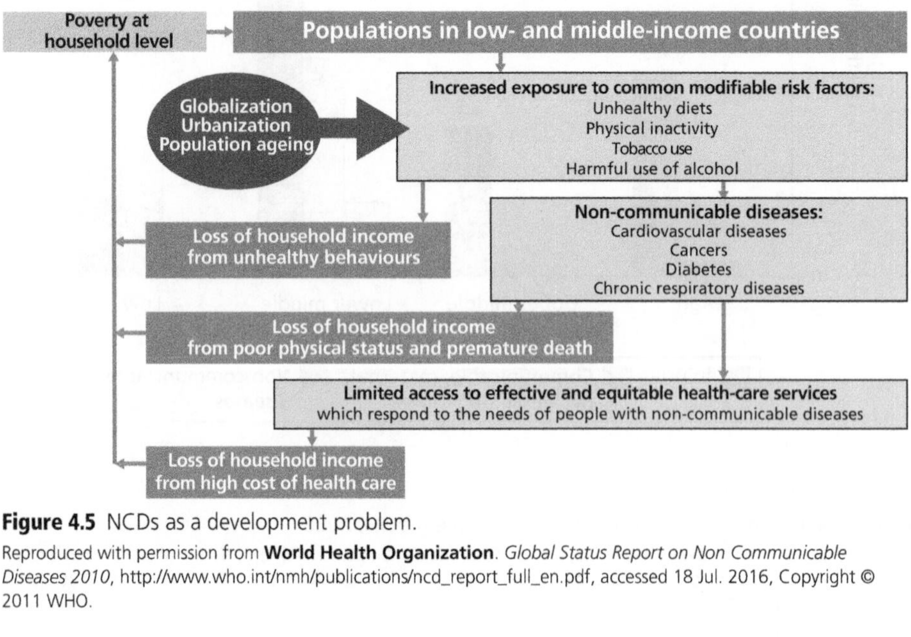

Figure 4.5 NCDs as a development problem.

Reproduced with permission from **World Health Organization**. *Global Status Report on Non Communicable Diseases 2010*, http://www.who.int/nmh/publications/ncd_report_full_en.pdf, accessed 18 Jul. 2016, Copyright © 2011 WHO.

burden attributed to malaria in the 1960s or to AIDS in the 1990s.[6] According to the World Health Organization (WHO) estimates, China, India, and Russia alone lost US $1 trillion cumulatively from diabetes, stroke, and coronary heart disease from 2005–2015.[7]

The social and economic impact of the premature death and disability caused by NCDs is certainly a hindrance to the development process, while the healthy population that can be achieved with effective NCD prevention drives forward economic development. The schema in Figure 4.5 illustrates that NCDs are a serious development issue by showing how NCDs exacerbate poverty and how poverty exacerbates the development of NCDs.

The prevention and control of NCDs, therefore, needs to be an integrated part of the development agenda. Health concerns need to be taken into account across the wide range of inter-related development issues, such as environmental, urban development, transport, and energy policies.

4.4 Competing voices and vested interests

Public health advocates must recognize that, in trying to make their voices heard in the policy-making process, they are competing with many different voices. Advocates and policy-makers in other areas of public policy will be pushing their own causes as higher—and sometimes competing—priorities. In addition, corporations and other vested interests that stand to be affected by public health policy are working hard to influence the agenda. Figure 4.6 shows the dramatic spread of tobacco and soft drinks in developing countries, illustrating why unhealthy commodity manufacturers and distributors have a great deal to lose if international efforts to cut consumption of their products succeed.

Public health advocates and policy-makers have much to learn from many decades of fighting to implement effective tobacco control and from the tactics of major tobacco companies

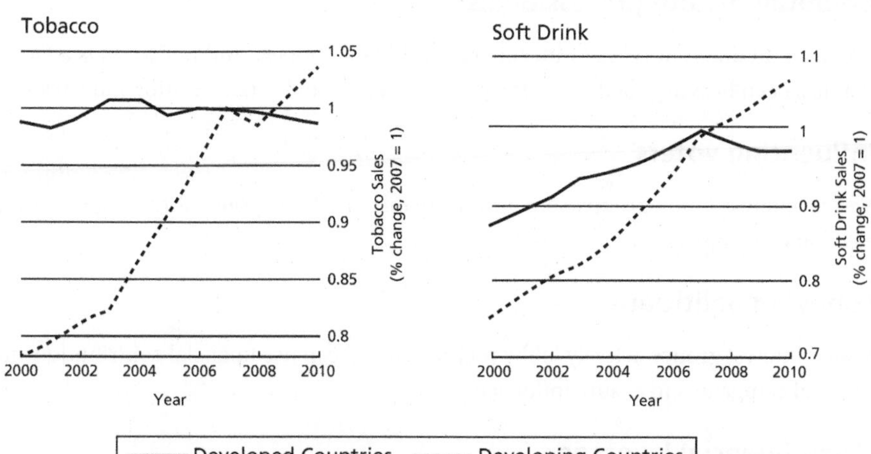

Figure 4.6 Vested interests in the NCD epidemic: the global spread of unhealthy commodities.

Reproduced from **Stuckler D** and **Nestle M**. Big food, food systems and global health. *PLoS Med*, Volume 9, Issue 6, e1001242, Copyright © 2012 Stuckler, Nestle.

('big tobacco') to derail those efforts. The extent of big tobacco's resistance is illustrated by the fact that the only 16% of the world's population are protected by comprehensive national smoke-free laws, despite the fact it is over half a century since evidence of harm from tobacco use emerged.[8] The public health fight against big tobacco is, nonetheless, decades ahead of similar challenges in relation to 'big food' and other vested interests (Box 4.2).

There is ongoing debate about the extent and nature of engagement with private sector actors, such as the food and pharmaceutical industries. There is a powerful case for multi-stakeholder solutions to problems like NCDs—a whole-of-society approach to tackling

Box 4.2 Vested interest tactics to hinder public health measures

Biasing science

This can be done by funding research studies. A meta-analysis of nutrition-related scientific articles found that the chances of a conclusion favourable to industry were nearly eight times higher when the study was completely funded by industry than when a study had no industry funding.[9]

Influencing media

A favoured tactic is to establish and fund front groups not transparently linked to industry interests. These groups then put forward media spokespersons, advocate positions favourable to industry, and create the appearance of schisms within the public health community.

Co-opting health professionals

Provision of different types of incentives for doctors, nurses, and midwives is a tactic that has been heavily relied on by the pharmaceutical and infant-feeding industries.

Influencing voters

Vested interest lobby groups sometimes organize or fund political messages during election campaigns.

Lobbying politicians

Vested interest groups actively lobby politicians and can use financial contributions to political campaigns to ensure influence.

Using financial leverage

Vested interests may also seek to influence international organizations by, for example, exerting pressure through member state governments.

issues that are detrimental to society as a whole. Voluntary action by enlightened companies could potentially be faster than the process of making new laws and ensuring that such laws are complied with. It also potentially has wider reach, whereby global companies could adopt global positions whereas laws or policies are limited by borders.

On the other hand, there are serious concerns that involving vested interests in the process can have a negative influence on the agenda—steering policies away from those which are optimal for public health. Moreover, the influence of such vested interests may be largely hidden.

This challenge of working with vested interests is one of the key issues on the global health agenda. WHO, for example, has developed a detailed framework for engagement with non-state actors.[10]

Case study: The Danish fat tax

Denmark's experience in introducing the world's first—albeit short-lived—tax on saturated fat illustrates clearly how competing voices and vested interests can block public health progress. It provides a particularly vivid example of how, even after measures have been introduced, vested interests can use lobbying, legal challenges, and public opinion to get them overturned. This underlines the role for public health advocates in defending public health action in the face of such opposition.

WHO recommends that governments consider using economic instruments—including targeted subsidies and taxes—to promote healthy eating.[11] In March 2011, the Danish parliament voted to introduce a tax on saturated fat in foods. From October 2011 an excise tax of DKr 16 (€2.15) per kg of saturated fat was charged on products with more than 2.3 g of saturated fat per 100 g. Although the tax was part of a package of fiscal reforms, it was presented as primarily a public health measure. In a nine-month period the tax raised around DKr 1 billion (approximately £100 million).[12]

Just over a year later the tax was abolished for economic reasons. During its short life, the tax had been the subject of intense criticism. Negative coverage in the media blamed the tax for rising inflation, a 10% increase in cross-border trade as Danes travelled to Sweden and Germany to do their shopping, and the loss of around 1,300 jobs. There were criticisms that the tax was expensive to administer and had been poorly designed for purpose.[13,14,15] It is important to note that the tax was introduced during a period of economic crisis and of political change—it was implemented two weeks after a general election.

In their analysis of the political processes behind the rise and fall of the tax, Bødker and colleagues report that many of the statistics cited in the media coverage did not correspond with official estimates (e.g. on the increase in cross-border trade) and/or no methodology for the calculations was presented (e.g. on job losses). Food industry stakeholders were quoted in more than a third (34%) of all media coverage of the tax between 2009 and 2013 (Figure 4.7).[16]

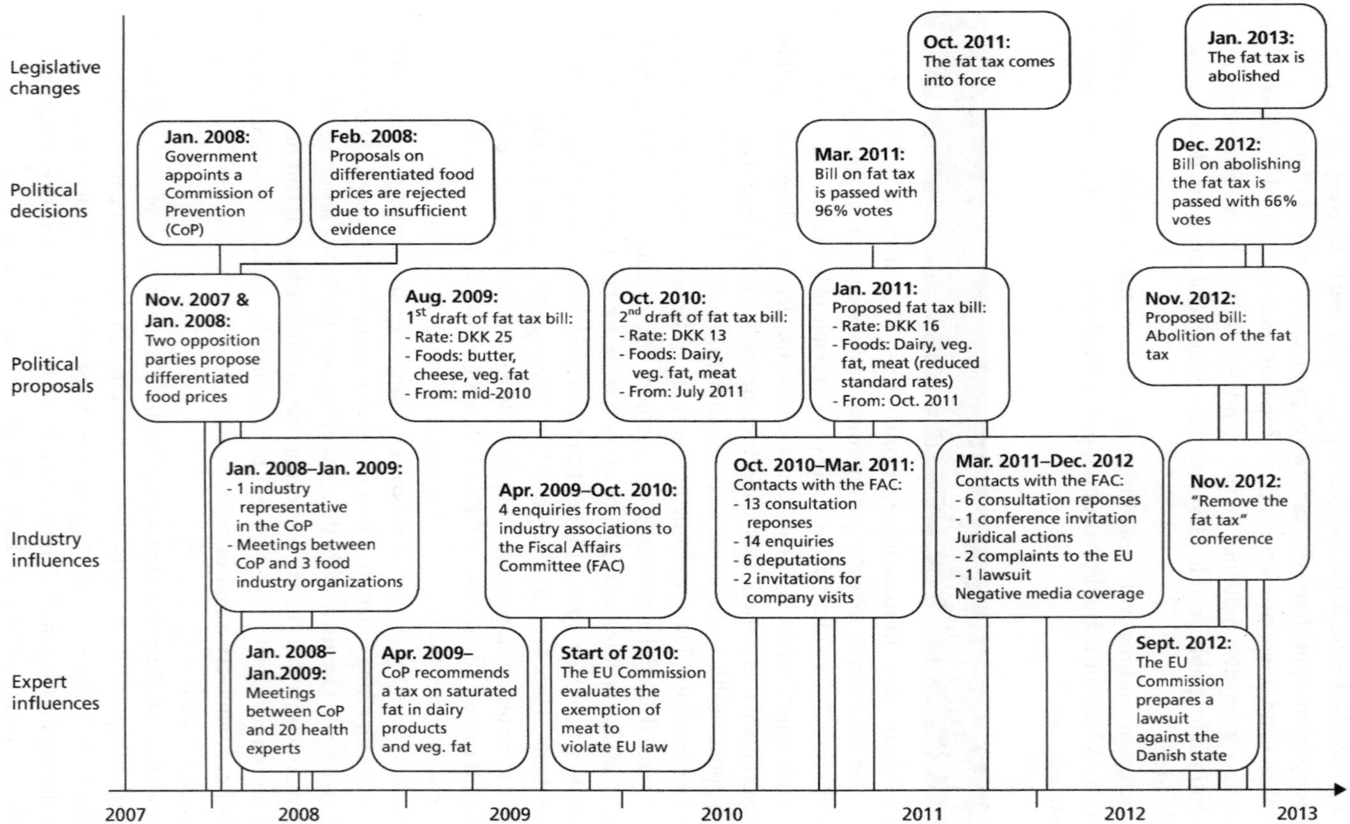

Figure 4.7 Political timeline of Denmark's saturated fat tax.

Reprinted from *The Lancet*, Volume 119, Issue 6, **Bødker M**, **Pisinger C**, **Toft U**, and **Jørgensen T.**, The rise and fall of the world's first fat tax, pp. 737–42, Copyright © 2015, with permission from Elsevier.

The bill to repeal the tax legislation did not make any reference to health, nutrition, or obesity. In fact, the tax was abolished far too soon for the impact on saturated fat intakes and, ultimately, on health to be clear. Research published since the tax was abolished has demonstrated that it did reduce fat consumption by between 10 and 15%.[16] Research published in 2016—using data from a representative panel of over 2,500 Danish households to estimate the changes in diet—suggests that, overall, the tax made a positive contribution to public health in Denmark.[17] The study found a reduction in saturated fat consumption after the introduction of the tax across all age and sex groups, with an average drop of 4%. This was accompanied by an increase in consumption of vegetables (up by 7.9%) and of fibre (3.7%). There was also, however, an undesirable increase in salt intakes in nearly all age groups. When all the dietary changes were entered into a risk assessment model to estimate the overall impact on health and mortality in Denmark, it was estimated that 123 deaths would be averted annually by the tax. Of these, 76 deaths would be averted in those aged under 75.

There are a number of lessons to draw from this Danish experience. Vallgårda and colleagues concluded that, contrary to the way the proposed tax had been framed, the main motivation for the majority of political parties to support the tax was really the revenue it would generate.[15] The authors suggest that if any similar tax is to survive 'it probably needs to be politically supported for health rather than fiscal reasons'. It is notable that plans for systematic monitoring of the effects of the tax on fat consumption, or on health, were not included in the measure. Impact on government revenue, however, was monitored from the outset.

Sectors of the food industry fought the tax, employing various tactics including intense lobbying, media briefing, requesting postponement, and threatening or filing legal challenges.[16] Crucially, their attacks on the tax continued *after* it had been implemented. The existence of some apparent problems with the design of the tax—such as the application of a standard rate of taxation on all the various cuts of meat (irrespective of fat content), which did not provide any incentive for consumers to choose healthier cuts of meat—created a window of opportunity for critics to attack the tax in the media, and public support waned. Once the tax had been introduced, public health voices to defend the measure were very weak. There is an important role for public health advocates, therefore, to be proactive in policy-making, and to continue to make the health case even after measures have been implemented.

Drawing on this experience and other examples of price policies, WHO highlights a number of valuable lessons for policy development—namely, the importance of identifying clear policy objectives, foreseeing unanticipated effects of the policy through smart policy design, and investing in monitoring and surveillance.[12]

Case study: Public health impacts of austerity

Austerity refers to a state of frugal spending where governments aim to reduce budget deficits by either raising taxes or reducing government spending.[18] Austerity measures are particularly common in the wake of a financial crisis, when governments, faced with the impending doom of a budgetary deficit, must take measures to stabilize the country's economy. While austerity may help governments avoid potential problems—such as the risk of default in cases when public debt is large—austerity has a direct effect on the health of a nation. Economic downturns have an association with substantial short-term rises in premature deaths associated with intentional violence. The fairly large and unexpected rises in unemployment following financial crises have a significantly worse effect on suicide and alcohol-related death than slow rises in unemployment in working age groups. According to Stuckler et al.,[19] a 1% increase in unemployment is associated with a 0.79% rise in suicides and a 0.79% rise in homicides among people under the age of 65 years. A more than 3% increase in unemployment had a greater effect on suicides at ages younger than 65 years and death from alcohol abuse. Active labour market programmes that keep people employed—or reintegrate the unemployed back into work—could prevent adverse health outcomes of economic downturns.

Research on the level of the individual also suggests that austerity may have adverse health effects. For example, the prevalence of psychological problems in unemployed people is more than twice that in employed people. Poor health in unemployed groups is a direct result of limited financial resources. Loss of income can lead to poor nutrition and greater barriers in accessing health care.[20] Jäntti and colleagues[21] showed that, when demographic and socioeconomic factors are controlled for, unemployed people have higher mortality than their employed counterparts. Morris and colleagues reported that duration of unemployment correlates with increased risk of mortality.[22] Unemployment is associated with increased unhealthy behaviours and affects mental health, leading to increased psychological and behavioural disorders and increased risk of psychosomatic diseases and suicides.[23]

The financial crisis in Europe in the late 2000s posed major threats for health. Immediate rises in suicides and HIV plagued nations that made cuts to public programmes. Greece, Spain, and Portugal adhered to strict fiscal austerity, resulting in alarming rates of suicides and outbreaks of infectious diseases. In comparison, Iceland, Finland, and Sweden declined taking on austerity measures and there have been no apparent effects on health care found. Though differences remain between countries, evidence suggests that fiscal austerity and weak social policies following economic catastrophes is what escalates health crises.

After receiving a loan of €252 billion from the International Monetary fund (IMF), the European Central Bank, and many European governments, Greece was forced to make severe cuts to its universal health-care system with 40% cuts in hospital budgets, resulting in crumbling health-care infrastructure. Citizens of Greece paid the price with the loss of access to care and preventative services, facing higher risks of HIV and sexually transmitted diseases. The Greek Ministry of Health reported a 40% rise in suicides between January and May 2011, compared to the previous year. The prevalence of major depressive disorders in 2008 and 2009 doubled during this period, evidence proving that those facing the most serious economic hardship were most at risk. Furthermore, an HIV outbreak in injecting drug users that started in 2011 worsened in 2012. Between 2007 and 2010, between 10 and 15 HIV infections were reported yearly in injecting drug users, a number that rose to 256 in 2011 and 314 in 2012. A low provision of preventative services, such as needle exchange programmes and other preventative initiatives has also contributed to increased HIV transmission.[21]

In stark contrast, in the mid-1990s Iceland faced economic downturn when taking huge risks in hopes of becoming a global financial centre. When the US mortgage market collapsed, Icelandic banks faced massive losses. The IMF was called in and offered Iceland a rescue package that included severe austerity measures and 50% of its national income being paid to the UK and Dutch governments between 2016 and 2023. After holding a referendum, 93% of the population rejected the rescue package which caused uproar among the Icelandic bank creditors and the Icelandic krona collapsed. However, the effects of the financial crisis on the nation's health were not discernible. There was a slight increase in cardiac emergencies but this peak subsided within a week. A national survey on health and well-being reaffirmed that the crisis has had few effects on the nation's happiness. Several factors resulted in the sustained level of Icelandic health. Firstly, rather than succumbing to austerity measures, Iceland chose to invest in social protection and pursued active measures to ensure employment. Secondly, the population's diet improved. Fast food chains, such as McDonalds, pulled out of the country because of the rising cost of importing ingredients. Icelanders began to cook more at home with local ingredients due to high import costs. Thirdly, Iceland kept its restrictive policies on alcohol contrary to the advice given by the IMF. Lastly, the population was driven by strong reserves of social capital, uniting together as they bore through this crisis.[21]

Austerity has continuously been an unpopular and severe measure to counteract a financial crisis. Cuts to public funding results in adverse health effects for the working population—potentially contributing to further economic instability. Strong social protection mechanisms can mitigate negative impacts of recession on health while austerity measures serve to exacerbate the short-term public health effects of economic crises. In times of economic downturn, it is key that public health voices emphasize the health outcomes of austerity (Figure 4.8).

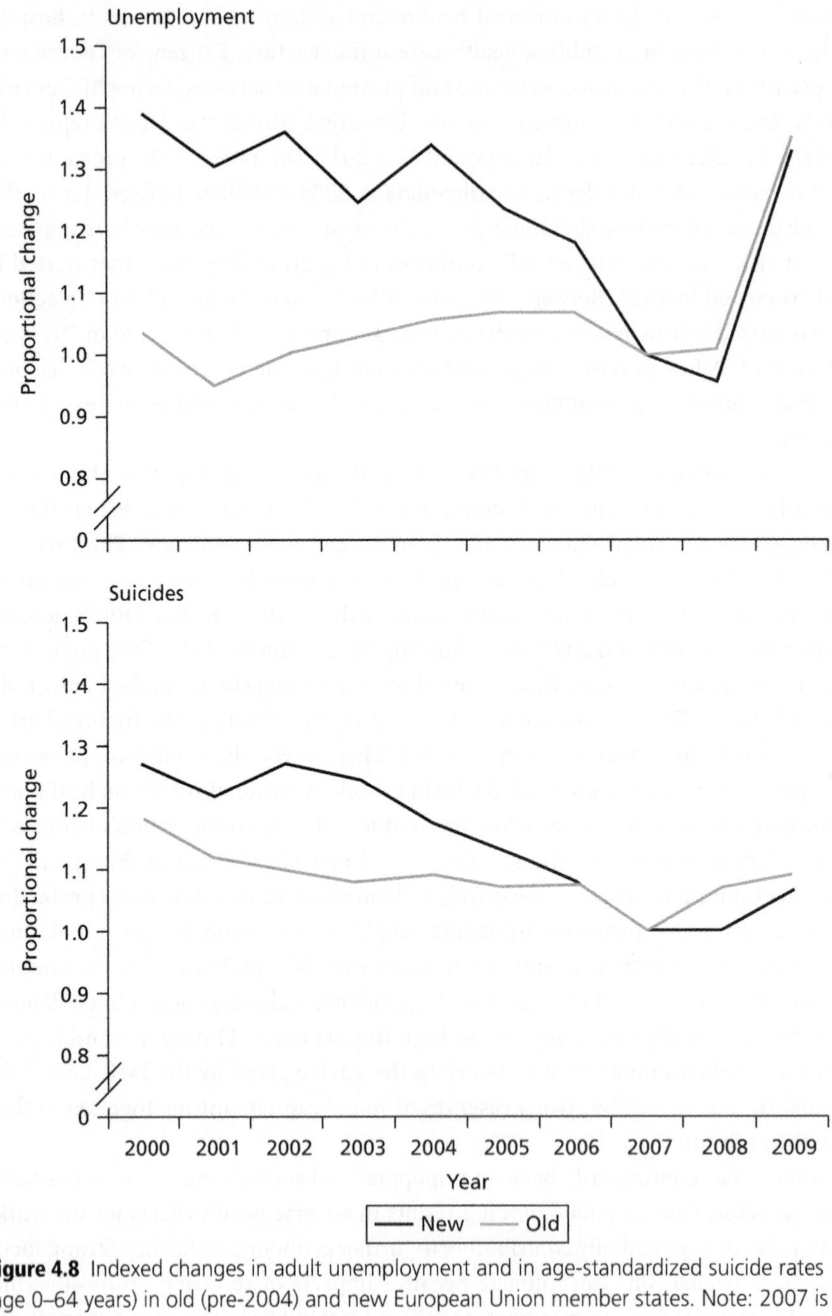

Figure 4.8 Indexed changes in adult unemployment and in age-standardized suicide rates (age 0–64 years) in old (pre-2004) and new European Union member states. Note: 2007 is the index year, and *y*-axis values represent proportional change relative to that year.

Reprinted from *The Lancet*, Volume 381, Issue 9874, Karanikolos M, Mladovsky P, Cylus J, Thomson S, Basu S, Stuckler D, et al. Financial crisis, austerity, and health in Europe, pp. 1323–31, Copyright © 2013, with permission from Elsevier.

Acknowledgements

This chapter is based on presentations by Professor KS Reddy and Dr David Stuckler with additional material provided by Nousin Hussain.

References

1. **Rayner G, Lang T.** Public health and nutrition. Our vision: Where do we go? *World Nutrition* 2012; 3(4):92–118.
2. **Reddy KS, Prabhakaran D, Jeemon P, Thankappan KR, Joshi P, Chaturvedi V, Ramakrishnan** L, et al. Educational status and cardiovascular risk profile in Indians. *Proceedings of the National Academy of Sciences* 2007; **104**(41):16263–68.
3. **United Nations Economic and Social Council.** Millennium development goals and post-2015 development agenda. Available at: http://www.un.org/en/ecosoc/about/mdg.shtml.
4. **Heeley E, Anderson CS, Huang Y, Jan S, Li Y, Liu M,** et al., **for the China Quest Investigators.** Role of health insurance in averting economic hardship in families after acute stroke in China. *Stroke* **2009; 40**(6):2149–56.
5. **World Health Organization.** Preventing chronic diseases: a vital investment: WHO global report. WHO: Geneva, 2005.
6. **Institute of Medicine.** Promoting cardiovascular health in the developing world: A critical challenge to achieve global health. Washington DC: Institute of Medicine of the National Academies, 2010. Available at: http://books.nap.edu/openbook.php?record_id=12815
7. **World Health Organization Western Pacific Region.** Prioritizing a preventable epidemic: a primer for the media on noncommunicable diseases. WHO: Manila, 2011.
8. **World Health Organization.** Tobacco Free Initiative: Implementing tobacco control. Available at: http://www.who.int/tobacco/control/en/
9. **Lesser L, Ebbeling CB, Goozner M, Wypij D, Ludwig DS.** Relationship between funding source and conclusion among nutrition-related scientific articles. *PLoS Med* 2007; 4(1):e5.
10. **World Health Organization.** Framework of engagement with non-State actors. World Health Assembly Resolution 69.10, 2016. Available at: http://www.who.int/about/collaborations/non-state-actors/en/
11. **World Health Organization Regional Office for Europe.** European Food and Nutrition Action Plan 2015–2020. Copenhagen: World Health Organization, 2015.
12. **World Health Organization Regional Office for Europe.** Using price policies to promote healthier diets. Copenhagen: World Health Organization, 2015.
13. **Snowdon C.** The Proof of the Pudding. Denmark's fat tax fiasco. London: Institute of Economic Affairs, May 2013. Available at: http://www.iea.org.uk/sites/default/files/publications/files/The%20Proof%20of%20the%20Pudding.pdf.
14. **Vallgårda S, Holm L, Jensen JD.** The Danish tax on saturated fat: why it did not survive. *European Journal of Clinical Nutrition* 2015; **69**(2):223–6.
15. **Bødker M, Pisinger C, Toft U,** et al. The rise and fall of the world's first fat tax. *Health Policy* 2015; **119**:737–42.
16. **Jensen K, Smed S.** Danish tax on saturated fat: short run effects on consumption and consumer prices of fats. Copenhagen: Institute of Food and Resource Economics, 2012.
17. **Smed S, Scarborough P, Rayner M, Jensen JD.** The effects of the Danish saturated fat tax on food and nutrient intake and modelled health outcomes: an econometric and comparative risk assessment evaluation. *European Journal of Clinical Nutrition* 2016; **70**(6):681–6.

18. **Austerity Definition** | Investopedia. (2010, May 13). Available at: http://www.investopedia.com/terms/a/austerity.asp. Accessed 5 July 2016.

19. **Stuckler D, Basu S, Suhrcke M, Coutts A, McKee M.** The public health effect of economic crises and alternative policy responses in Europe: an empirical analysis. *Lancet* 2009; **374**:315–23.

20. **Karanikolos M, Mladovsky P, Cylus J, Thomson S, Basu S, Stuckler D**, et al. Financial crisis, austerity, and health in Europe. *Lancet* **381**(9874):1323–31.

21. **Jäntti M, Martikainen P**, and **Valkonen T**. When the welfare state works: unemployment and mortality in Finland. In: **A Cornia, R Paniccia** (Eds.), *The Mortality Crisis in Transitional Economies*. Oxford: Oxford University Press, 2000: 351–69.

22. **Morris J, Cook D, Shaper, G.** Loss of employment and mortality. *BMJ* 1994; **308**:1135–9.

23. **Moser KA, Jones DR, Fox AJ, Goldblatt PO.** Unemployment and mortality: further evidence from the OPCS longitudinal study 1971–81. *Lancet* 1986; **327**:365–67.

Chapter 5

The sociopolitical landscape of NCDs, Part II

5.1 Tackling NCDs: towards a global response

Following decades of neglect and inaction, the issue of non-communicable disease (NCD) has finally grabbed the attention of policy-makers globally.

As described in Chapter 4, NCDs were for decades regarded as being of little relevance to low- and middle-income countries (LMICs). NCDs were excluded from the global health agenda and neglected in development discussions.

Between 2000 and 2011, however, this apathy gradually dissipated as increasing attention focused on NCDs as a global issue. This was achieved through a number of global strategies and action plans, culminating in the UN High-Level Meeting on NCDs—and its resulting political declaration—in September 2011.

Recent events give grounds for optimism that the world has moved beyond these periods of, first, apathy and, subsequently, attention into a period of action (Box 5.1). In May 2013, the WHO Global NCD Action Plan for 2013–2020 was adopted by 194 ministries of health at the sixty-sixth World Health Assembly.

This action plan sets out nine voluntary targets on NCDs (Figure 5.1). Countries are committed to working towards the achievement of these targets by 2025. Four of these targets relate to behavioural risk factors (alcohol, physical inactivity, salt/sodium, tobacco), two relate to intermediate outcomes (blood pressure and diabetes/obesity), and two relate to health systems. The overall target of a 25% reduction in premature mortality by 2025 is considered to be ambitious on a global scale.

It is important to stress that countries are expected to set their own national targets, adapted to the national context. Many high-income countries already have falling mortality rates, for example, so it may be appropriate to set a more ambitious overall target.

5.2 NCD control and prevention to achieve the sustainable development goals

Further evidence of this building global momentum is provided by the incorporation of NCDs into the latest global development agenda. At the United Nations Sustainable Development Summit on 25 September 2015, world leaders adopted the *2030 Agenda*

Box 5.1 Global milestones in NCD prevention and control

2000	Global strategy for the prevention and control of non-communicable diseases
2003	WHO Framework Convention on Tobacco Control
2004	Global strategy on diet, physical activity, and health
2008	Action Plan 2008-2013 on the Global Strategy for the Prevention and Control of NCDs
2009	Global strategy to reduce the harmful use of alcohol
2010	WHO Global Status Report on NCDs
2011	Political Declaration of the High-Level Meeting of the United Nations General Assembly on NCDs
2013	WHO Action Plan for the Prevention and Control of NCDs for 2013-2020 and adoption of nine voluntary global targets for 2025
2014	Second Global Status Report on NCDs
2014	Establishment of the WHO Global Coordination Mechanism on NCDs
2015	2030 Agenda for Sustainable Development adopted, setting out 17 sustainable development goals (SDGs)

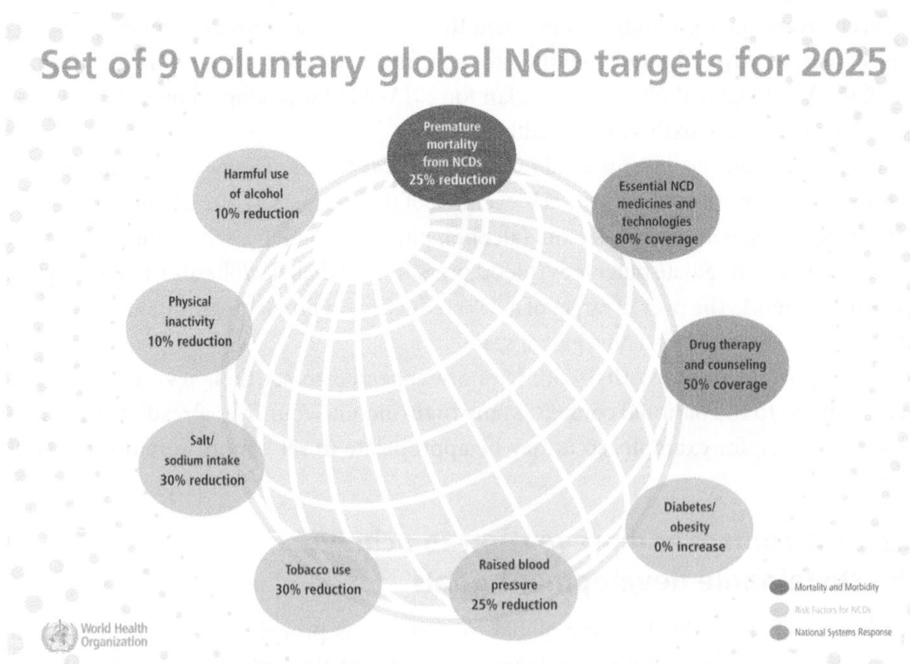

Figure 5.1 WHO Global NCD Action Plan—nine voluntary targets for 2025.

Reproduced with permission from **World Health Organization**. 'NCD Global Monitoring Framework: Ensuring progress on noncommunicable diseases in countries'. Geneva: World Health Organization, Copyright © 2016 WHO, http://www.who.int/nmh/global_monitoring_framework/en/, accessed 16 Nov. 2016.

for Sustainable Development, which includes a set of 17 sustainable development goals (SDGs) to end poverty, fight inequality, and injustice, and tackle climate change by 2030.[1] The sustainable development agenda incorporates a number of targets directly related to NCDs (see Box 5.2).

More broadly, efforts to address NCDs and their risk factors are closely aligned with this sustainable development agenda. Prioritizing NCD prevention and control will ensure that each country achieves these 17 goals in an efficient manner, simultaneously protecting human health and the environment, ultimately leading to widespread sustainable development. Furthermore, partnered approaches to the prevention and control of NCDs resonates with the 'integrated and indivisible' nature of the 2030 Agenda for Sustainable Development. The NCD-related targets may reside under the health goal, but approaches to achieving these targets cut across many of the other goals, most of which deal with social, economic, and environmental determinants of health.[2] There are, therefore, many direct and indirect links between decreasing the NCD burden and achieving a nation's SDGs.

Box 5.2 Direct NCD targets incorporated in the 2030 Agenda for Sustainable Development Targets

- **Target 3.4:** By 2030, reduce by one-third premature mortality from NCDs through prevention and treatment and promote mental health and well-being.
- **Target 3.5:** Strengthen the prevention and treatment of substance abuse, including narcotic drug abuse and harmful use of alcohol.
- **Target 3.8:** Achieve universal health coverage, including financial risk protection, access to quality essential health-care services, and access to safe, effective, quality, and affordable essential medicines and vaccines for all.
- **Target 3.a:** Strengthen the implementation of the World Health Organization Framework Convention on Tobacco Control in all countries, as appropriate.
- **Target 3.b:** Support the research and development of vaccines and medicines for the communicable and NCDs that primarily affect developing countries, provide access to affordable essential medicines and vaccines, in accordance with the Doha Declaration on the TRIPS Agreement and Public Health, which affirms the right of developing countries to use to the full provisions in the Agreement on Trade-Related Aspects of Intellectual Property Rights regarding flexibilities to protect public health, and, in particular, provide access to medicines for all.

Source: data from United Nations. Sustainable Development Knowledge Platform, 'Transforming our world: the 2030 Agenda for Sustainable Development', https://sustainabledevelopment.un.org/post2015/transformingourworld, accessed 18 Jul. 2016, Copyright © 2015 United Nations.

Goal 1—End poverty in all its forms everywhere.

NCDs are a development issue because of loss of household income from unhealthy behaviours, from loss of productivity (due to disease, disability, and premature death), and from the high cost of health care, which can drive families below the poverty line. Additionally, people's exposure to tobacco use, unhealthy diets, physical inactivity, and the harmful use of alcohol is much higher in developing countries than in high-income countries where people tend to be protected by comprehensive interventions. The cost of buying tobacco and alcohol also diverts household income and resources from ensuring food and nutrition security. Spending on tobacco and alcohol is more detrimental to the poor as their resources are limited.[3] It is important that those involved in poverty eradication and development consider not only the economic impacts of their interventions, but also their impacts on health. Linking NCD prevention with the development agenda is one of the key actions recommended by the WHO.

Goal 2—End hunger, achieve food security and improved nutrition, and promote sustainable agriculture.

One of the 169 proposed targets of the SDGs is to reduce premature deaths from NCDs by one-third; another is to end malnutrition in all its forms.[2] Many poorer countries are now beginning to suffer from a double burden of undernutrition and obesity. Nutrition-related NCDs stand at the intersection between malnutrition and NCDs (see section 5.4 later in this chapter for more information on malnutrition and NCDs).

NCD risks often stem from unsustainable environmental systems and practices, such as those related to agriculture and urbanization. Industrialized agriculture and food systems can be a contributing factor in unhealthy diets that are low in fruits, vegetables, pulses, nuts, and whole grains. An increasingly commercialized food system has led to greater availability of processed foods that are high in fats, sugar, and salt—often at the expense of localized food production. People in LMICs are increasingly exposed to these NCD risks as their environments around them change faster than their resources and capacities can protect them.[4]

Enabling sustainable agriculture can play a role in providing people healthy diets that can help prevent NCDs. A diverse diet with access to healthy food, including fruits and vegetables, and one that is limited in processed foods is important for preventing NCDs. A 'sustainable food system' is 'one that provides healthy food to meet current food needs while maintaining healthy ecosystems that can also provide food for generations to come with minimal negative impact to the environment'. [5]

Ensuring food security—when all people have access at all times to sufficient, nutritionally adequate and safe food—is a precondition for preventing NCDs. Policies and programmes to improve maternal and infant health and nutrition can reduce a child's susceptibility for developing NCDs later in life, particularly diabetes and cardiovascular disease. Policies to encourage shifts in agricultural production from commodities such as meat, dairy, palm oil, and tobacco to more fruits and vegetables would reduce greenhouse gas emissions and protect the environment, while also contributing to NCD prevention efforts.

Goal 3—Ensure healthy lives and promote wellbeing for all at all ages.

This SDG directly encompasses NCDs by targeting reducing premature mortality from NCDs by a third through prevention and treatment (target 3.4). Other targets under this goal address the various risk factors of NCDs, including targets to strengthen the prevention and treatment of alcohol abuse and implementing the WHO Framework Convention on Tobacco Control in all countries. The targets also address the interdependency of health outcomes; often communicable diseases and other acute conditions when left untreated can lead to NCDs. Hence, achieving universal health coverage allows access to quality essential health care, and investment in, and access to safe, effective, quality, and affordable essential medicines is of the utmost importance (target 3.8).

Goal 4—Ensure inclusive and equitable quality education and promote lifelong learning opportunities for all.

NCD prevention starts with education. Schools play an important role in encouraging healthy lifestyles, including physical activity, healthy diet, and avoiding alcohol and tobacco. School feeding programmes are associated with increased school enrolment and attendance can be extended to educate students about healthy dietary practices. As discussed in chapter 4, NCDs have economic costs which have consequences for sectors such as education. The cost of treating NCDs related to tobacco use and harmful alcohol use may mean that fewer resources are available for educating children, especially girls. Reducing tobacco use and the harmful use of alcohol, especially in lower income populations, provides more resources for education.[6] Education, in turn, may provide an individual with job opportunities and a potential path to improving their socioeconomic status, which, in turn, may improve their health and the health of their families.

Goal 5—Achieve gender equality and empower all women and girls.

NCDs are a significant cause of poor health and premature death for women in their potentially productive years, particularly in developing countries. As the prevalence or incidence of NCDs rises, young women are increasingly led to assume caregiving roles, which diverts their time and attention away from investing in their education and career.[5]

Goal 6—Ensure availability and sustainable management of water and sanitation for all.

Over 663 million people worldwide still lack access to safe water.[7] At the same time there is an increasing dependency on sugar-sweetened beverages (SSBs). There has been rapid expansion of the SSB industry in LMICs where large portions of the population remain deprived of safe water. The widespread distribution and low cost of these products has led to a scenario in which SSBs are frequently substituted for water. Ensuring the availability of safe water will lead to the decreased consumption and distribution of SSBs, which will help countries attempting to address rising rates of obesity and other fatal chronic illnesses.[8]

Goal 7—Ensure access to affordable, reliable, sustainable, and modern energy for all.

Around 3 billion people still cook and heat their homes using solid fuels (i.e. wood, crop wastes, charcoal, coal, and dung) in open fires and leaky stoves. This unsustainable and harmful form of energy is more prevalent in LMICs. The use of these inefficient cooking fuels and technologies produces high levels of household air pollution with a range of health-damaging pollutants, including small soot particles that penetrate deep into the lungs. Swapping these methods with cleaner cooking stoves and sources of energy can help prevent illness and death from respiratory and cardiovascular diseases, especially in women and children, who traditionally spend more time at home.

Goal 8—Promote sustained, inclusive, and sustainable economic growth, full and productive employment, and decent work for all.

Economic costs imposed by NCDs are expected to soar over the next two decades. NCDs are estimated to cause cumulative global economic losses of US$47 trillion by 2030. This constitutes a huge strain on the development process as there is a huge loss of productivity. NCDs strike people in LMICs during their prime working years—much younger than in high-income countries. Close to half of all NCD deaths in LMICs occur below the age of 70, and nearly 30% occur under age 60. Most NCD deaths are preceded by long periods of ill health. Prolonged illness and early death of the main income earner result in loss of productivity, which leads to slowed economic growth and development. There is also an indirect productivity impact when people limit their economic engagement to care for family members with NCDs.[9] Economic and employment growth impacts individuals and their wider environments. In some instances, the impacts may be positive. For example, the growth may provide individuals with the resources that they need to take better control of their lifestyle choices. Such growth may also lead to positive changes in their environment, such as improved access to health care. However, as described in Chapter 4, economic growth can also have negative impacts on health. For example, it may correspond with environmental changes that lead to a more sedentary lifestyle and a more unhealthy diet. Therefore, policymakers should take a more balanced approach to promote both the economy and the population's health.

Goal 9—Reduce inequality within and among countries.

Social determinants, such as education and income, influence vulnerability to NCDs and exposure to their modifiable risk factors. People of lower education and economic status are increasingly exposed to NCD risks and are disproportionately affected by NCDs. For example, in countries such as Bangladesh, India, Philippines, and Thailand, tobacco use is highest among the least educated and poorest segments of the populations.[10] At the same time, NCDs may also contribute to social inequalities. The costs associated with NCDs increase the risk of children missing school and becoming at risk of poverty for the rest of their lives. Addressing the social determinants of NCDs and health more broadly will augment progress towards poverty eradication and foster a more equitable society that supports sustainable development.[11]

Goal 11—Make cities and human settlements inclusive, safe, resilient, and sustainable.

Rapid unplanned urbanization in developing countries also creates conditions in which people are more exposed to unhealthy goods and physical inactivity.[12] Improved urban planning and transport policies can support a shift from private motorized transport to walking, cycling, and public transport—helping to prevent heart disease, diabetes, some cancers, depression, and dementia through increased physical activity. The shift away from motorized transport can also help prevent respiratory and cardiovascular diseases through reductions in air pollution.

Goal 13—Take urgent action to combat climate change and its impacts.

Poor air quality from greenhouse gas emissions increases the risk of developing NCDs such as cancer, cardiovascular disease, and chronic respiratory diseases. Cities account for more than 70% of global carbon dioxide emissions,[13] and almost one-quarter of carbon dioxide emissions from global energy use are due to transport. Urban development and transport systems that are not built at a communal scale and pace can also discourage physical activity, which increases a person's risk of developing cardiovascular disease, diabetes, and some cancers. Climate change can also have direct impacts on health. Extremely high air temperatures contribute directly to deaths from cardiovascular and respiratory disease. Climate change can also impact agriculture, food production, and diets.

Goal 15—Protect, restore, and promote sustainable use of terrestrial ecosystems, sustainably manage forests, combat desertification and halt and reverse land degradation, and halt biodiversity loss.

NCDs are linked to the exploitation of natural resources. The rise in palm oil consumption—a risk factor for cardiovascular disease—has been responsible for destruction of rain forests and for soil and water pollution, especially in key palm oil-producing countries, such as Malaysia and Indonesia. Tobacco farming, which contributes to deforestation and soil degradation, has also been responsible for displacing food crops, such as vegetables and pulses in Bangladesh and cassava, millet, and sweet potatoes in Kenya.[4]

Goal 16—Promote peaceful and inclusive societies for sustainable development, provide access to justice for all, and build effective, accountable, and inclusive institutions at all levels.

National policies in sectors other than health have a major bearing on the risk factors for NCDs. Policy decisions related to agriculture, trade, finance, taxation, food production, pharmaceutical production, industry, education, transportation, and urban development can have a major influence on the population levels of risk factors like tobacco use, unhealthy diet, physical inactivity, overweight and obesity, and harmful alcohol use. Therefore, gains can be achieved much more readily by influencing public policies in these sectors than by making changes in health policy alone. The health system, like many institutions, is negatively affected by war, disaster, and political upheaval. In war and disaster situations, primary health care and NCD prevention activities are often displaced by the more urgent need to manage acute conditions and emergencies. Such changes have a significant impact on prevention and control of NCDs.

5.3 **Current global action plans and targets for NCD control**

The WHO Global Action Plan For the Prevention and Control of Non-communicable Diseases 2013–2020 (hereafter referred to as the 'Global NCD Action Plan' or 'the Action Plan') aims to put into practice the promises of the 2011 political declaration on NCDs, which emerged from the high-level meeting at the UN General Assembly in New York.

The Action Plan has six overall objectives (see Box 5.3) and sets an overall global target of reducing premature mortality from NCDs by 25% by 2025.

In addition to the nine global goals, 25 indicators have been selected for the global monitoring framework. Countries will then select which monitoring indicators are

Box 5.3 Objectives of the Global NCD Action Plan

Objective 1: To strengthen international cooperation and advocacy to raise the priority accorded to the prevention and control of NCDs in the development agenda and in internationally agreed development goals.

Objective 2: To strengthen national capacity, leadership, governance, multisectoral action, and partnerships to accelerate country response for the prevention and control of NCDs.

Objective 3: To reduce exposure to modifiable risk factors for NCDs through the creation of health-promoting environments.

Objective 4: To strengthen and reorient health systems to address the prevention and control of NCDs through people-centred primary health care and universal coverage.

Objective 5: To promote and support national capacity for high-quality research and development for the prevention and control of NCDs.

Objective 6: To monitor trends and determinants of NCDs and evaluate progress in their prevention and control.

Reproduced with permission from **WHO**. *Global Action Plan: For the prevention and control of noncommunicable diseases 2013-2030*. Geneva: World Health Organization, Copyright © 2016 WHO, http://apps.who.int/iris/bitstream/10665/94384/1/9789241506236_eng.pdf?ua=1, accessed 19 Jul. 2016.

relevant to their particular context and report their progress towards targets through the global monitoring framework (see Chapter 14).

An important resource for policy-makers is the menu of policy options and cost-effective interventions for NCD prevention and control set out in the Action Plan. (For more information, see Chapter 10.)

The Action Plan seeks to involve a wide range of sectors and stakeholders in NCD prevention and control. This will require collaboration between a wide range of UN agencies, policy-makers, members of civil society, and, where appropriate, the private sector. A key challenge for NCD prevention is to engage policy-makers and stakeholders from non-health sectors such as agriculture, food, transport, urban planning, finance, education, employment, environment, sports, energy, housing, foreign affairs, social welfare, justice, socioeconomic development, tax and revenue, trade and industry, and youth affairs.

With up to 24 UN organizations potentially involved in tackling NCDs, the World Health Assembly asked WHO to work on the division of tasks and responsibilities for international organizations. A UN Interagency Task Force on the Prevention and Control of Noncommunicable Diseases has been formed, by expanding the mandate of the existing United Nations Ad Hoc Interagency Task Force on Tobacco Control, and in 2014, a Global Coordination Mechanism on NCDs was established. This mechanism is led by member states and other participants include UN organizations, private sector and non-governmental organizations (NGOs), and civil society.

5.4 **Another element of the global response: Preventing all forms of malnutrition**

Global action to tackle NCDs is complemented by international commitments to eradicate hunger and prevent malnutrition in all its forms. Undernutrition remains a major global challenge, directly affecting one in three people. In 2015, while 42 million children under the age of 5 were overweight or obese, 156 million children were stunted by malnutrition. Similarly, 1.9 billion adults were overweight, while at the same time 462 million people were underweight and over 2 billion people suffer from micronutrient deficiencies. These different—and inter-related—forms of malnutrition now coexist in the same countries, communities, households, and even individuals.

There have been a number of important recent global commitments on nutrition, seeking to tackle the multifaceted challenge of malnutrition and this devastating double burden.

On 1 April 2016 the United Nations General Assembly agreed a resolution proclaiming the UN Decade of Action on Nutrition from 2016 to 2025. The resolution aims to trigger intensified action to end hunger and eradicate malnutrition worldwide, and ensure universal access to healthier and more sustainable diets—for all people, whoever they are and wherever they live. It endorses the Rome Declaration on Nutrition and Framework for Action[14] issued when ministers and top officials from over 170 countries assembled at the Second International Conference on Nutrition in Rome in November 2014. The Rome Declaration included a number of important commitments (Box 5.4).

The Framework for Action sets out a set of 60 recommended policy programme options for countries to be able to translate the commitments of the Rome Declaration into action. Many of these policy areas are specifically aimed at reversing the rising trends in overweight and obesity and reducing the burden of diet-related NCDs. Given the inter-related nature of the different forms of malnutrition, however, *all* of the policy areas set out in the Framework for Action have implications for diet-related chronic diseases, reflecting the multifactorial nature of malnutrition and the multisectoral approach required.

Box 5.4 Summary of the commitments of the Rome Declaration on Nutrition

1. Eradicate hunger and prevent all forms of malnutrition worldwide.
2. Increase investments for effective interventions and actions to improve people's diets and nutrition.
3. Enhance sustainable food systems by developing coherent public policies from production to consumption and across relevant sectors.
4. Raise the profile of nutrition within relevant national strategies, policies, action plans, and programmes and align national resources accordingly.
5. Improve nutrition by strengthening human and institutional capacities through relevant research and development, innovation, and appropriate technology transfer.
6. Strengthen and facilitate contributions and action by all stakeholders and promote collaboration within and across countries.
7. Develop policies, programmes, and initiatives for ensuring healthy diets throughout the life course.
8. Empower people and create an enabling environment for making informed choices about food products for healthy dietary practices and appropriate infant- and young child-feeding practices through improved health and nutrition information and education.
9. Implement the commitments of the Rome Declaration on Nutrition through the Framework for Action.
10. Give due consideration to integrating the vision and commitments of the Rome Declaration on Nutrition into the post-2015 development agenda process, including a possible related global goal.

Reproduced with permission from Food and Agriculture Organization of the United Nations. © FAO 2014, *Second International Conference on Nutrition, Rome, 19-21 November 2014—Conference Outcome Document: Rome Declaration on Nutrition*, http://www.fao.org/3/a-mm215e.pdf, accessed 18 Jul. 2016.

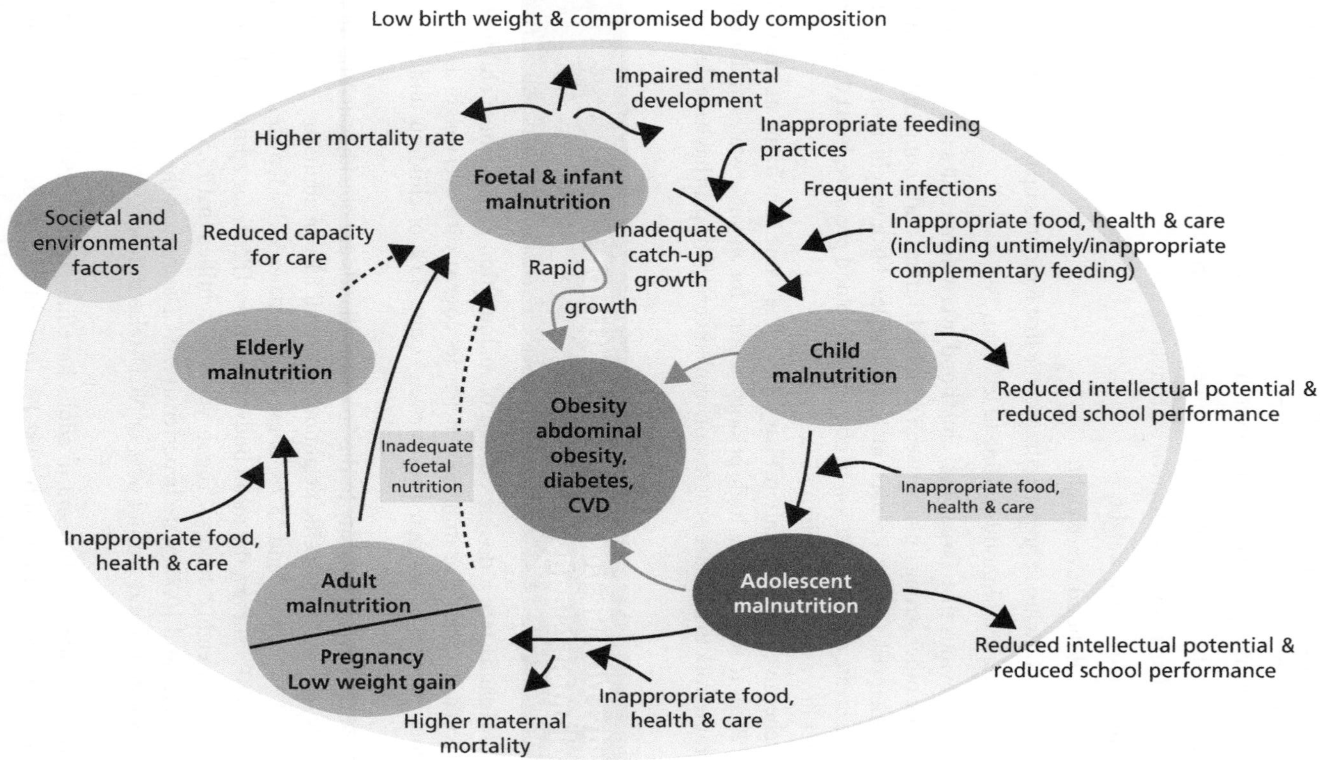

Figure 5.2 Links between NCDs and maternal, infant, and young child nutrition.

Adapted with permission from **Darnton-Hill I**, **Nishida C**, and **James WPT**. A life-course approach to diet, nutrition and the prevention of chronic diseases. *Public Health Nutrition*, Volume 7, Issue 1A, pp. 101–21, Copyright © 2004 I Darnton-Hill, C Nishida, and WPT James.

The Framework for Action encourages governments to establish nutrition targets and milestones and endorsed the six global nutrition targets to be achieved by 2025 set out in the Comprehensive Implementation Plan on Maternal, Infant, and Young Child Nutrition, endorsed by the World Health Assembly (WHA) in May 2012.

The six global nutrition targets to be achieved by 2025 are:

- 40% reduction in the number of children under 5 who are stunted;
- 50% reduction of anaemia in women of reproductive age;
- 30% reduction in low birth weight;
- No increase on childhood overweight;
- Increase the rate of exclusive breastfeeding in the first 6 months up to at least 50%; and
- Reduce and maintain childhood wasting to less than 5%.

It is immediately obvious that Target 4 on childhood overweight relates to NCDs. In fact, however, there are other strong links between maternal, infant, and young child nutrition and NCDs and their risk factors. Prenatal malnutrition, low birth weight, and undernutrition in early life create a predisposition to obesity, high blood pressure, heart disease, and diabetes in later life, as shown in Figure 5.2.

The Comprehensive Implementation Plan follows the same timeframe as the Global NCD Action Plan. It sets out five high-priority actions for member states and a global monitoring framework to measure progress on implementing the plan has been developed.

Case study: Double burden of malnutrition in the Solomon Islands

The Solomon Islands face a double burden of malnutrition exists, where childhood undernutrition and vitamin or mineral deficiencies coexist with overweight and obesity. Sixty-four percent of women are overweight and 33% of children under 5 are stunted.

Levels of overweight and obesity in the Solomon Islands are quickly catching up to the high levels seen in their Pacific neighbours. Overall 55% of adults are overweight (47.3% male, 63.9% female) and 23.7% obese (17.9% male, 30.1% female). According to the 2005–6 STEPS survey, the mean body mass index (BMI) for adults aged 15–64 is 26.7 (in the overweight category). The survey also identified that 13.5% of the population had diabetes and 10.7% were hypertensive. NCDs are now the leading cause of death in the Solomons and around 60% of NCD-related deaths occur in those aged under 70 years.[15]

While levels of undernourishment in adults have halved since 1990 to 11.3%, the prevalence of under-5 stunting fell by just 1% from 34 to 33% despite being a millennium development target.[16] Table 5.1 shows the regional breakdown in childhood undernutrition taken from the Demographic and Health Survey (DHS).[16]

Table 5.1 Prevalence of under nutrition in children under 5 years

	Low birth weight (% <2.5 kg)	Under-5 mortality rate (2012)	% of under-5s (2007–11) suffering from:					
			Stunting[a]	Severe stunting[b]	Wasting[c]	Severely wasted[d]	Underweight[e]	Overweight[f]
Total	12.5	22	33 (h)	9	4 (l)	1	12 (m)	3
Honiara (capital)	11		24 (m)	6	4 (l)	0	10 (m)	
Guadalcanal	12		34 (h)	12	5 (l)	2	14 (m)	
Malaita	17		34 (h)	10	6 (l)	3	12 (m)	
Western Province	13		33 (h)	10	6 (l)	3	17 (m)	

Severity of malnutrition by WHO classification based on prevalence: (h) high, (m) medium, (l) low.[16]

[a] Stunting: height-for-age < -2 SD from the mean height of the WHO reference population at the same age.

[b] Severe stunting: height-for-age < -3 SD from the mean height of the WHO reference population at the same age.

[c] Wasting: weight-for-height < -2 SD from the mean of the WHO reference population at the same age.

[d] Severe wasting: weight-for-height < -3 SD from the mean of the WHO reference population at the same age.

[e] Underweight: Weight-for-age < -2 SD from the mean of the WHO reference population at the same age.

[f] Overweight: Weight-for-height > +2 SD from the mean of the WHO reference population at the same age.

Source: data from **National Statistics Office (SISO)**, Secretariat of the Pacific Community (SPC), and Macro International Inc. *Solomon Islands Demographic and Health Survey 2006-2007*, http://www.pacificdisaster.net/pdnadmin/data/original/SLB_NSO_2006_DHS06_07.pdf, accessed 01 Aug. 2016, Copyright © 2009 Secretariat of the Pacific Community (SPC).

All forms of undernutrition are more common among rural children, children whose mothers have no education or only a primary education, and children in lower wealth quintiles. Stunting and wasting were also found to be almost twice as likely in children classified as 'very small' at birth, which is associated with exposure to malaria, mother's nutritional status, and betel nut chewing.[17]

The high prevalence of stunting in relation to wasting suggests chronic undernutrition and hidden hunger within the first 1000 days of life. This can be caused by inadequate dietary intake and/or as a consequence of repeated exposure to illnesses such as malaria. Stunting is a serious health concern as it impairs physical and mental development throughout the life course. In fact, undernutrition is attributable for up to 50% of cases of childhood mortality as it weakens the immune system, leaving children susceptible to infectious diseases such diarrhea, tuberculosis, and pneumonia.[18] Figures from 2012 show an under-5 mortality rate of 30 per 1000 live births in the Solomon islands, twice that of the millennium development target.[19]

While initiatives supporting breastfeeding have helped ensure 74% of infants are exclusively breastfed for the first 6 months,[20] issues surrounding complementary feeding prevail. Around 60% of children have a minimally diverse diet (meaning they are fed foods from the minimum number of food groups), and about 60% are fed the minimum number of times appropriate for their age.[17] Financial restraints and food availability mean complementary feeds consist primarily of carbohydrate-rich foods, which are typically low in protein and essential nutrients.

Hidden hunger is also evident within the Solomons as the women and children face severe levels of anaemia. Anaemia affects 44% of women and 49% of children under 5 and is often caused by a combination of a chronic lack of dietary iron intake and infectious diseases such as malaria.[21]

Dietary patterns in the Solomon Islands

Subsistence agriculture accounts for 60% of dietary intake in rural areas and is usually sufficient to put daily food consumption above the poverty line. Despite this, the Solomon Islands shows one of the highest levels of food poverty in the Pacific at 10.6%.[22]

Food balance sheets show that dietary energy consumption was adequate at 2,400 cal, although 73% of those calories were from carbohydrates and only 18% from fats and 9% protein. This equates to just 53 g protein, which is not enough to meet the average adult's requirements.[23]

Locally produced staple foods such as root crops (sweet potato, taro), vegetables, and fruits are rich in vitamin C, calcium, and iron but traditional sustenance gardening practices are threatened by increasingly severe weather events and degradation of soils.[24]

Rapid urbanization has also left the urban poor without access to land and in the urban centre of Honiara just 10% of food is grown at home. Driven by taste preferences, ease of preparation, cost, and availability, the consistent demand for imported foods has expanded markets and increased reliance across the Solomon Islands. As a result, over 90% of Solomon Islanders are not consuming the recommended five servings of fruits and vegetables each day.[15] In place of local root crops, the consumption of rice and wheat has doubled since 1990 and the Solomon Islands is now one of the highest per capita consumers of rice.[21] While fish is the primary source of protein in the diet, consumption of fresh fish has also declined due to the high cost. Fresh fish is now more commonly sold to fund popular canned fish and rice. Even in rural areas communities, 'wantoks' (family members who live in urban areas) provide supplies of imported foods and local foods are often planted solely to sell in exchange for rice, canned tuna, noodles, and sugar.[21]

Another contributory factor may be betel nut chewing, with over 60% of adults in the Solomon Islands chewing this psychostimulant (30% chewing daily).[15] As well as creating a high, it is also commonly used to starve off hunger pangs when food and money are short and may, therefore, reduce dietary intake. Betel nut chewing can also impair the absorption of nutrients and is often bought in preference to nutritious foods. Commonly chewed by pregnant women to prevent morning sickness—76% of pregnant mothers have been found to partake in chewing[25]—habitual betel nut chewing has been shown to cause a statistically significant reduction in birth weight.[26]

The nutrition transition in the Solomons has been caused and compounded by issues such as globalization, urbanization, climate change, gender inequalities, poverty, and betel nut chewing. Consequently, the Solomon Islands now face a double burden of malnutrition and coordinated, multisector action to specifically address malnutrition and food security is required. Without urgent and sustained action to improve nutritional status this burden will continue to hinder the country's social and economic development.

Acknowledgements

This chapter is drawn from the presentations by Dr Shanti Mendis and Kaia Engesveen, with additional material provided by Jessica Pullar and Nousin Hussain.

References

1. **United Nations Development Program**. *World leaders adopt Sustainable Development Goals*. Retrieved 1 December 2016, from: http://www.undp.org/content/undp/en/home/presscenter/press-releases/2015/09/24/undp-welcomes-adoption-of-sustainable-development-goals-by-world-leaders.html
2. **Transforming our world: The 2030 Agenda for Sustainable Development**. *Sustainable Development Knowledge Platform*. Retrieved 1 December 2016, from: https://sustainabledevelopment.un.org/post2015/transformingourworld.

3. **World Health Organization.** *Equity, Social Determinants and Public Health Programmes.* Geneva: World Health Organization, 2010.
4. **Hawkes C, Popkin BM.** Can the sustainable development goals reduce the burden of nutrition-related non-communicable diseases without truly addressing major food system reforms?. *BMC medicine* 2015; **13**(1):143.
5. **American Public Health Association.** *APHA policy statement 2007–12: Toward a healthy, sustainable food system,* 2017. Available at: http://www.apha.org/advocacy/policy/policysearch/default.htm?id=1361.
6. United Nations high-level meeting on noncommunicable disease prevention and control. http://www.who.int/nmh/events/un_ncd_summit2011/en/ Accessed 1 December 2016.
7. **World Health Organization.** *Drinking water fact sheet,* 2016. Accessed online: http://www.who.int/mediacentre/factsheets/fs391/en/ Accessed on 1 December 2016.
8. **Popkin BM, Adair LS, Ng SW.** Global nutrition transition and the pandemic of obesity in developing countries. *Nutrition reviews* 2012; **70**(1):3–21.
9. **NCD Alliance.** *Tackling non-communicable diseases to enhance sustainable development.* NCD Alliance Briefing Paper. Geneva: The NCD Alliance, 2012. https://ncdalliance.org/sites/default/files/NCD%20Alliance%20-%20NCDs%20and%20Sustainable%20Development%20Brief_0.pdf. Accessed 1 December 2016.
10. **Palipudi KM, Gupta PC, Sinha DN, Andes LJ, Asma S, McAfee T,** and GATS Collaborative Group. Social determinants of health and tobacco use in thirteen low and middle income countries: evidence from Global Adult Tobacco Survey. *PloS one* 2012; 7(3):e33466.
11. **Alwan A.** *Global status report on noncommunicable diseases 2010.* World Health Organization, 2011.
12. **World Health Organization.** *Noncommunicable diseases fact sheet,* 2015. http://www.who.int/mediacentre/factsheets/fs355/en/. Accessed 1 December 2016.
13. **Overview of Greenhouse Gases.** *Environmental Protection Agency. Environmental Protection Agency.* https://www3.epa.gov/climatechange/ghgemissions/gases/co2.html. Accessed 1 December 2016.
14. **Food and Agriculture Organization of the United Nations.** *Second International Conference on Nutrition, Conference Outcome Document: Framework for Action,* 2014. Available at: http://www.fao.org/3/a-mm215e.pdf. Accessed 1 December 2016.
15. **Solomon Islands Ministry of Health** and **Medical Services** and **WHO Western Pacific Region.** *Solomon Islands NCD Risk Factors STEPS Report [Internet].* WHO: Manila, 2010. Retrieved from: http://www.who.int/chp/steps/reports/en/
16. **National Statistics Office (SISO), SPC and Macro International Inc.** *Solomon Islands 2006–2007 Demographic and Health Survey.* 2007. Retrieved: http://www.pacificdisaster.net/pdnadmin/data/original/SLB_NSO_2006_DHS06_07.pdf
17. **Cafaro J, Randle E, Wyche P, Higgins M, Fink J, Jones PD.** An assessment of current antenatal care practices and identification of modifiable risk factors for prematurity and low birth weight infants in pregnancy in Solomon Islands. *Rural and Remote Health* 2015; **15**: 3230. Available at: http://www.rrh.org.au/articles/subviewnew.asp?ArticleID=3230. Accessed 1 December 2016.
18. **World Health Organization.** *Achieving the Health Related Millennium Development Goals in the Western Pacific Region.* Geneva: World Health Organization, 2014. Accessed online: http://www.wpro.who.int/health_information_evidence/documents/mdg2014leaflet_final.pdf?ua=1
19. **World Bank Development Indicators.** *Solomon Island Development Indicators: Under 5 Mortality Rate.* 2015. Available at: http://databank.worldbank.org/data/views/variableselection/selectvariables.aspx?source=world-development-indicators

20. **Secretariat of the Pacific Community.** Child Health: Solomon Islands. Solomon Island 2007 Demographic and Health Survey. 2007. Available at: http://www.spc.int/prism/solomons/index.php/sinso-documents?view=download&fileId=5

21. **World Health Organization.** *What is the Double Burden of Malnutrition—Backgrounder 4 for the Child Growth Standards.* Geneva: World Health Organization, 2006. Available at: http://www.who.int/nutrition/media_page/backgrounders_4_en.pdf

22. **United Nations Development Programme.** *Final Report on the Estimation of Basic Needs Poverty Lines, and the Incidence and Characteristics of Poverty in Solomon Islands.* Solomon Islands National Statistics Office and UNDP Pacific Centre Suva, Fiji, 2008.

23. **FAO.** Food Security and Nutrition profile, Solomon Islands. 2014. Available at: http://www.fao.org/fileadmin/templates/rap/files/nutrition_profiles/DI_Profile_-_Solomon_Islands_280714.pdf

24. **Andersen AB, Thilsted SH, Schwarz AM.** *Food and Nutrition Security in Solomon Islands.* Working paper. 2012. Available at: http://pubs.iclarm.net/resource_centre/WF_3544.pdf

25. **World Health Organization.** Review of Areca (betel) nut and tobacco use in the pacific—a technical report. 2012. Available at: http://www.wpro.who.int/tobacco/documents/betelnut.pdf

26. **Senn M, Baiwog F, Winmai J, Mueller I, Rogerson S, Senn N.** Betel nut chewing during pregnancy, Madang province, Papua New Guinea. *Drug and Alcohol Dependence* 2009; **105**(1–2):126–31.

Further Reading

WHO strategies:

World Health Organization. *Framework Convention on Tobacco Control.* Available at http://www.who.int/fctc/en/

World Health Organization. *Global Strategy on Diet, Physical Activity, and Health.* Geneva: World Health Organization; 2004. Available at http://www.who.int/dietphysicalactivity/strategy/eb11344/strategy_english_web.pdf

World Health Organization. *Global Strategy to Reduce the Harmful Use of Aclcohol.* Geneva: World Health Organization; 2010. Available at http://www.who.int/substance_abuse/alcstratenglishfinal.pdf

World Health Organization. *Global Action Plan for the Prevention and Control of Non-communicable Diseases, 2013–2020.* Geneva: World Health Organization; 2013. Available at http://apps.who.int/iris/bitstream/10665/94384/1/9789241506236_eng.pdf

World Health Organization. *Global status report on Noncommunicable diseases.* Geneva: World Health Organization, 2014. Available at http://www.who.int/nmh/publications/ncd-status-report-2014/en/

World Health Organization. Noncommunicable Diseases Progress Monitor 2015. Available at http://www.who.int/nmh/publications/ncd-progress-monitor-2015/en/

Chapter 6

Public health advocacy for the prevention of NCDs

6.1 Introduction

The realities of the sociopolitical landscape relating to non-communicable diseases (NCDs) described in Chapters 4 and 5 mean that sustained advocacy is a necessary element of the policy cycle, often required to achieve policy action. This means, in addition to defining the problem, it is important to communicate about the problem and the need for change.

This chapter explores the role and effectiveness of advocacy for the prevention of NCDs. While advocacy may be undertaken by a number of different actors ranging from governments, to industry and civil society, this chapter focuses on advocacy carried out by civil society (non-governmental agencies (NGOs), charities, academia, and professional organizations). These groups of actors have formidable strengths and powers including facts, integrity, popular appeal, consumer support, and trust.

The role of advocacy in the pursuit of better public health, including in the prevention of NCDs, was first formally recognized in the 1986 World Health Organization Ottawa Charter for Health Promotion as an important component of health improvement.[1]

At its heart, advocacy is about communicating a viewpoint in relation to a decision or action and taking steps towards trying to achieve a particular change. Advocacy encompasses a wide range of tools, tactics, and techniques to influence the setting and implementation of policies, guidelines, laws, regulations, and other decisions that affect people's lives.[2] While much advocacy invokes legal and quasi-legal notions of rights, justice, and equity, advocates for better health and environment and consumer rights are often depicted as killjoys, nannies, risk-averse, or against personal choice and freedom. Thus, advocacy in public health involves the delicate task of charting the route to improvements for the public good while deflecting attacks of being called a protectionist, an interfering busybody, or worse.

6.2 The need for public health advocacy in NCD prevention

Efforts to tackle the growing burden of NCDs and obesity cannot ignore the relative ease of access to and acceptability of harmful commodities such as tobacco and alcohol, and the shift from nutritional insufficiencies towards excess consumption of calories, salt, sugar, and saturated fat.

These patterns are a result of undeniable changes to society. Entire behaviours and lifestyle patterns, methods of food production, access to medicines, and cultural preferences have all shifted. Laws have been passed, trade rules liberalized, some choices increased while others declined, multinational companies expanded, and prices changed. These changes have resulted from a combination of factors and pressures coming from a range of interests. Policies at local, national, and international levels have played an important role in shaping these environments, whether it be related to food supplies, physical activity, tobacco, alcohol, or awareness and education amongst the public. However, environments and policies are also shaped by markets and the commercial operators who promote the overconsumption of products which undermine healthy behaviour patterns and raise the risk of NCDs.

In the past, public health advocacy relied on genteel, expert-led domination by professional perspectives within social democracies. Public health data and proposals from a medical and health elite were taken seriously and shaped public policy. But with the loosening of such politics, and the rise of neoliberal more market-oriented policy thinking from the 1980s, these old styles of advocacy have both diminished and lost their impact. Change is now more complex and involves many more actors and intervention points, something which is exemplified in the NCDs world.[2,3] The opening-up of opportunities for market actors with priorities in conflict with public health, to also influence and be involved in policy, presents an added challenge for public health advocacy which advocates need to overcome.

These issues are applicable across all three of the main NCD risk factors which are underpinned by consumption of unhealthy products: unhealthy food (high in fat, salt and sugar), alcohol, and tobacco. These products are all socially acceptable, are often consumed in excess, and have a known impact on health. The lessons from tobacco show the extent of power and influence that business interests often have in resisting change to the status quo,[4] and just as 'Big Tobacco' was deemed an 'evil' business in that fight, increasingly 'Big Food' is being seen in the same light, playing by the same 'corporate play book' to protect their business.[2]

Improving population health and reducing NCDs requires public health advocacy to reframe societal and economic ground rules to maximize good health for all, with an emphasis on prevention. Public health advocacy has a role in ensuring that the public's health is prioritized, that the required action is taken, and that, in the face of often significant challenge, the public good is protected.

6.3 The theory of advocacy

Advocacy is not something that is done or occurs in isolation of contextual surroundings; it is a product of both the issue context and the political context at a specific moment in time. This might be linked to the political will to act, the desirability of the solutions being advocated, a response to a specific crisis that has emerged, or the challenges related to opposition from market interests.

Case study: The UK's salt reduction programme 2000–2010

Under the leadership of the Food Standards Agency, the UK's 'groundbreaking' salt reduction programme achieved salt reductions of 20–30% in food products, and a 1.5-g reduction in population salt intake between 2000 and 2010, which is estimated to have prevented 20,000 CVD cases each year.[5,6] As one of just five countries (alongside the USA, France, Ireland, and Malaysia) to report salt reductions across a broad range of foods,[7] the UK's salt reduction programme has been hailed a global success by a diverse range of stakeholders, ranging from the World Health Organization (WHO) to food companies, NGOs, and academics.[8,9,10,11,12,13,14] Public health advocacy played a role in this success—from agenda setting to ensuring successful policy implementation in the face of a variety of political challenges.[15]

Raising the political priority of salt reduction in the UK

Most of the 1980s and 1990s were characterized by government inaction on salt and sections of the food industry actively sought to undermine progress on salt reduction. In keeping with policy network theory, members of the public health community played a key role in the political prioritization and subsequent implementation of the salt reduction programme.[16,17] Their power was demonstrated by their ability to draw attention to issues, shape public opinion, and hold government and industry actors to account through public naming, shaming, and praising approaches. Academics and health and consumer actors collaborated on a process of agenda setting to raise the profile of the links between poor diet (including salt) and cardiovascular disease and to stimulate action. Academics produced research on the rising prevalence of hypertension[18] and evidence that processed foods were the major contributor of salt to UK diets,[19] and shaped the policy agenda by ensuring that salt and health was considered by expert advisory committees to government.[20,21,22,23] Health NGOs used the evidence generated by academics to campaign for government action on salt reduction.[24,25]

The global scandal of the bovine spongiform encephalopathy (BSE) crisis changed the political climate and, shortly after publication of the official inquiry report into the origins and handling of the crisis, members of the public health community collaborated with the British Medical Journal (BMJ) on a series of papers which drew attention to similar conflicts of interest in the area of salt and health. The papers included new analyses confirming the link between salt intake and population blood pressure,[26,27] an article highlighting the extent of industry tactics in blocking effective policy on salt, for example, through threats to withdraw funding from political parties,[28] a letter from the industry-funded 'front group' the Salt Institute to illustrate how industry sought to undermine the evidence,[26] and an article announcing the establishment of the NGO Consensus Action on Salt and Health (CASH). CASH's objectives were to counteract the industry 'propaganda' and misinformation on salt, raise awareness of its harms, advocate for government action, and in the absence of government leadership, take on the role of working with and persuading the food industry to reduce the salt content in food.[29] The organization was spearheaded by Graham MacGregor, a blood pressure doctor and professor of cardiovascular medicine.[30,31] CASH worked with progressive food companies in the late 1990s on salt reduction. The supermarket Asda adopted comprehensive salt reduction targets and cut 900 tonnes of salt from its food between 1998 and 2003.[32] These early efforts provided important evidence on technical feasibility and provided the basis for the model which was subsequently developed by the Food Standards Agency's salt reduction programme.[31,33]

Implementation of the Food Standards Agency Salt Reduction Programme

The public health community's resources were significantly boosted by the change of government in 1997 which prioritized salt reduction within its health policies[34,35,36] and established an independent Food Standards Agency (FSA) in 2000.

The FSA adopted a *strong leadership* role in which it brought together actors from all sectors to collaborate on salt reduction. Industry actors were particularly keen to cooperate in order to restore the reputational damage from the BSE crisis.

Through the process of 'negotiated agreements' the FSA facilitated a process of communication, openness, and information sharing, which helped to build trust and improve collaboration among the diverse actors from industry and public health who were involved in the salt reduction programme. The process led to the FSA developing an inclusive *salt reduction model* which identified salt reduction targets for different food groups based on their contribution to the population's salt intake. The model was broadened to cover 85 food groups, creating a level playing field for the food industry. The process supported knowledge sharing and learning on the feasibility of reformulation among the different actors involved. Those food companies who had embarked on salt reduction initiatives from the late 1990s provided valuable evidence and information on technical feasibility which further supported the programme.

The FSA complemented the salt targets with four *public awareness raising campaigns*, which informed consumers of the role of salt in health, highlighted the fact that 75% of salt came from processed foods, and urged consumers to check the labels and choose products with less salt.

The FSA also developed an open and *transparent monitoring mechanism* for assessing progress on salt reduction. Data were collected through a number of monitoring mechanisms[37] including a standardized self-reporting form for industry completion and independent data from a processed foods database. This provided essential motivation for companies, as it publicly exposed those who were doing well and those who were lagging behind. Public health actors were also able to target their advocacy and naming and shaming efforts. FSA's data were complemented by information generated by CASH, which also undertook surveys of salt levels and ensured the issue retained a high profile. Urinary sodium data from the national diet and nutrition survey demonstrated a reduction in salt intakes in the population and provided a further source of motivation and reward for all actors.

The robustness of the salt reduction programme's monitoring mechanism and public, open, and transparent approach led the FSA to be praised by the Better Regulation Authority for its innovative alternative approach to 'traditional' regulation and enforcement.[38] The 'soft regulation' approach is supported by the evidence that successful voluntary agreements include those with 'substantial and financially important incentives and sanctions for non-participation or non-fulfilment of targets'.[15,39]

Advocacy is largely driven by the policy process. Understanding what causes change and applying that to advocacy actions, opportunities, process, and strategy is therefore valuable to understand the role advocacy can play in the policy world we are in. Political scientists have theorized policy change extensively and well and thus drawing attention to this literature should be of interest and value to academics and advocates alike when exploring the role of public health advocacy.

Political theorists have outlined a number of models of policy change. Advocacy carried out by civil society, including NGOs and academics, plays an important role in these policy processes, using a range of actions to frame issues, set agendas, influence discourse, stimulate policy change, and ensure adequate policy implementation so as to protect the public good and promote public health. An overview of each theory and a suggestion of the types of advocacy linked to each are described in Table 6.1.

6.4 **Advocacy in practice**

Advocacy takes place in a complex and often fluid and unpredictable context which nonetheless needs to be understood as much as possible. Time must be assigned to understanding, not only the perspectives and arguments to be used by the advocate, but the context, the issue, the actors, the perspectives, the arguments, the counter-lobby, the opportunity(ies) for change, where the movement might come from, where advocates should push, and so on. The best advocacy will take these in turn and work out the best methods and tactic for each as part of a wider strategy.

Strategies for advocacy require consideration of the agenda setting, framing, and awareness-raising processes identified in the political theory, through to whether advocacy should be targeted 'inside' or 'outside' formal processes, who else should be engaged, and whether actions will be reactive or proactive. Due to the fact that advocates have little power to make changes themselves, instead relying on their power to influence the policy elite,[40] advocacy often reflects the nature of the relationship that exists between the advocate and the policy-maker. A relationship may be cooperative, where views on goals and strategies are similar; concurrent or complementary, where the goals are the same but strategies differ; or competitive/confrontational, where the goals and strategies are different.[40,41,42]

Table 6.1 Theorizing advocacy

Theory/framework	Description	The role of advocacy	Examples of advocacy methods
Advocacy coalition framework (ACF)	ACF is rooted in the political sciences and argues that policy change happens as a result of coordinated activities by coalitions with shared beliefs which are resistant to change, unless exposed to external events or new learning. Coalitions compete for sympathetic policy-makers and opportunities to inform popular thinking. A change will occur, not due to an event or external factor, but due to the exploitation of that event by a coalition. This theory puts a lot of value on research to support the coalition's beliefs and argues that the non-dominant coalitions must invest time in altering and challenging this dominant way of thinking in order to increase the likelihood of change occurring.	◆ Share resources such as expertise, knowledge, and people-power across sectors to help increase power and leverage change. ◆ Focus on changing public opinion/norms using a range of tactics ◆ Targeting different stakeholders, rather than just focusing on the policy-makers themselves ◆ Undertaking research	◆ Policy analysis ◆ Forming coalitions and networks ◆ Using social media ◆ Consumer awareness ◆ Watchdog role (governments and industry) ◆ Undertaking research
Punctuated Equilibrium Theory (PET)	PET infers that significant changes in policy can occur abruptly when the right conditions take place, such as following a crisis, research development, new perceptions, new governments, increased media attention, public interest, new stakeholders. This theory assumes that government policies typically maintain a status quo, that redefining a problem helps to mobilize new people, and that media can play an integral role in this. Under periods of stability, opposition to the status quo can arise amongst policy-makers and key decision-makers, thus increasing opportunity for change. This theory may be useful for looking at large-scale policy.	◆ To increase the likelihood of change occurring ◆ Prepare to respond quickly when such a change does occur ◆ Framing, mobilization, attention to policies at fundamental level	◆ Securing media coverage ◆ Stakeholder meetings ◆ Expert advice at hearings and committees ◆ Consumer awareness ◆ Undertaking research

Policy window	Policy window theory focuses on three independent streams—policies, politics, and problems—and argues that change occurs when 'windows of opportunity' arise due to two or more of these streams aligning. The 'problem' refers to how a policy issue is framed, and the relevance of policy to address it; 'policy' refers to the different policy options available to do this; 'politics' refers to the political climate, stakeholders, and national mood on the issue.	◆ Ensuring the problem is framed in a palatable way for politicians ◆ Suggesting a range of policy options with evidence that they will work ◆ Prepare to respond quickly when such a change does occur ◆ Raising awareness amongst citizens and stakeholders to create demand ◆ Advocates need knowledge, time, relationships, good reputations	◆ Policy analysis ◆ Publishing reports and briefings ◆ Use of social media ◆ Consumer awareness ◆ Watchdog role (governments and industry) ◆ Calls to action/manifestos
Social movement theories and grassroots/ community organizing	Social movement theories focus on the processes required to stimulate change, such as the coalitions, framing, and sustained action. Collective action is defined as 'collective challenges, based on common purposes and social solidarities, in sustained interaction with elites, opponents, and authorities'[11] while grassroots and community organizing theories suggest that policy change is made through collective action of those affected by the problem. Social movement and grassroots organizing theories suggest that power is changeable and dynamic, rather than being held by elites. Power comes as a result of capacity building and coalitions which focus on the need for change by institutions not individuals.	◆ Building social networks ◆ Share resources such as expertise, knowledge, and people power ◆ Frame the issue ◆ Seek support and empower others ◆ Facilitating collaborations	◆ Securing media coverage ◆ Publishing reports and briefings ◆ Forming coalitions and networks ◆ Use of social media ◆ Training and capacity building ◆ Protests and media stunts

(*continued*)

Table 6.1 Continued

Theory/framework	Description	The role of advocacy	Examples of advocacy methods
Contextual Interaction Theory	Contextual interaction theory is a social process theory which builds on networks and governance frameworks to focus on the interactions among the actors involved in the policy process. It suggests that the policy process is dependent on the characteristics of the actors involved in relation to their attempts to support, hinder, or alter the character of the implementation process. Actors have a set of three core constructs which contribute to implementation and through which all other factors operate: motivation, information, and power. Collaboration is most likely when an actor perceives the policy as a priority, is convinced there is a solution, concludes that action in its own interest, and has the capacity to implement interventions.	◆ Build networks and alliances with other stakeholders ◆ Undertake advocacy between organizations to enable collaboration to achieve shared goals ◆ Synthesizing, framing, and disseminating information and communicating this between actors	◆ Forming coalitions and alliances ◆ Information sharing and dissemination ◆ Message framing ◆ Joint actions
Narrative theories	Narrative theory is about communicating an argument and telling a story in order to stimulate policy change. At the heart of narrative theories is framing to aid agenda setting. Reasoned arguments, with justifications, are the basis of policy decisions and can therefore be viewed as a result of the communication of ideas. The justifications are critically assessed by different actors. Policies based on justification from narratives can be criticized for serving a small number of people only.	◆ Framing and communicating a problem and a solution ◆ Carry out research that supports the story	◆ Stakeholder meetings ◆ Expert advice at hearings and committees ◆ Publishing reports and briefings ◆ Use of social media ◆ Conferences and events

Adapted with permission from Brinsden H and Lang T. *An Introduction to Public Health Advocacy: Reflections on Theory and Practice*, 12 October 2015. London: Food Research Collaboration Brief, http://foodresearch.org.uk/wp-content/uploads/2015/10/BrinsdenLang_PublicHealthAdvocacy_FRC_briefing_FINAL2_19_10_15.pdf, accessed 11 Aug. 2016,

A package of actions targeted in the right way will increase the chances of goals being achieved. Common methods used as part of advocacy to influence policy include conducting and disseminating research,[43,44,45,46] generating public support through campaigns and education,[45,47,48] the use of media to communicate and frame messages,[44,49,50,51] electoral-based lobbying or campaigning and direct targeting of policy-makers or other decision-makers, evaluating policies,[48,52] legislative action and litigation,[44,47,53] and taking on an independent watchdog role.[54,55,56] Some of these strategies are discussed further later, and illustrated in the case studies on salt reduction and nutrition labelling.

6.4.1 The media

Using media is a powerful tool for communication, and has been defined as a 'blend of science, politics and activism',[57] which is 'in a large part about making sure the story gets told from a public health point of view'.[58] The media can have a number of functions in public health advocacy, including to share evidence and research, raise awareness and concern amongst the public, demonstrate public support to decision-makers, and expose practices which undermine health. The media are commonly cited as having played a key role in tobacco control advocacy and policy,[59,60] as well as in advocacy related to food and nutrition.

Any NCD media strategy—whether for advocacy, health promotion, or other aspects of NCD prevention—needs to recognize the important role of social media, and the differences from traditional mass media (see Box 6.1).

Box 6.1 Social media—a new tool in the prevention of NCDs

The rapid rise in social media has dramatically changed how we communicate and access information. Since 2005 an information and communication technology revolution has seen the number of internet users triple to over 3.3 billion.[61] Historically, online presence was in the form of websites for the one-way broadcasting and dissemination of information. Today, social media has changed the monologue to a dialogue by creating forums for instant social interaction, exchange, and collaboration.

Social media describes webpages and applications which enable people to participate in social networking and the creation or sharing of content (videos, picture, web links).[62] Popular social media sites include Twitter, YouTube, and Instagram, though the most well-known and utilized site is Facebook with an estimated 1.59 billion users logging on each month.[63] Over 70% of internet users now engage in social media. Thanks to the rapid growth of mobile internet this boom is not isolated to developed countries. India, Indonesia, Vietnam, and the Philippines are now some of the world's most active social media users.[64]

This revolution in communication and information sharing has had a significant impact in the health arena. The two-way nature of social media creates a new interface among the public, patients, and health-care professionals. We now live in a generation that is more likely to go online to answer general health questions than ask a doctor and a health message can spread via twitter faster than a virus.

Social media in health

In 2009 health organizations began to realize the potential of social media when it was utilized to geographically locate the presence of flu based on people's search terms during the H1N1 influenza pandemic.[65] WHO also harnessed social media to counteract a dangerous rumour following the 2011 Japan earthquake and Fukushima disaster that consuming large amounts of iodized table salt would reduce the effects of radiation, triggering people in China to begin stockpiling salt.[66] Delivering coordinated messages alongside local health agencies over social media channels they were able to bring clarification to this misconception and warn of excessive salt intakes effect on blood pressure. Within a few days the message had spread, the number of tweets spreading the rumour reduced, and reports came through of people trying to refund their bulk salt purchases.[66] In Afghanistan too, social media has been a crucial element of communication campaigns to improve transparency and dispel rumours that have previously hindered the success of vaccinations for the eradication of polio.[67]

In the area of NCDs, social media is playing an increasing role in health awareness. In fact, WHO has declared mass media campaigns which promote healthy eating and physical activity as a 'best buy' for the prevention and control of non-communicable diseases.[68] Within mass media campaigns, social media offers an affordable and rapid avenue to reach far greater audiences than previously achieved with traditional media. A 2016 review of social media's impact on behavioural risk factors of NCDs revealed the need for strengthened action in the area.[69] While a small, significant improvement in physical activity, body weight, and eating habits was found in social media-based interventions, the potential impact was limited by the quality of both the social media itself and the evaluation conducted.

Barriers to social media in health

While the potential benefits of social media in both informing and delivering health programmes are countless, barriers can limit progress and must be adequately addressed.

Social media requires constant updating and engagement to ensure readership. Its rapid rise has created new workloads, and many health professionals lack experience, knowledge, and training around its successful delivery. This has caused a current gap in health-related social media experts. Social media also places health-care professionals under greater public scrutiny and the current lack of training or formal guidelines and procedures also places them at risk of unintentionally violating professional regulations.

Lack of content regulation on social media sites has also increased the risk of misconceptions and rumours surrounding personal health as non-experts can quickly gain popularity and audience reach. This was witnessed in the Ebola outbreak were the rapid spread of rumours caused mass panic. Increased social media engagement by the public also leads to greater exposure to food marketing. The Coca-Cola company is now the most popular food and beverage marketer on Facebook and its heavy investment in marketing has gained over 95 million followers. The extent to which social media exacerbates health inequalities is also unknown, as previous research has indicated that social media users are more likely to have higher levels of education and income.

Future potential

While social media may not achieve world health, it does create invaluable points of contact between professionals and the public to provide accurate health information and promote sustained behaviour change. As the United Nations vows, 'to connect villages … health centres and hospitals with Information Communication Technologies', the influence of social media in health is only set to rise and warrants a larger investment in NCD prevention and control programmes. Through increased utilization and training of health professionals, social media creates a novel, affordable tool for health promotion in low-, middle-, and high-income countries.

6.4.2 Research

The use of research information by advocates is frequently highlighted as an important component of advocacy,[44,70] especially when focusing on evidence-based advocacy[71] where advocates want to ensure they establish themselves as having expertise and credibility.[72] Where there have been public health wins, a clear evidence base on the problem, intervention effectiveness, and exposure of industry tactics can be seen,[73] which allowed for a clear public health policy to be implemented. Strong research not only equips the public health advocates themselves, but also helps equip government officials with the necessary armour to defend industry advocacy which often challenges the evidence base, as seen in tobacco, salt reduction, and alcohol.

6.4.3 Networks, alliances, and coalitions

Networking and coalitions[45,48,74] are common in advocacy not only because they allow the pooling of resources, but because they allow advocates to work together and synthesize a view point which can signal to policy-makers that an issue has a large amount of support.[75] Public health policies are more likely to be adopted and implemented when government policy-makers, academics, professional groups, and health and consumer NGOs collaborate and pool resources in the pursuit of public health policy goals. There are numerous examples of effective advocacy networks—from global (e.g. the NCD Alliance[76] or

World Obesity[77]) to regional (e.g. the European Heart Network[78]) to local (e.g. UK Health Forum[79] and Sustain, the alliance for better food and farming[80], in the UK).

The nutrition labelling case-study illustrates the potential benefits associated with collaborations between public health practitioners and willing food companies, as well as the potential risks. Where there is significant divergence in missions, there is the risk that such collaborations can divert attention from effective public health action, help to 'whitewash' a corporation's tarnished image, and/or risk damaging the reputation of the public health actors. Public health actors will therefore need to carefully weigh up the benefits and risks of partnerships with private sector companies as an approach to improving public health.

6.4.4 Challenging commercial interests

The tobacco advocacy which culminated in the Framework Convention on Tobacco Control (FCTC)[81] and also the advocacy to get the International Code of Marketing of Breast-milk Substitutes[82] showed that effective advocacy can emerge through monitoring and challenging commercial activity and power, raising awareness of this and also getting consensus on what needs to happen, especially where there are significant commercial and economic interests at stake. If health advocates are to win against powerful industry interests, they must argue for government to govern, using the full range of policy measures, not just the lowest hanging fruit. They are also going to have to be prepared to target very powerful commercial interests and convince the public of the necessity of change, thus being 'thought leaders' and 'policy listeners'.

6.4.5 Advocates as watchdogs

Civil society organizations often take on the role of independent 'watchdogs'[54,55,56] who monitor policies and practices, and challenge the status quo[83,84,85] to accelerate change. The shift towards multilevel governance, self-regulation, and government deregulation has meant these mechanisms of monitoring as part of advocacy are increasingly pertinent in NCDs policy. Such activities form part of an accountability framework[86] and can be directed both at governments[87,88] to highlight where progress is and is not being made and therefore where government regulation is required and at businesses to put pressure on them directly to make changes.[89]

The specific methods used by NGOs and academia to explore the performance of government policies or industry action vary.[90] In relation to food companies, for example, Which?, a UK based consumer organization, compares companies' (in)action on food and nutrition;[91] surveys carried out by Consensus Action on Salt & Health (CASH) in the UK and The Rudd Centre in the USA compare and rate company progress in product reformulation;[92] the Obesity Policy Coalition compares local governments in Australia as part of an Obesity Action Award;[93] while the International Network for Obesity/NCD Research, Monitoring and Action Support (INFORMAS) takes a more comprehensive approach and aims to monitor public and private sector action that influences food environments in the context of rising levels of NCDs and obesity.

6.5 Measuring the effectiveness of public health advocacy

The impact that advocacy has and the extent to which it is effective are under-researched in public health. The relative absence of evidence on how, when, and why the different advocacy methods may (or may not) be effective tools for advocates to use presents a major gap in the advocacy literature.

There is increasing interest from organizations to better understand the impact that their advocacy has so as to identify best practice, how advocacy works at different levels and in different arenas, and where funding would be best spent to stimulate the desired change and to help shift the balance of power towards the public interest. A number of organizations have developed frameworks to aid individuals and organizations in their ability to influence agendas and to highlight levels at which advocacy should be assessed.[94] The frameworks provided cover a range of dimensions to assess the results of a campaign, for example, civil society capacity building (e.g. the role of networks/coalitions), empowerment, and participation (e.g. of communities and organizations) on the one hand and policy change or development on the other.

A hierarchy of measures which includes awareness, contribution to the debate, changed opinions, policy change, implemented policy, and, finally, health outcomes have been suggested.[95,96] They have also been described in relation to the following:

- Access (the voices of previously excluded stakeholders are now heard);
- Agenda (desired policy change is supported by powerful decision makers);
- Policy (desired change is translated into policy);
- Output (new policy is implemented);
- Impact (new policy has intended consequences); and
- Structural changes (when new policy is widely accepted as the new norm).[45]

Each of these factors should be considered when planning and undertaking advocacy and it is important to recognize that, in a complex and evolving space, the end goal of improved health or the implementation of a policy is not, or may not be, the only way you can measure the effectiveness of advocacy. It might be that support has grown, that a key figure has supported the cause, that the standard framing and discourse on the topic has changed, or that the topic has become a mainstream topic of consideration.

6.6 Challenges

As previously discussed, the policy options sought for addressing the main NCD risk factors—food, alcohol, and tobacco—are rarely favourable to market actors as they are likely to damage either the profits or market share that they are mandated to generate.[73,97] In the case of food, products high in fat, sugar, and salt are often the most profitable and thus any policies seeking to reduce their consumption to protect health are often challenged. In the case of tobacco and alcohol, reducing demand and consumption is high risk for entire businesses. Finding ways to make the healthy option also the most profitable is therefore one important, yet challenging, consideration in advocacy.

Another major challenge for public health advocates is the power and influence held by industry lobby(ies) to protect their own sectoral goals. This power can be a major barrier to successful, rational public health advocacy outcomes.[98] Unlike businesses who produce and market products, public health advocates have few direct opportunities to shape the environment. Instead they are often forced to act as 'outsiders' whose only strength is in influencing,[99] rather than directly shaping events and environment themselves. This often means that, even with the best advocacy, change can be slow and even elusive. But good advocacy must be built on full understanding of wider factors outside of the control of advocates and their remit.

Furthermore, approaches to preventing and tackling NCDs increasingly rely on models involving industry self-regulation and/or partnerships such as the Global Coordination Mechanism on NCDs.[100] So what are public health advocates to do? Are these examples of NCD advocacy having been captured by market dynamics and distracted by market players? Or have public health advocates had to make calculated decisions based on what's possible, given the market dynamics, and in order to progress the thinking in this space? The public–private partnership approach to food and alcohol policy can lead to conflicts of interest[101] and ineffective action. Advocates must carefully manage, negotiate, and deal with these issues in their pursuit of their goals and the greater good.

Another key, and not unrelated, challenge faced by public health advocates is a lack of funding. The capacity required for research, to run campaigns, and to monitor policy development is extensive, but more often than not very little funding is available for these sorts of activities. This problem is exacerbated by the fact that businesses have significant resource for their own advocacy, thus putting public health advocates on the back foot. Grappling with the idea of advocacy impact and better defining the changes and outcomes that advocacy may realistically expect to see may help with this in the future.

6.7 Recommendations

A number of recommendations can be made to increase the effectiveness of public health advocacy in the prevention of NCDs.

6.7.1 Practical recommendations

1. Advocates need to work together, and with other likeminded individuals, in pursuit of their goals and to enhance their strength and power. They would also benefit from building alliances within the health sector to speak with a unified voice.
2. The public–private partnership approach to food and alcohol policy can lead to conflicts of interest[101] and ineffective action. Public health practitioners and policy-makers would benefit from training and tools on identifying, avoiding and mitigating conflicts of interest in their interactions with industry actors.[15]
3. Governments need to recognize the important contribution of civil society in supporting NCD prevention policy, including their role in holding actors to account. Given the central role of public health advocates to supporting the public interest and public

good, independent funding should be made available to support these activities by governments and foundations.

6.7.2 Recommendations on education

1. To strengthen awareness of advocacy, education on political science theories and skills should be incorporated within the core curriculum and competencies of the public health workforce to ensure that practitioners have a better understanding of the political contexts and dimensions which are key to influencing public health policies.[102]
2. Public health practitioners should work with policy analysts to develop strategies which help to create and/or make the most of political windows.[103]
3. Training on how to deal with the 'corporate playbook' of common strategies adopted by manufacturers of unhealthy products should be incorporated within core public health training curricula.[104]

Case study: Traffic light nutrition labelling in the UK

One example of successful public health advocacy from agenda setting to policy implementation in the face of a variety of political challenges is the introduction of front-of-pack colour-coded nutrition labelling ('traffic light labelling') in the UK to make it easier for consumers to choose healthy foods.

Traffic light nutrition labels were first recommended by the UK's Food Standards Agency in 2006, and were finally adopted as part of the official national nutrition labelling scheme in 2012 following a change in EU rules to formally allow member states to adopt voluntary national schemes. The official format of the UK scheme is a hybrid label with both traffic lights and guideline daily amounts. Around 75% of products in the UK now carry voluntary traffic light labelling on the front of their packs.[105] The UK scheme is the first to be adopted by a national government in the EU region,[106,107] despite strong opposition to the traffic light element by some sections of the food industry. It is the culmination of nearly three decades of advocacy by members of the public health community who pooled resources to push for action.[16,17] The process has been described in more detail elsewhere and is outlined briefly below.[15]

Public health attempts to raise the political priority

Nutrition labelling first came to prominence in the UK policy scene in the early 1980s through the agenda-setting activities of members of the public health community. They promoted labelling of public health nutrients including fats, salt, and sugar on food products as a key policy to help consumers choose healthier options and address the emerging concern of cardiovascular disease. These public health actors adopted a mix of advocacy activities and strategies to promote nutrition labels during the 1980s and 1990s:

- Academic and expert advisers ensured that nutrition labelling recommendations were included within the reports of influential national expert advisory groups.[108,109]
- A public health consensus report on tackling coronary heart disease recommended the adoption of traffic light food labels.[110]
- The health NGO Coronary Prevention Group (CPG) developed a 'high, medium, low' nutrition labelling scheme.[111,112,113,114] This was then subsequently adopted by the Coop supermarket.[115]
- CPG worked with sympathetic parliamentarians to advocate for mandatory nutrition labels through reports, letters to ministers, and parliamentary debates.[116,117]
- Consumer NGOs worked with the Ministry of Agriculture, Fisheries and Food (MAFF) on consumer research to identify what formats of food label worked best.[111,118]
- MAFF published a consumer facing leaflet with guideline daily intakes for fat, saturated fat, total sugars, and salt to help consumers to interpret nutrition labels.[119]
- Well-connected individual and organizational 'policy entrepreneurs' ensured coordination across the different efforts and actor groups.[15]

EU and industry block efforts on nutrition labels

These early attempts to get the government to adopt a national nutrition labelling scheme were unsuccessful, but they nevertheless helped to 'soften up the system' for future action on labelling.[120] A half-hearted attempt by government to introduce mandatory fat labelling in the late 1980s was abandoned when the European Commission considered but then abandoned mandating nutrition labels across Europe.[121] In 1994, the government's Nutrition Task Force made a commitment to introduce a comprehensive graphic nutrition labelling scheme by 1996.[122] In line with previous findings, research to inform this process concluded that consumers would benefit from additional information on a wide range of nutrients.[44,122,123] However, vocal industry actors were hostile to the concept of comprehensive nutrition labels. They adopted a number of strategies to thwart efforts on nutrition labelling:

- They denied there was evidence linking poor diet and health. Sympathetic right-wing journalists promoted these ideas in the media;[124]
- They argued that by providing information on the 'Big 4' nutrients (protein, carbohydrate, fat, energy) they were already providing nutrition information for consumers;

- They argued that, as consumers did not understand what fats, salt, and sugars were, providing this information was not a priority;[114]
- They argued that comprehensive nutrition labels would result in reduced sales and damage businesses;[125,126]
- They directly lobbied government and ministers against action on nutrition labelling;[124] and
- They also used their financial muscle by withdrawing their funding from the Conservative Party, which was in government at the time, in protest at the 'radical' proposals on healthy eating such as nutrition labelling and product reformulation.[127]

As a result of these activities, the Nutrition Task Force's efforts to introduce a comprehensive unified scheme was abandoned[125,126] in favour of labelling which was 'simple and focused on one or two nutrients' (total fat and saturated fat).[123] The Task Force was prematurely disbanded in 1995 as a result of the industry hostility towards it. Responsibility for developing a nutrition labelling scheme was then transferred to the Institute of Grocery Distribution on behalf of the food industry.[123]

The policy windows of the BSE crisis and change of government

In 1996, a political 'window' was opened up by the global scandal of the BSE crisis and the new Labour government elected in 1997 was thus highly motivated to take the necessary actions to address major diet-related public health problems, including by shaping the environment to support individuals to improve their health.[128] The government fulfilled its pre-election manifesto pledge to establish a Food Standards Agency which would provide leadership on food and bring state responsibility for food matters under one roof[129] and ensured the new FSA had sufficient power and independence.

The development of the UK traffic light nutrition labelling scheme

The FSA became operational in 2000 and committed to improve food labelling to support consumers.[130] FSA commissioned an extensive number of qualitative and quantitative consumer research projects between 2000 and 2010 to inform the development of the front-of-pack nutrition sign-posting scheme.[131–134] The findings were consistent with earlier studies, namely that consumers wanted consistent, clear, and comprehensive nutritional information[134] and preferred the inclusion of traffic light and 'high, medium, low' guidance on nutritional values. This was found to enhance performance, facilitate rapid judgements and comparisons between products, enhance interpretation of numerical information such as guideline daily amount, and be better suited to those from lower socioeconomic backgrounds.[131–134] The development of the FSA's front-of-pack nutrition labelling scheme was supported by extensive engagement and consultation with food companies, health and consumer bodies, and researchers.[130] Certain food companies began to adopt traffic light labels from 2004 onwards in light of the emerging consumer evidence.[135] This provided important evidence on technical feasibility which encouraged more companies to adopt the scheme and helped dispel hostile arguments from the scheme's opponents.[32,33]

The FSA Board recommended the use of voluntary front-of-pack traffic light labels in March 2006.[136] FSA established a traffic light 'adopters and supporters group', including industry adopters and NGO supporters.[137] The group agreed common communication messages and advice to consumers, and provided positive recognition to companies adopting the scheme.[138,139] Examples of actions adopted by public health NGOs included:

- Watchdog activities such as highlighting misleading nutrition labels and publicity stunts to name and shame companies who failed to adopt traffic lights;[140,141]
- Informing and educating consumers on how to use front-of-pack nutrition labels;[142,143]
- Undertaking advocacy to policy-makers in support of traffic lights in the UK and Europe, such as joint letters and statements;[144] and
- Galvanizing and demonstrating public opinion, e.g. parent surveys which demonstrated overwhelming support for traffic light labels.[145]

A significant group of manufacturers remained vehemently opposed to traffic light labels, and embarked on a parallel process to develop a rival guideline daily amount (GDA) scheme without traffic light colours. In addition, the food industry exported the GDA scheme to Europe, where it was presented as a commitment to the public–private partnership EU Platform on diet,[146] and also embarked on a comprehensive campaign against traffic lights in the EU.[15]

The UK's nutrition labelling scheme proved hugely controversial in Europe following its announcement in October 2012, owing to the traffic light colours. Members of the food industry galvanized complaints against traffic lights from a myriad of actors ranging from EU member states, to parliamentarians and the EU trade directorate.[147,148,149,150] At the time of writing, these challenges were ongoing. However, the UK's struggles on nutrition labelling policy are not unique. Similar efforts to introduce consumer-friendly nutrition labels have been challenged and/or overturned in several other countries.[151,152,153,154]

Acknowledgements

This chapter was written by Hannah Brinsden, Modi Mwatsama, and Tim Lang. It draws on Brinsden H and Lang T, 2015. *An introduction to public health advocacy: reflections on theory and practice*. 12 October 2015. Food Research Collaboration Policy Brief. Case study material provided by Modi Mwatsama and Jessica Pullar.

References

1. **World Health Organization.** The Ottawa Charter for Health Promotion [Internet]. [cited 2/8/2013]. Available from: http://www.who.int/healthpromotion/conferences/previous/ottawa/en/.
2. **Lang T, Heasman M.** *Food Wars: The Global Battle for Mouths, Minds and Markets.* 2nd edn. Abingdon: Routledge, 2015.
3. **Rayner G, Lang T.** *Ecological Public Health: Reshaping the Conditions for Good Health.* Abingdon: Routledge, 2012.
4. **Lobstein T, Brinsden H.** Symposium report: the prevention of obesity and NCDs: challenges and opportunities for governments. *Obesity Reviews* 2014; **15**(8):630–9.
5. **CASH (Consensus Action on Salt and Health).** Press Release: UK leading the world in salt reduction London: CASH, 2012 [updated 21/06/12; cited 2013 4 May]. Available from: http://www.worldactiononsalt.com/news/saltnews/2012/78091.html.
6. **Wyness LA, Butriss JL, Stanner SA.** Reducing the population's sodium intake: the UK Food Standards Agency's salt reduction programme. *Public Health Nutrition* Feb; **15**(2):254–61.
7. **Webster J, Trieu K, Dunford E, Hawkes C.** Target Salt 2025: A global overview of national programs to encourage the food industry to reduce salt in foods. *Nutrients* 2014; **6**(8):3274–87.
8. **World Health Organization.** *Creating an Enabling Environment for Population-Based Salt Reduction Strategies: Report of a Joint Technical Meeting Held by WHO and the Food Standards Agency, United Kingdom, July 2010.* Geneva: World Health Organization, 2010.
9. **Better Regulation Executive.** *Voluntary Salt Reduction Strategy Reformulation Targets.* London: Better Regulation Executive, 2010.
10. **Department of Health.** *The Public Health Responsibility Deal.* London: Department of Health; 2011 [cited 2016 6 March]. Available at: https://responsibilitydeal.dh.gov.uk/about/.
11. **Quinn I.** *Study Shows 'Reformulation Efforts Paying Off'.* London: The Grocer, 2012 [cited 2014 19 August]. Available from: http://www.thegrocer.co.uk/topics/health/salt-study-shows-reformulation-efforts-paying-off/230162.article.
12. **Arnold B.** *Gradually Grinding Down Salt Intake.* London: Institute of Grocery Distribution; 2012 [cited 2013 5 May]. Available at: http://www.igd.com/our-expertise/Nutrition-food-and-farming/Sugar-salt-fat/5228/Gradually-grinding-down-salt-intake/.
13. **Appel LJ, Angell SY, Cobb LK, Limper HM, Nelson DE, Samet JM,** et al. Population-wide sodium reduction: the bumpy road from evidence to policy. *Annals of Epidemiology* 2012; **22**(6):417–25.
14. **Cappuccio FP, Capewell S, Lincoln P, McPherson K.** Policy options to reduce population salt intake. *British Medical Journal* 2011; **343**:d4995.
15. **Mwatsama M.** *Public health policy struggles: Comparison of salt reduction and nutrition labelling in the UK, 1980–2015.* DrPH Thesis. London: LSHTM, 2016.
16. **Borzel TA.** Organizing Babylon—on the different conceptions of policy networks. *Public Administration* 1998; **76**(2):253.
17. **Thatcher M.** The development of policy network analyses: from modest origins to overarching frameworks. *Journal of Theoretical Politics* 1998; **10**(4):389–416.
18. **Hawthorne VM, Greaves DA, Beevers DG.** Blood pressure in a Scottish town. *British Medical Journal* 1974; **3**(5931):600–3.
19. **Sanchez-Castillo CP, Warrender S, Whitehead TP, James WP.** An assessment of the sources of dietary salt in a British population. *Clinical Science* 1987; **72**(1):95–102.
20. **Health Education Council.** *A Discussion Paper on Proposals for Nutritional Guidlines for Health Education in Britain: Prepared for the National Advisory Committee on Nutrition Education by*

an ad hoc Working Party under the Chairmanship of Professor WPT James. London: The Health Education Council, 1983.

21. **World Health Organization**. *Prevention of Coronary Heart Disease: Report of a WHO Expert Committee*. WHO Technical Report Series 678. Geneva: World Health Organization, 1982.
22. **COMA**. *Dietary Reference Values for Food Energy and Nutrients for the United Kingdom*. London: Her Majesty's Government, 1991.
23. **Department of Health**. *Nutritional Aspects of Cardiovascular Disease*. Report on Health and Social Subjects no 46. London: HMSO 1994.
24. **Coronary Prevention Group**. *Nutritional Labelling of Foods: A Rational Approach to Banding*. London: Coronary Prevention Group, 1986.
25. **Rose G, Ball K, Catford J, James P, Deryck L, Maryon-Davis A**, et al. *Coronary Heart Disease Prevention: Plans for Action*. London: Pitman Publishing, 1984.
26. **Hanneman RL**. INTERSALT: Hypertension rise with age revisited. *British Medical Journal* 1996; **312**(7041):1283–4.
27. **Intersalt Cooperative Research Group**. INTERSALT: An international study of electrolyte excretion and blood pressure. Results for 24 hour urinary sodium and potassium excretion. *British Medical Journal* 1988; **297**(6644):319–28.
28. **Godlee F**. The food industry fights for salt. *British Medical Journal* 1996; **312**(7041):1239–40.
29. **MacGregor GA, Sever PS**. Salt—overwhelming evidence but still no action: Can a consensus be reached with the food industry? *British Medical Journal* 1996;**312**(7041):1287–9.
30. **Macgregor G, Best F, Cam J, Markandu N, Elder D, Sagnella G**, et al. Double-blind randomised crossover trial of moderate sodium restriction in essential hypertension. *The Lancet* 1982; **319**(8268):351–5.
31. **Cappuccio FP, Markandu ND, Carney C, Sagnella GA, MacGregor GA**. Double-blind randomised trial of modest salt restriction in older people. *The Lancet* 1997; **350**(9081):850–4.
32. **Just Food**. UK: Asda says it has removed 900 tonnes of salt from the nation's diet: just-food.com; 2002 [cited 2014 13 August]. Available at: http://www.just-food.com/news/asda-says-it-has-removed-900-tonnes-of-salt-from-the-nations-diet_id73230.aspx.
33. **Galston W**. Political feasibility: Interests and power. In: **Moran M, Rein M, Goodin RE**, editors. *The Oxford Handbook of Public Policy*: 319. Oxford: Oxford University Press, 2006.
34. **Department of Health**. *The NHS Plan: A Plan for Investment, a Plan for Reform*. London: Department of Health, 2000.
35. **Department of Health**. *Saving Lives: Our Healthier Nation*. London: Department of Health, 1999.
36. **Department of Health**. *Reducing Health Inequalities: An Action Report*. London: HMSO, 1999.
37. **Food Standards Agency**. *Salt self-reporting framework London*. FSA, 2007. Updated 14 April 2009; cited 9 June 2014. Available from: http://collections.europarchive.org/tna/20100927130941/http://food.gov.uk/healthiereating/salt/selfreport/
38. **Better Regulation Executive**. *Effective Inspection and Enforcement: Implementing the Hampton Vision in the Food Standards Agency*. London: National Audit Office, 2008.
39. **Bryden A, Petticrew M, Mays N, Eastmure E, Knai C**. Voluntary agreements between government and business: A scoping review of the literature with specific reference to the Public Health Responsibility Deal. *Health Policy* 2013; **110**(2–3):186–97.
40. **Najum A**. The four-c's of third sector government relations—cooperation, confrontation, complementary and co-optation. *Nonprofit Management and Leadership* 2000; **104**(4):375–96.

41. **Young DR.** Complementary, supplementary, or adversarial? A theoretical and historical examination of nonprofit-government relations in the United States. In: **Boris ET, Steuerle CE**, editors. *Nonprofits and Government: Collaboration and Conflict*: 31–67. Washington, DC: Urban Institute Press, 1999.

42. **Coston J.** A model and typology of government-NGO relationships. *Nonprofit Voluntary Sector Q* 1998; **27**(3):358, 382.

43. **Onyx J, Armitage L, Dalton B, Melville R, Casey J, Banks R.** Advocacy with gloves on: The 'manners' of strategy used by some third sector organizations undertaking advocacy in NSW and Queensland. *Voluntas* 2010; **21**(1):41–61.

44. **Raynor J, York P, Sim S.** What makes an effective advocacy organization? A framework for determining advocacy capacity. *California Endowment* 2009.

45. **Casey J.** *Understanding Advocacy: A Primer on the Policy Making Role of Nonprofit Organizations*. New York: Center for Nonprofit Strategy and Management; 2011.

46. **Christoffel KK.** Public health advocacy: process and product. *American Journal of Public Health* 2000; **90**(5):722.

47. **Freudenberg N.** Public health advocacy to change corporate practices: implications for health education practice and research. *Health Education and Behavior* 2005; **32**(3):298–319.

48. **Gen S, Wright AC.** Policy advocacy organizations: a framework linking theory and practice. *Journal of Policy Practice* 2013;**12**(3):163–93.

49. **Lane CH, Carter MI.** The role of evidence-based media advocacy in the promotion of tobacco control policies. *Salud Pública de México* 2012; **54**(3):281–8.

50. **Reams RR, Odedina FT, Pressey S.** Advocacy resource: engaging the media and promoting your cancer program in Africa. *Infectious Agents and Cancer* 2013; **8**:S5–S11.

51. **Chapman S.** *Public Health Advocacy and Tobacco Control: Making Smoking History*. Oxford: Blackwell Publishers; 2007

52. **Nelson P.** New agendas and new patterns of international NGO political action. *Voluntas* 2002; **13**(4):377–92.

53. **Hopkins B.** *Charity, Advocacy, and Law*. New York: Wiley, 1992.

54. **Norman DJ.** From shouting to counting: civil society and good governance reform in Cambodia. *Pacific Review* 2014; **27**(2):241–64.

55. **Szper R, Prakash A.** Charity watchdogs and the limits of information-based regulation. *Voluntas* 2011; **22**(1):112–41.

56. **Cnaan RA, Jones K, Dickin A, Salomon M.** Nonprofit watchdogs: do they serve the average donor? *Nonprofit Management and Leadership* 2011; **21**(4):381–97.

57. **Pertshuck M.** Forward. In: **Wallack L**, editor. Media *Advocacy and Public Health: Power for Prevention*: vii. New York: Sage, 1993.

58. **Wallack L**, editor. *Media Advocacy and Public Health: Power for Prevention*. New York: Sage; 1993.

59. **Chapman S, Wakefield M.** Tobacco control advocacy in Australia: reflections on 30 years of progress. *Health Education and Behavior* 2001; **28**(3):274–89.

60. **Dorfman L, Wilbur P, O'Lingus E, Woodruff K, Wallack L.** *Accelerating Policy on Nutrition: Lessons from Tobacco, Alcohol, Firearms and Traffic Safety*. Berkeley media publishing group; 2005.

61. **Internet Society.** *Global Internet Report 2015: Mobile evolution and development of the internet*. Available at: http://www.internetsociety.org/globalinternetreport/assets/download/IS_web.pdf

62. **Perrin A.** *Social media usage: 2005–2015*. Pew Research Centre—Internet, Science and Technology, 2015. Available at: http://www.pewinternet.org/2015/10/08/social-networking-usage-2005-2015/

63. **Facebook.** Our Mission. Facebook News Room, 2016. Available at: http://newsroom.fb.com/company-info/

64. **Kemp S.** *Digital, social, and mobile in APAC 2015.* We are Social, 2015. Available at: http://wearesocial.com/uk/blog/2015/03/digital-social-mobile-apac-2015

65. **Freberg K, Palenchar MJ, Veil SR.** Managing and sharing H1N1 crisis information using social media bookmarking services. *Public Relations Review* 2013; **39**(3):178–84.

66. **Jones B.** Mixed uptake of social media among public health specialists. *World Health Organisation Bulletin* 2011; **89**(11):784–5. Available at: http://www.who.int/bulletin/volumes/89/11/11-031111/en/

67. **Polio Eradication Initiative.** *Strengthening momentum for eradication: a polio eradication initiative communication action plan for Afghanistan.* 2015. Available at: http://www.polioeradication.org/Portals/0/Document/Aboutus/Governance/IMB/13IMBMeeting/4.4_13IMB.pdf

68. **WHO and World Economic Forum.** *From burden to 'best buys': reducing the economic impact of non-communicable diseases in low- and middle-income countries.* 2011. Available at: http://www.who.int/nmh/publications/best_buys_summary.pdf

69. **Mita G, Ni Mhurchu C, Jull A.** Effectiveness of social media in reducing risk factors for noncommunicable diseases: a systematic review and meta-analysis of randomized controlled trials. *Nutrition Reviews* 2016; 74(4):237–47.

70. **Lobstein T, Brinsden H, Landon J, Kraak V, Musicus A, Macmullan J.** INFORMAS and advocacy for public health nutrition and obesity prevention. *Obesity Reviews* 2013; 14:150–6

71. **Start D, Hovland I.** *Tools for Policy Impact: A Handbook for Researchers.* London: ODI, 2004

72. **Berry JM.** *Effective Advocacy for Nonprofits: Nonprofit advocacy and the policy Process: A Seminar Series, Volume 2, Exploring Organizations and Advocacy.* The Urban Institute; 2000

73. **Stanley F, Daube M.** Should industry care for children? Public health advocacy and law in Australia. *Public Health* 2009; 123(3):283–6

74. **Reid E.** Nonprofit advocacy. In: **Boris ET, Steuerle CE**, editors. *Nonprofits and Government: Conflict or Collaboration?*: 291–328. Washington, DC: Urban Institute Press, 1999

75. **Mahoney C.** *Brussels versus the Beltway: Advocacy in the United States and the European Union.* Washington, DC: Georgetown University Press; 2008

76. NCD Alliance. Available at: https://ncdalliance.org/

77. www.worldobesity.org

78. European Heart Network. Available at: http://www.ehnheart.org/

79. www.ukhealthforum.org.uk

80. www.sustainweb.org

81. **About the Framework Convention on Tobacco Control.** Geneva: World Health Organization, 2016. Available at: http://www.who.int/fctc/about/en/

82. **World Health Organization.** *International Code on Marketing of Breast-milk Substitutes.* Geneva: World Health Organization, 1981

83. **Wiist WH.** Public health and the anticorporate movement: rationale and recommendations. *American Journal of Public Health* 2006; 96(8):1370–5.

84. **Phillips R.** Is corporate engagement an advocacy strategy for NGOs? The community aid abroad experience. *Nonprofit Management and Leadership* 2002; 13(2):123–37.

85. **Freudenberg N, Galea S.** The impact of corporate practices on health: implications for health policy. *Journal of Public Health Policy* 2008; 29(1):86–104.

86. **Kraak VI, Swinburn B, Lawrence M.** Distinguishing accountability from responsibility: an accountability framework. *American Journal of Public Health* 2014; 104(6):e2–3.

87. **Glanz K.** Measuring food environments: a historical perspective. *American Journal of Preventive Medicine* 2009; 36(4, Supplement):S93–8.

88. **Vandevijvere S, Swinburn B,** for the International Network for Food and Obesity/non-communicable diseases (NCDs) Research, Monitoring and Action Support (INFORMAS). Towards global benchmarking of food environments and policies to reduce obesity and diet-related non-communicable diseases: design and methods for nation-wide surveys. *British Medical Journal Open* 2014; 4(5).

89. **Cashore B.** Legitimacy and the privatization of environmental governance. *Governance* 2002; 15(4):503–29.

90. **Brinsden H, Lobstein T, Landon J, Kraak V, Sacks G, Kumanyika S,** et al. Monitoring policy and actions on food environments: rationale and outline of the INFORMAS policy engagement and communication strategies. *Obesity Reviews* 2013; 14:13–23.

91. Which?. *A Taste for Change: Food Companies Assessed for Action to Enable Healthier Choices.* London: Which?, 2012.

92. **Brinsden HC, He FJ, Jenner KH, MacGregor GA.** Surveys of the salt content in UK bread: progress made and further reductions possible. *British Medical Journal Open* 2013; 3(6).

93. **Martin J, Peeters A, Honisett S, Mavoa H, Swinburn B, de Silva-Sanigorski A.** Benchmarking government action for obesity prevention—An innovative advocacy strategy. *Obesity Research and Clinical Practice* 2014; 8(4):e388–98.

94. **Chapman J, Wameyo A.** Monitoring and evaluating advocacy: a scoping study. Online: ActionAid; 2001.

95. **Keck ME, Sikkink K.** *Activists beyond Borders: Advocacy Networks in International Politics.* Ithaca: Cornell University Press; 1998.

96. Oxfam. Monitoring, evaluation, accountability and learning. London: Oxfam GB, 2014. Available at: http://policy-practice.oxfam.org.uk/our-work/methods-approaches/monitoring-evaluation.

97. 'Eat less': A difficult message for industry. Food Navigator USA; 2011 [updated 08 Feb 2011]. Available at: http://www.foodnavigator-usa.com/Suppliers2/Eat-less-A-difficult-message-for-industry.

98. **ETC Group.** *Oligopoly, Inc. 2005. Concentration in Corporate Power.* Online: ETC Group; 2005.

99. **Hehenberger L, Harling A, Scholton P.** *A Practical Guide to Measuring and Managing Impact.* Online: European Venture Philanthropy Association; 2013.

100. About the WHO Global Coordination Mechanism on NCDs (WHO GCM/NCD). 2016. Available at: http://www.who.int/global-coordination-mechanism/about-coordination-mechanism/en/.

101. **AAMC (American Association of Medical Colleges).** *The Scientific Basis of Influence and Reciprocity: A Symposium.* 2007.

102. **Hunter DJ.** Role of politics in understanding complex, messy health systems. *British Medical Journal* 2015; 350(h1214).

103. **Buse K.** Addressing the theoretical, practical and ethical challenges inherent in prospective health policy analysis. *Health Policy and Planning* 2008; 23(5):351–60.

104. **Brownell KD, Warner KE.** The perils of ignoring history: big tobacco played dirty and millions died. How Similar Is Big Food? *Milbank Quarterly* 2009; 87(1):259–94.

105. **House of Commons Health Committee.** *Childhood Obesity—Brave and Bold Action. First Report of Session 2015–16.* London: TSO, 2015. Available at: http://www.publications.parliament.uk/pa/cm201516/cmselect/cmhealth/465/465.pdf.

106. **EUFIC (The European Food Information Council).** *Global Update on Nutrition Labelling.* Brussels: EUFIC, 2013.
107. **Kerr MA, McCann MT, Livingstone MB.** Food and the consumer: Could labelling be the answer? *Proceedings of the Nutrition Society* 2015;74(2):158–63.
108. **The Health Education Council.** *A Discussion Paper on Proposals for Nutritional Guidelines for Health Education in Britain. Prepared for the National Advisory Committee on Nutrition Education by an Ad Hoc Working Party under the Chairmanship of Professor WPT James.* London: The Health Education Council, 1983.
109. **Department of Health.** *Diet and Cardiovascular Disease—Report of the Panel on Diet in Relation to Cardiovascular Disease of the Committee on Medical Aspects of Food Policy. Report on Health and Social Subjects 28.* London: HMSO, 1984.
110. **Rose G, Ball K, Catford J, James P, Deryck L, Maryon-Davis A, et al.** *Coronary Heart Disease Prevention. Plans for Action.* London: Pitman Publishing, 1984.
111. **MAFF (Ministry of Agriculture FaF, Consumers Association, National Consumer Council).** *Consumer Attitudes to and Understanding of Nutrition Labelling: Summary Report.* London: Ministry of Agriculture, Fisheries and Food, 1985.
112. **Coronary Prevention Group.** *Nutritional Labelling of Foods: A Rational Approach to Banding.* London: CPG, 1986.
113. **Black A.** *Coronary Prevention Group. Just read the label: Understanding Nutrition Information in Numeric, Verbal and Graphic Format.* London: HMSO, 1992.
114. **Luba A.** *The Food Labelling Debate: A report for the London Food Commission.* London: London Food Commission, 1985.
115. **CooP.** *Expert Papers 6a and 6b: Evidence from the Co-operative Group.* In: *NICE (National Institute of Health and Care Excellence), editor. NICE Guidelines [PH25] Prevention of Cardiovascular Disease.* London: 2010.
116. **UK Parliament.** *Nutritional Labelling in the EC.* House of Lords Debate. *Hansard.* 1988; 493:738–48.
117. **Shannon B.** Nutrition labelling: putting the consumer first. *British Food Journal.* 1994; 96(4):40–4.
118. **CooP.** *Food Crimes. A consumer perspective on the ethics of modern food production.* Manchester: CooP Food, 2000.
119. **Rayner M, Williams C, Myatt M, Boaz A.** *Use your label: Making sense of nutrition information.* London: MAFF (Ministry of Agriculture, Fisheries and Food), 1996.
120. **Kingdon JW.** *Agendas, Alternatives, and Public Policies.* London: Longman Publishing Group, 2002.
121. **European Commission.** Council Directive 90/496/EEC of 24 September 1990 on nutrition labelling for foodstuffs Brussels: Eur-Lex Access to European Law; 1990 [cited 2014 6 July]. Available from: http://eur-lex.europa.eu/legal-content/EN/ALL/;ELX_SESSIONID=0KKCT5cC21Y47X1qlgszdhNwNGRVrlhm3MgcLVNtPJfZZ8JgXxr6!472874858?uri=CELEX:31990L0496
122. **Department of Health.** *Eat Well: An action plan from the Nutrition Task Force to achieve the Health of the Nation targets on diet and nutrition.* London: Department of Health, 1994.
123. **Department of Health.** *Eat Well II: A progress report from the Nutrition Task Force on the action plan to achieve the Health of the Nation targets on diet and nutrition.* London: Department of Health, 1996.
124. **Young R.** Food firms fear healthy eating campaign. *The Times.* 9 August 1994.
125. **Hope J.** The plates of wrath: Food industry and healthy eating experts at odds over new guidelines. *Daily Mail.* 11 November 1994.

126. Food label shortcomings 'cost 500 lives a week'. *The Guardian*. 27 March 1992.
127. **Jones J**. Nutrition: Weight of evidence forces government ministers to eat their words. *The Observer*. 16 October 1995.
128. **Department of Health.** *Saving Lives: Our Healthier Nation*. London: HMG, 1999.
129. **Krebs J.** Establishing a single, independent food standards agency: The United Kingdom's experience. *Food and Drug Law Journal* 2004; **59**(3):387–97.
130. **Food Standards Agency.** *Strategic plan 2001-2006. Putting consumers first*. London: FSA, 2001.
131. **Food Standards Agency.** *Development timeline of front-of-pack nutrition labelling*. London: FSA, 2009 [updated 8 August 2010; cited 2013 4 March]. Available from: http://tna.europarchive.org/20100815112448/http://www.food.gov.uk/foodlabelling/signposting/devfop/signposttimeline/
132. **Malam S, Clegg S, Kirwan S, McGinigal S.** BMRB Social Research. *Comprehension and use of UK nutrition signpost labelling schemes*. London: British Market Research Bureau, 2009.
133. **Synovate.** *Quantitative Evaluation of Alternative Food Signposting Concepts*. London: Synovate, 2005 [cited 2015 29 June]. Available from: http://webarchive.nationalarchives.gov.uk/20131104005023/http://www.food.gov.uk/multimedia/pdfs/signpostquanresearch.pdf
134. **Food Standards Agency.** *Nutritional Labelling Qualitative Research: Final Report*. London: FSA, 2001.
135. **Foodmanufacturer.co.uk.** *Manufacturers adopt traffic lights*. London: Foodmanufacturer.co.uk, 2006 [cited 2014 25 August]. Available from: http://www.foodmanufacture.co.uk/Business-News/Manufacturers-adopt-traffic-lights
136. **Food Standards Agency.** Press Release: Food Standards Agency Board agrees principles for front of pack signposting labelling. London: FSA, 2006 [updated 29/09/2010; cited 2013 15 March]. Available from: http://collections.europarchive.org/tna/20100927130941/http://www.food.gov.uk/news/newsarchive/2006/mar/signpostnewsmarch
137. **Food Standards Agency.** *Supporters of FSA's approach to front-of-pack labelling*. London: FSA, 2008 [updated 24 September 2008; cited 2013 14 March]. Available from: http://tna.europarchive.org/20100815112448/http://www.food.gov.uk/foodlabelling/signposting/supportfsasignp
138. **Food Standards Agency.** Board meeting minutes, 9 March. London: FSA, 2006 [cited 2013 15 March]. Available from: http://tna.europarchive.org/20100815112448/http://www.food.gov.uk/aboutus/ourboard/boardmeetings/boardmeetings2006/boardmeeting90306/boardmins9mar06
139. **Food Standards Agency.** *Retailers, manufacturers, importers/suppliers and service providers that use signpost labelling*. London: FSA, 2009 [cited 2013 4 March]. Available from: http://tna.europarchive.org/20100815112448/http://www.food.gov.uk/foodlabelling/signposting/
140. **Lobstein T, Landon J, Lincoln P.** *Misconceptions and misinformation: The problems with Guideline Daily Amounts (GDAs)*. London: National Heart Forum, 2007.
141. **Sustain Children's Food Campaign.** *Labelling wall of shame*. London: Sustain, 2013 [cited 2014 13 July]. Available from: http://labellingwallofshame.tumblr.com/.
142. **Food Standards Agency.** *Labelling claims*. London: FSA, 2002.
143. **Rayner M, Scarborough P, Williams C.** The origin of Guideline Daily Amounts and the Food Standards Agency's guidance on what counts as 'a lot' and 'a little'. *Public Health Nutrition*. 2004; 7(4):549–56.
144. **British Heart Foundation, National Heart Forum, Diabetes UK, CASH, Which?, Faculty of Public Health, et al.** Joint NGO briefing: Traffic Light Nutrition Labelling. London: British Heart Foundation, 2012.
145. **Brimelow A.** Public want food 'traffic lights'. *BBC News Corporation*, 2007 [cited 2015 04 May]. Available from: http://news.bbc.co.uk/1/hi/health/6397187.stm

146. **CIAA (Confederation of the Food and Drink Industries of the EU).** *Promoting balanced diets and healthy lifestyles. Europe's food and drink industry in action.* Brussels: CIAA, 2010.

147. **De Castro P, Scottà G, Dorfmann H, La Via G, Silvestris SPF, García Pérez I, et al.** Written question—Food labelling: UK traffic-light system—E-011011/2013. Brussels: European Parliament, 2013 [cited 2014 13 July]. Available from: http://www.europarl.europa.eu/sides/getDoc.do?pubRef=-//EP//TEXT+WQ+E-2013-011011+0+DOC+XML+V0//EN

148. **Council of the European Union.** Note from Italian delegation to Council. 'Hybrid' nutrition labeling system recommended in some Member States—Information from the Italian delegation 16575/13. Brussels: European Council, 2013.

149. **Voss A.** Written question—UK traffic light system for nutrition labelling of foodstuffs—E-010157/2013. Brussels: European Parliament, 2013 [cited 2014 13 July]. Available from: http://www.europarl.europa.eu/sides/getDoc.do?type=WQ&reference=E-2013-010157&language=EN.

150. **Scott-Thomas C.** *EU to reassess UK traffic light food labels.* Montpellier: FoodNavigator.com, 2014 [cited 2014 13 July]. Available from: http://www.foodnavigator.com/Legislation/EU-to-reassess-UK-traffic-light-labels.

151. **Thow AM, Snowdon W, Labonte R, Gleeson D, Stuckler D, Hattersley L, et al.** Will the next generation of preferential trade and investment agreements undermine prevention of noncommunicable diseases? A prospective policy analysis of the Trans Pacific Partnership Agreement. *Health Policy* 2015; **119**(1):88–96.

152. **Rimpeekool W, Seubsman S-a, Banwell C, Kirk M, Yiengprugsawan V, Sleigh A.** Food and nutrition labelling in Thailand: a long march from subsistence producers to international traders. *Food Policy* 2015; **56**:59–66.

153. **Nestle M, Ludwig DS.** Front-of-package food labels: public health or propaganda? *JAMA* 2010; **303**(8):771–72.

154. **Lachat C, Tseng M.** A wake-up call for nutrition labelling. *Public Health Nutrition* 2013 Mar; **16**(3):381–82.

Chapter 7

Screening and surveillance

7.1 Screening, surveillance, and the differences between them

Screening and surveillance play an important role in tackling non-communicable diseases (NCDs)—particularly as part of defining the problem. The differences between the two approaches—screening and surveillance—are mainly in relation to the overall aim. Screening is an activity that includes intention to treat and, generally, involves feedback of results to the individuals concerned. Surveillance, in contrast, aims to quantify prevalence and does not generally include feedback to individuals, nor is it linked to treatment. Other differences are highlighted in Table 7.1 and further details of both screening and surveillance are provided in the next section.

There are advantages and disadvantages to both screening and surveillance, and their respective utilities will depend on a programme's specific goals, the available resources, and the broader context. A third option exists—monitoring, which can combine elements of surveillance and screening.

7.2 Screening

As outlined in section 7.1, screening aims to identify condition(s) prior to onset and/or symptoms of disease as an attempt to prevent onset or delay progression of the condition (Table 7.2).

There are some long-standing criteria, set out by WHO in 1968, for health conditions suitable for screening (Box 7.1).[1]

For some NCDs it is not clear that they meet the criteria for screening. For example, although screening has been implemented for obesity there has been considerable debate about the value of screening for this condition, with some reviews concluding that there is not enough evidence to support such a practice. However, the increasing size of this epidemic and the need for time-urgent action may have influenced decisions to introduce screening (Box 7.2).

Table 7.1 Differences between surveillance and screening

Surveillance	Screening
◆ Refers to monitoring of a given condition ◆ Principal aims • Quantify prevalence • Analyse trends over time ◆ Data are anonymized ◆ Does not include: • Feedback of individual results • Formal link to treatment	◆ Includes intention to treat ◆ Aim: identify condition prior to onset ◆ Allows for: • Complete prevention • Earlier treatment • Delayed progression ◆ Feedback of individual results typically provided

Table 7.2 Advantages and disadvantages of screening

Advantages	Disadvantages
Complete prevention, earlier treatment, or delayed progression of illness.	There is not always a detectable early stage.
Typically provides feedback of results to individuals.	The natural history of the condition is not always well understood.
Can promote change in lifestyle behaviours.	Costs and risks are not always outweighed by benefits.
Can increase awareness of an issue among health-care professionals.	Hawthorne effect may apply, i.e. that which is being measured may be affected by the very fact of it being measured in the first place.
May enhance communication between health-care providers and the general public; may reduce misperceptions and provide support or reassurance.	

Box 7.1 Criteria for conditions which are suitable for screening

1. The condition being screened for should be an important health problem.
2. The natural history of the condition should be well understood.
3. There should be a detectable early stage.
4. Treatment at an early stage should be of more benefit than at a later stage.
5. A suitable test should be devised for the early stage.
6. The test should be acceptable.
7. Intervals for repeating the test should be determined.
8. Adequate health service provision should be made for the extra clinical workload resulting from screening.
9. The risks should be less than the benefits.
10. The costs should be balanced against the benefits.

Source: data from Wilson JMG and Jungner G. Principles and practice of screening for disease. *Public Health Papers*, Issue 34, Geneva: World Health Organization, Copyright © 1968 World Health Organization, http://apps.who.int/iris/bitstream/10665/37650/17/WHO_PHP_34.pdf, accessed 15 Jul. 2016.

Box 7.2 Effect of organized cervical cancer screening on incidence of invasive cervical cancer in England, UK

A good example of how screening can impact on incidence and mortality is the experience of introducing a national call and recall system for cervical screening in England. Cervical screening in England had started in the mid-1960s, but with limited impact—over 90% of women over 40 with invasive cervical cancer had never been screened. To increase coverage a national call and recall system for cervical smears was introduced in 1988 and financial incentives for family doctors were introduced in 1990. As Figure 7.1 shows, coverage of cervical screening increased greatly and a 35% fall in incidence of invasive cervical cancer was recorded. Although there was a fall in mortality among women over 55 this could not be solely attributed to screening (because relatively few in this group would have been screened). Screening was, however, estimated to have prevented 800 deaths in younger women (25 to 54) in 1997.[2]

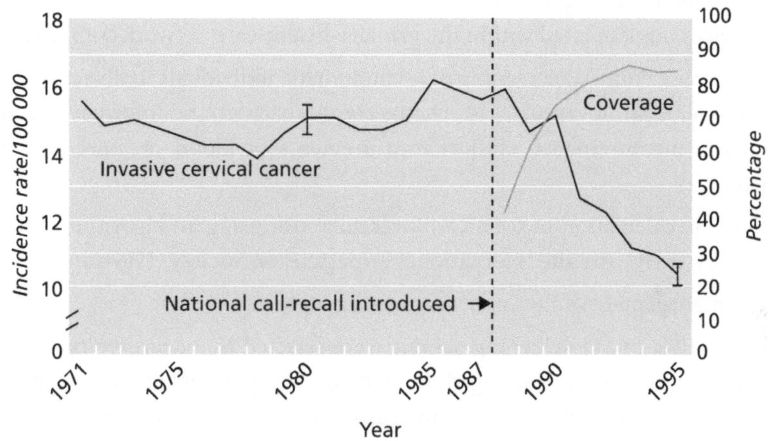

Figure 7.1 Age-standardized incidence of invasive cervical cancer and coverage of screening, England, 1971–95.

Reproduced with permission from **Quinn M, Babb P, Jones J, Allen A**. Effect of screening on incidence of and mortality from cancer of the cervix in England: evaluation based on routinely collected statistics. *British Medical Journal*, Volume 318, Issue 7188, pp. 904–8, Copyright © 1999 BMJ Publishing Group Ltd.

Case study: Cardiovascular risk screening in Lebanon

Following the epidemiological transition of the past two decades, NCDs are the leading causes of death and illness in Lebanon, accounting for 84% of all deaths in 2010. CVD alone accounts for almost half of all deaths in the country, and the prevalence of modifiable cardiovascular risk factors is high.[3]

The Lebanese government subsidizes access to secondary and tertiary care for those who are uninsured. Primary health-care services, in contrast, are not subsidized, and there is little funding for preventive measures. This has resulted in overdependence on hospitalization and advanced medical care, at the expense of primary care. Specifically in relation to CVD, a major amount of public spending goes to subsidizing costly diagnosis and treatment related to CVD and there is insufficient early detection of risk factors.

In order to address this imbalance and encourage CVD prevention, the Ministry of Public Health (MOPH) decided to launch a two-step initiative of cardiovascular risk factor screening, based on a total cardiovascular risk approach implemented within the network of 220 primary health-care centres. This initiative—which was conceived in late 2012 and presented as an assignment during the University of Oxford's short course on Introduction to Population-Level Prevention Strategies for NCDs—was piloted in late 2013 and has since been implemented across the whole network as an integral part of primary health care in Lebanon. This approach was designed to address cardiovascular risk as a multifactorial condition, instead of dealing with cardiovascular risk factors separately.

The services implemented within the primary health-care network comprised:

- massive opportunistic screening of asymptomatic individuals to detect simultaneously several cardiovascular risk factors (health background information, anthropometric measurements, clinical measurements of blood pressure, and blood sugar);
- systematic calculation of total cardiovascular risk using an algorithm developed jointly by WHO and the International Hypertension Society (IHS); and
- active management of the cohort presenting higher risk.

The beneficiaries of the screening service were selected by purposive opportunistic recruitment, focusing on those aged 40 or older. The participants were approached while attending the health centre for any reason or, as part of the outreach component of the initiative, were approached in their homes or places of work.

There are three consecutive steps of the service, as summarized in Table 7.3.

Table 7.3 Consecutive steps in the cardiovascular risk prediction and management service in Lebanon

Step	Eligibility	Output	Outcome
Screening	All	Suspected metabolic impairment/ CV risk detected	Referral to diagnostic step
Diagnostic	Referred to diagnostic step	Confirmed metabolic impairment/confirmed CV risk	Eligible for management step
Management	Confirmed cases	Treatment	Controlled cases

Table 7.4 Definition of risk categories based on screening

Risk definition	History of cardiovascular event	DM	AHT	TCVR ≥ 10%	RBS+	BP +	Elevated WC	History of DL	FH	Smoker	Obese
Null	No	No	No	No	No	No	No	No	No	No	No
Gen/ Behav.	No	No	No	No	No	No	No	No	At least any of three		
Metabolic	No	No or controlled		No	No	No	At least any of two				
Probable	No	No or controlled		At least any of three							
Definite	Yes	Any Uncontrolled									

Abbreviations: TCVR, total cardiovascular risk by WHO/ISH charts; DM, previously diagnosed diabetes mellitus; AHT, previously diagnoses arterial hypertension; RBS+, impaired results for random blood sugar screening; BP+, impaired results for blood pressure screening; Elevated WC, elevated waist circumference (≥ 99 cm in men and ≥ 92 cm in women); DL, dyslipidemia; FH, family history of premature CVD.

The MOPH, in collaboration with the WHO country office, funded the training and the electronic management of the initiative. For the pilot phase, only the screening step—which was performed by non-physician health workers—was subsidized by the MOPH, whereas fees were charged as usual for the diagnostic and the management steps in the health centres.

After the completion of the screening step, screened individuals were assigned to one of five mutually exclusive risk groups, as set out in Table 7.4.

Patients in the 'metabolic' and 'probable' risk groups were directed to the diagnostic step for verification of the screening results and additional investigations under the supervision of a doctor. Those with confirmed diagnosis were directed to the management step and followed up for risk-lowering management, including pharmaceutical and non-pharmaceutical treatment, preferably by a doctor.

The Null Group cohort was advised to repeat the screening in one year's time, while those presenting solely with behavioural risk factors benefited from information and education from non-physician health workers.

Those having undergone a major cardiovascular event, or who presented uncontrolled metabolic disorders, were referred to secondary care to adjust their treatment.

Analysis of the results demonstrates the value of the screening (Table 7.5). For every six people screened, one was detected with impaired blood sugar or elevated blood pressure. Over 60% of the screened population had one or more metabolic impairments, whether previously diagnosed or just detected.

Table 7.5 Risk assessment for men and women screened

Assigned risk group	Men		Women		Men and Women	
	N	%	N	%	N	%
Definite	244	11.8	353	9.3	597	10.2
Probable	706	34.1	949	25.0	1655	28.2
Metabolic	467	22.5	1187	31.2	1654	28.2
Genetic/Behavioural	371	17.9	608	16.0	979	16.7
Null Risk	284	13.7	706	18.6	990	16.9

The findings that two-thirds of the metabolically impaired population were unaware of the risk before participating in the screening justifies the inclusion of this service at the primary care level in Lebanon.

Those screened benefited not only from knowledge of their metabolic status and cardiovascular risk, but also became more aware about the combination of risks. Such awareness can trigger decisions to modify behaviour. Moreover, since the service did not exclude those known to have a metabolic condition, the screening could detect those with uncontrolled conditions.

In addition to the direct benefits of the service, health workers have been introduced to the notion of total cardiovascular risk, and this is expected to improve the quality of health information delivered to patients.

Adapted from **Yamout R**, **Adib SM**, **Hamadeh R**, **Freidi A**, and **Ammar W**. Screening for cardiovascular risk in asymptomatic users of the primary health care network in Lebanon, 2012–2013. *Preventing Chronic Disease*, Volume 11, Article 140089, July 17, 2014, http://www.cdc.gov/pcd/issues/2014/14_0089.htm, accessed 01 Aug. 2016.

7.3 **Surveillance**

Public health surveillance, as defined by WHO, is the continuous, systematic collection, analysis, and interpretation of health-related data needed for the planning, implementation, and evaluation of public health practice.

The fundamental importance of surveillance to the prevention and control of NCDs is widely recognized. WHO cites public health surveillance as an essential function of any public health system. Surveillance can serve as an early warning system, document the impact of interventions, track progress towards goals, and monitor and clarify the epidemiology of health problems. Crucially, surveillance data should provide accountability for local health status and should form the basis for public health decision-making. Some advantages and disadvantages of surveillance are set out in Table 7.6.

Table 7.6 Advantages and disadvantages of surveillance

Advantages	Disadvantages
Highlights particular health condition	May prompt unnecessary worry or give false reassurance
Provides forum for increasing public engagement	Data collected for epidemiological purposes alone may be inefficient
Raises and maintains political exposure and support	Data collection may be unethical in some contexts
Fewer concerns around privacy/confidentiality than with screening	
Lower requirement for time/resources than with screening	

7.3.1 What type of surveillance?

There are two broad categories of surveillance. *Active surveillance* involves employing staff to deliberately seek information about health conditions, whereas *passive surveillance* relies on routine reporting of cases that reach health-care facilities.

Active surveillance is expensive, but can be carefully targeted, providing timely information to assess the effectiveness of interventions. This often involves repeated surveys of health-related behaviours, the largest example being the US Centers for Disease Control and Prevention's Behavioral Risk Factor Surveillance System of ongoing telephone health surveys.[4]

Passive surveillance is less costly because it uses data that are collected routinely and, increasingly, information technology can be used to harvest information from routine data. Information about disease and programmes can be collected through a country's routine health information system. Alternatively, routine financial, logistic, or administrative data can be gathered through health information and management systems.

A third type of surveillance is sometimes considered—*sentinel surveillance* can be either passive or active, but uses key individuals or locations/sites to provide information. Sentinel surveillance is based on selected institutions or individuals that provide regular, complete reports on one or more diseases.

The precise goals of any surveillance programme—and what it seeks to measure—will impact on exactly what type of system to introduce. Surveillance aims can be considered under three broad headings:

- **Categorical surveillance** is focused on one or more diseases or behaviours.
- **Integrated surveillance** uses a single infrastructure to gather information about multiple diseases or behaviours of interest to several intervention programmes.
- **Syndromic surveillance** uses case definitions based entirely on clinical features without any clinical or laboratory diagnosis.

Table 7.7 Implementing surveillance

Stage in implementing surveillance	Key issues to consider
Establish goals	Be clear about what the surveillance aims to measure. The precise goals of any programme will impact on the type of surveillance to implement.
Develop case definitions	It is very important to develop well-defined definitions for cases and cut-off points. These must be accurate and clear.
Select appropriate personnel	Make sure there are personnel in place for all the stages of implementation, including analysis as well as data collection.
Acquire tools and clearance	WHO and others have developed tools for surveillance. These include WHO's STEPwise approach to surveillance[5] and CDC's Field Epidemiology Training Program.[6] Legal and ethical clearance is very important. The type of clearance obtained can have significant implications for the way information can be used and disseminated.
Implement surveillance system	Try not to take too long to implement the surveillance system—remember the ultimate goal of the surveillance is to be able to take public health action.
Evaluate surveillance system	Evaluation of how the surveillance system is working, how much it is costing etc., should be ongoing and should feed back into the implementation process.

7.3.2 Implementing surveillance

Table 7.7 shows the various steps involved in setting up surveillance systems and some key issues to consider at each stage.

Sample size is another important issue to consider when setting up a surveillance system. In practice, sampling is a balance between what is feasible or affordable and ensuring the sample is big enough to achieve meaningful results. To decide how big a sample will need to be, it is important to consider what kind of changes are sought and what will be done with the data. The required sample size depends on a variety of factors (see Box 7.3).

The WHO *STEPS Manual* provides detailed guidance, and worked examples, on sample size calculations. The manual also provides guidance on a number of other issues related to setting up a surveillance system.

7.3.3 Using surveillance data

In its definition of surveillance, WHO has emphasized that surveillance means more than simply collecting data—information must be analysed and interpreted to be of value in controlling disease. There is, in fact, often a gap between the production of data and the ability to convert the data into usable information that initiates appropriate public health action. Some of the different uses of surveillance data are shown in Table 7.8.

A related issue is the question of how best to disseminate surveillance information. It is important to tailor the information to the desired target audience. Policy-makers, for example, need information in a very concise and accessible format. Graphic representations,

Box 7.3 Factors affecting the required sample size

Approaches for determining the appropriate sample size will depend upon the purpose of the study, the study design, and the main outcome measure of the study. The calculations require a measure of variance, which may be proportions (for discrete measures) or means (for continuous measures). When data are collected to measure a significant change, the degree of change should be measured.

What is the desired level of significance of the results? What is the acceptable margin of error?

Regarding stratification, the more age/sex/socioeconomic status categories to be reported, the bigger the sample size required. It is also important to take into account the anticipated non-response rate.

Cluster sampling underestimates standard errors and so must be increased accordingly. A design effect can be calculated to adjust for this and allows the required number of clusters and number of cases to be calculated.

If analysis of the outcome measure will include a number of confounding factors, the sample size must be increased. A general rule of thumb is that a 10% increase should be included for every confounding factor.

Table 7.8 Variety of uses for surveillance data

Immediate detection of	Annual dissemination for	Archival information for
◆ Epidemics ◆ New health problems ◆ Changes in health practices ◆ Changes in treatment effectiveness ◆ Change in distribution of population at risk of disease	◆ Estimating magnitude of problem ◆ Assessing control activities ◆ Setting research priorities ◆ Determining risk factor for disease ◆ Facilitating planning ◆ Monitoring risk factors ◆ Monitoring changes in health practices ◆ Documenting impact of disease	◆ Describing natural history of disease ◆ Facilitating research ◆ Validating use of preliminary data ◆ Setting research priorities ◆ Documenting distribution and spread of disease

Source: data from **Thacker SB** and **Stroup DF**. 'Public health surveillance and health services research'. In: **Armenian HK** and **Shapiro S** (eds.), *Epidemiology and Health Services*. New York: Oxford University Press, Copyright © 1998 Oxford University Press.

such as maps, can have greater impact than a series of tables or figures. Experience in the USA, for example, found that while tables presenting the data on overweight and obesity had been largely ignored, a series of maps to illustrate prevalence figures managed to attract a lot of attention and ignited public concern.

7.3.4 Implementing surveillance in low- and middle-income countries

Until relatively recently, surveillance has tended to be associated with high-income countries. Poorer countries have rarely had the necessary resources to allocate to surveillance in the face of many competing health challenges and a weak public health infrastructure. As a result, many have been dependent on knowledge gleaned from third parties' research. Increasing attention is now focused on the importance of surveillance in efforts to tackle NCDs in all countries.

WHO has described strengthening surveillance at national and global levels as a priority for tackling NCDs.[7] The first global strategy for the prevention and control of NCDs, endorsed by the World Health Assembly in 2000, highlighted 'surveillance to track and monitor the major risk factors' as a key priority. WHO has also, however, recognized the serious deficiencies that currently exist in relation to surveillance of NCDs, and set out four key steps to remedy these deficiencies (see Box 7.4).

WHO and others have developed tools and programmes to enable and support NCD surveillance in low- and middle-income countries (LMICs). WHO has also introduced the STEPwise approach to surveillance (STEPS) as a simple, standardized method for collecting, analyzing, and disseminating data that can be used globally (Figure 7.2). To date, there are two primary STEPS programmes: for risk factor surveillance and for stroke surveillance.

Box 7.4 Key steps necessary to strengthen surveillance for NCDs

- NCD surveillance systems should be strengthened and integrated into existing national health information systems.
- All three components of the NCD surveillance framework should be established and strengthened.
- Monitoring and surveillance of behavioural and metabolic risk factors in low-resource settings should receive the highest priority.
- A significant acceleration in financial and technical support is necessary for health information system development in LMICs.

Reproduced with permission from **WHO**. *Global status report on noncommunicable diseases 2010*, Geneva: World Health Organization, Copyright © 2011 World Health Organization, p. 3, http://apps.who.int/iris/bitstream/10665/44579/1/9789240686458_eng.pdf, accessed 01 Jul. 2016.

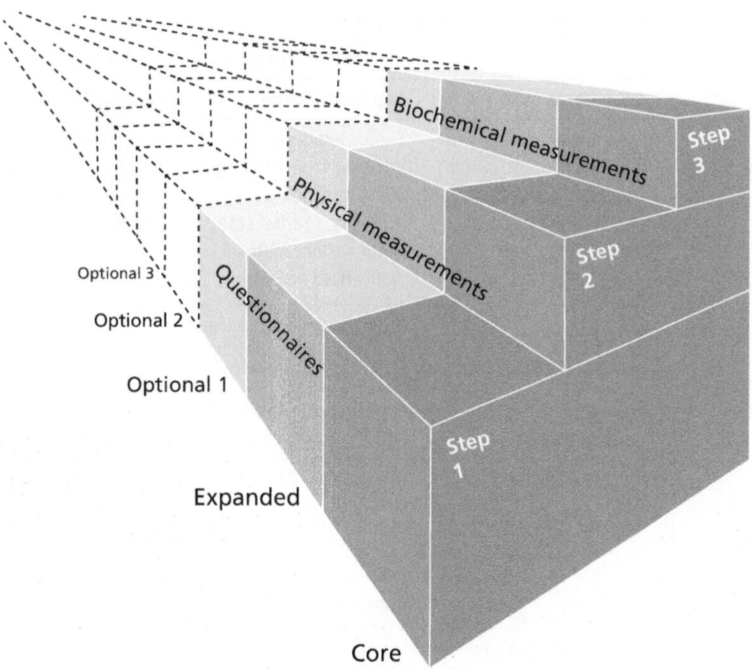

Figure 7.2 Elements of WHO's STEPwise approach to surveillance.

Reproduced with permission from **WHO**. *STEPS Manual*, Geneva: World Health Organization, Copyright © 2008 World Health Organization, p. 15, http://www.who.int/chp/steps/Part1.pdf?ua=1, accessed 15 Jul. 2016.

The risk factor surveillance approach is designed to be an entry point for LMICs to start chronic disease surveillance. The instrument covers three types of measurement—behavioural, physical, and biochemical—and for each defines three modules which set out lists of core, expanded, and optional variables, respectively (see Table 7.9). In this way, countries can implement surveillance depending on the resources available and the information required.

As countries progress through the STEPwise approach, the process becomes more demanding and more skilled staff will be needed. It is important that a cadre of competent, motivated health workers is developed for LMICs.

It is possible to implement surveillance in resource-limited, rural settings (see Box 7.5), and the growing use of electronic data systems and the availability of the internet may provide further opportunities for more timely and comprehensive surveillance in all parts of the world. Given sufficient political will and organizational commitment, data could be collected as an automatic by-product of any electronic system used to support clinical care.

Table 7.9 Variables included in WHO STEPwise approach to risk factor surveillance

	STEPS risk factors		
	Core items	**Expanded items**	**Optional modules**
Step 1 Behavioural	Basic demographic information, including age, sex, literacy, and highest level of education	Expanded demographic information including years at school, ethnicity, marital status, employment status, household income	Mental heath, intentional and unintentional injury and violence, and oral health
	Tobacco use	Smokeless tobacco use	
	Alcohol consumption	Past 7 days drinking	
	Fruit and vegetable consumption	Oil and fat consumption	
	Physical activity		Objective measure of physical activity behaviour
		History of blood pressure, treatment for raised blood pressure	
		History of diabetes, treatment for diabetes	
Step 2 Physical measurements	Weight and height, waist circumference, blood pressure	Hip circumference. Heart rate	Skin fold thickness, assessment of physical fitness
Step 3 Biochemical measurements	Fasting blood sugar Total cholesterol	Fasting HDL cholesterol and triglycerides	Oral glucose tolerance test, urine examination, salivary cotinine

Reproduced with permission from **WHO**. *STEPS Manual*, Geneva: World Health Organization, Copyright © 2008 World Health Organization, p. 15, http://www.who.int/chp/steps/Part1.pdf?ua=1, accessed 15 Jul. 2016.

Box 7.5 Establishing a surveillance system in Nepal

Through a collaboration between the Nordic School of Public Health NHV in Sweden, Kathmandu Medical College, and Nepal Medical College a Health Demographic Surveillance System (HDSS) was established in the peri-urban villages Jhaukhel and Duwakot (JD-HDSS), in Bhaktapur district outside Kathmandu in Nepal.[8] These are two adjacent, rapidly urbanizing villages with similar geo-ecological, ethnic, and cultural characteristics. There were many administrative, political, geographical, and social challenges to overcome during the establishment of the JD-HDSS. These included securing commitment from the authorities, recruiting an appropriately qualified workforce, and dealing with external political pressure applied to the recruitment process. Access to households was difficult, given the poor transport system and that there is no systematic numbering of houses or any list of addresses.

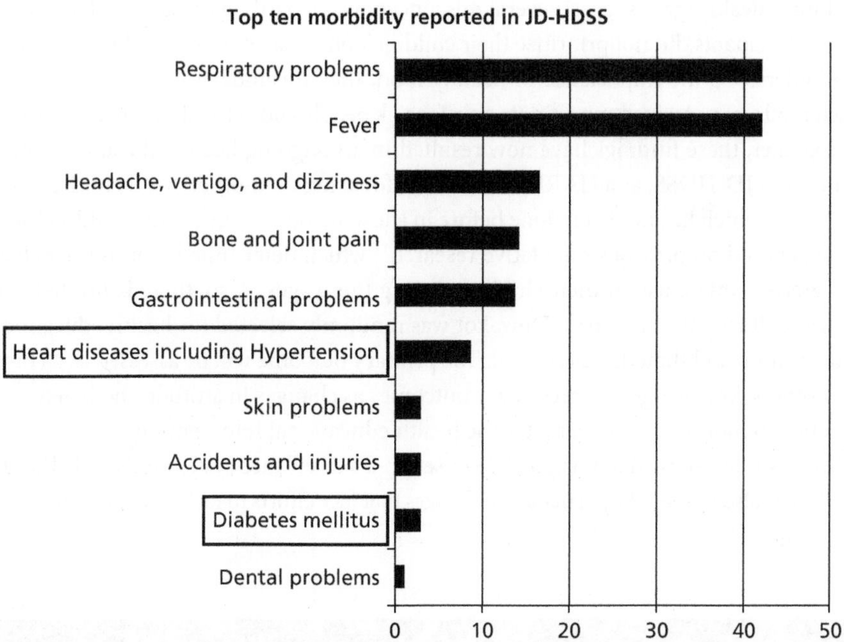

Figure 7.3 Double burden of disease in the Jhaukhel-Duwakot Health Demographic Surveillance System.

Reproduced from **Aryal UR**, **Vaidya A**, **Shakya-Vaidya S**, **Petzold M**, and **Krettek A**. Establishing a health demographic surveillance site in Bhaktapur district, Nepal: initial experiences and findings. *BMC Research Notes*, Volume 5, pp. 489. Copyright © 2012 Raj Aryal et al.

The initial baseline survey identified that NCDs were prevalent, existing alongside communicable diseases (see Figure 7.3). A similar pattern was evident, but more pronounced, at the two-year follow-up.[9]

As part of the JD-HDSS, a more specific cardiovascular health survey was also initiated in Bhaktapur district. The Heart-Health Associated Research and Dissemination in the Community (HARDIC) project is a longitudinal study to assess cardiovascular health knowledge, attitudes, practices, and behaviours in the district. This survey identified a high burden of cardiovascular risk factors (20% are current smokers, 43% have low physical activity levels, and 22% are hypertensive).[10] The survey also highlighted poor knowledge of heart disease causes and of heart attack symptoms (60% could not name any heart attack symptoms) and identified that there was no difference in health-related behaviours between people with diagnosed heart disease and those without.[10] In-depth interviews among people with cardiometabolic conditions, about perceptions regarding cause and prevention of cardiovascular disease, show that respondents embraced the importance of lifestyle modification only after receiving their diagnosis. Furthermore, they remarked that community awareness of heart disease was inadequate.[11] Similarly, an exploration of Nepalese mothers' perceptions regarding diet and physical activity for children's health again suggest several misconceptions regarding cardiovascular risk factors. Participants did not prioritize their children's physical activity and although mothers understood the importance of healthy food, they misunderstood its composition. Such food was perceived appropriate only for sick people and generally as unappetizing.[12]

Together, these findings have now resulted in an ongoing health educational intervention in JD-HDSS, as a HARDIC initiative, focusing on mothers with children aged 1–7 years which has not been done before in a low-income country. The children's age-span is based on previous qualitative research[12] which determined that mothers have the greatest influence on their children during these ages. Also, there is limited peer pressure during this age span. Duwakot was randomly selected for health educational intervention and Jhaukhel as control. The primary outcome will be assessed as changes in mothers' knowledge and secondary outcomes as changes in attitude and behaviour/practices 6 months and 1 year after the health educational intervention.

These studies show that it is possible to set up a surveillance system in Nepal. The JD-HDSS has also scoped the particular challenges that face efforts to tackle NCDs in this area.

Case study: Behavioural risk factor surveillance in Jordan

Jordan has experienced the health transition from infectious to chronic, degenerative diseases, and non-communicable diseases are now the leading causes of death and illness in the country. In order to adapt to this changing situation—and to be able to reduce exposure to risk factors for NCDs—the country has needed timely and ongoing information to track trends in prevalence of both diseases and risk factors. In 2002, therefore, Jordan conducted a population-based survey on behavioural risk factors associated with the most common NCDs. The Jordan Behavioural Risk Factor Surveillance Survey (BRFSS) was an early element in the country's NCD surveillance system.

The survey was implemented by the Jordan Ministry of Health, in cooperation with the Jordan Department of Statistics, WHO, and the US Centers for Disease Control and Prevention (CDC). The survey was modelled on the CDC's BRFSS tool. The BRFSS was established in the USA in 1984, with the participation of 15 states, and became a nationwide surveillance system in 1993. It is now the largest continuously conducted health survey in the world, collecting data in all 50 states through interviews with more than 400,000 adults each year.[7]

For the first BRFSS in Jordan in May 2002, 28 questions about behavioural risk factors and NCD prevalence were added to the Jordan Department of Statistics' quarterly, multistage, cross-sectional employment, and unemployment survey.

The sample was based on a nationally representative sampling frame, stratified by governorate, major city, and other urban and rural areas. People living in remote areas and those living in collective dwellings such as hotels, hospitals, work camps, and prisons were excluded. From every household in the sample one adult (aged 18 or over) was selected to be interviewed.

From the sample of 9,601 households, a total of 8,791 questionnaires were completed, with a response rate of 92%. The questionnaire included questions on smoking, self-reported height and weight, participation in weekly moderate or vigorous activity, when respondents had last sought health care from a professional, whether respondents had ever had their blood pressure or cholesterol checked by a health-care professional, and whether a health-care professional had ever told them that they had high blood pressure, high cholesterol, asthma, or diabetes or that they had had a heart attack (Table 7.10).

The survey documented substantial levels of overweight (32%) and obesity (13%), based on body mass index (BMI) calculations from self-reported height and weight data (Table 7.10). It also revealed very low levels of physical activity in both sexes—just over half of respondents (53%) reported taking part in any weekly physical activity (moderate or vigorous) and under a third (32%) reported any weekly vigorous physical activity. Physical activity levels were particularly low in women—less than a quarter (24%) reported any vigorous activity on a weekly basis and less than half (48%) reported any weekly physical activity at all.

Factors proposed as contributing to these low levels of physical activity include a reduction in school physical activity classes, a lack of encouragement and motivation to use school playgrounds after school hours, and—specifically for women—a lack of appropriate places for women to practice physical activity.[13] Small-scale strategies being implemented to change the physical environment include a multisectoral partnership in Greater Amman Municipality to support walking by opening four public gardens at specific times for women only.

The first BRFSS in Jordan was the first step in regular collection of data on risk factors. In order to use population-based surveys for surveillance it is important to ensure that factors such as the protocols, sampling, interviews, and questionnaires are comparable. It is important to be particularly attentive to the sample size and maintenance of a high response rate, in order to ensure that population changes do not affect the results.[14]

The BRFSS was repeated in 2004 and 2007 in Jordan. For the third survey in 2007, a sample of respondents were invited to participate in a medical examination. Standardized measurement of height, weight, waist circumference, blood pressure, cholesterol, and blood glucose took place. The self-reported prevalence of obesity increased from 12.8 to 19.5% between 2002 and 2004. In the 2007 survey, based on the measured heights and weights from the medical examination subsample, the prevalence of obesity was 36%, and 30.5% were overweight. In 2007, physical activity levels remained low—only 38% of respondents reported that they engage in any recreational moderate physical activity.[15]

The use of the BRFSS tool in Jordan, therefore, highlighted substantial prevalence of risk factors for NCDs and proved valuable for planning public health interventions. As part of its response, the Government of Jordan published a *National Strategy and Plan of Action against Diabetes, Hypertension, Dyslipidemia, and Obesity in Jordan* in 2011.[16]

Adapted from **Centers for Disease Control and Prevention (CDC)**. Prevalence of selected risk factors for chronic disease—Jordan, 2002. *Morbidity Mortality Weekly Report (MMWR)*, October 31, 2003, Volume 52, Issue 43, pp. 1042–4, http://www.cdc.gov/mmwr/preview/mmwrhtml/mm5243a3.htm, accessed 01 Aug. 2016.

Table 7.10 Prevalence of selected risk factors for chronic diseases, by sex and age group—Behavioural Risk Factor Surveillance Survey

Risk factor	Sex				Age group (yrs)								Total	
	Men		Women		18–34		35–49		50–84		>65			
	%	(95% CI[a])	%	(95% CI)	%	(95% CI)	%	(95%CI)	%	(95% CI)	%	(95% CI)	%	(95% CI)
High blood pressure	21.0	(±2.4)	23.2	(±2.1)	8.8	(±1.4)	22.8	(±2.5)	44.3	(±4.5)	43.8	(±6.3)	22.2	(±1.6)
High blood cholesterol	21.2	(±4.0)	20.5	(±4.4)	8.8	(±5.0)	18.3	(±4.5)	32.1	(±5.8)	34.0	(±9.9)	20.9	(±3.0)
Diabetes	6.5	(±1.0)	6.2	(±1.2)	0.7	(±0.3)	6.2	(±1.4)	19.9	(±3.5)	23.3	(±4.7)	6.4	(±0.8)
Heart attack history	3.2	(±0.7)	1.5	(±0.6)	0.2	(±0.1)	1.5	(±0.7)	8.2	(±2.4)	10.8	(±3.0)	2.4	(±0.5)
Asthma	3.7	(±0.7)	6.4	(±1.1)	3.7	(±0.8)	6.6	(±1.6)	6.8	(±2.0)	6.6	(±2.7)	5.1	(±0.7)
Smoking														
Ever smoker[b]	64.4	(±2.0)	10.9	(±1.7)	33.3	(±2.9)	44.5	(±3.8)	42.9	(±4.8)	45.5	(±6.0)	38.2	(±2.8)
Current smoker[c]	50.5	(±2.2)	8.3	(±1.4)	29.0	(±2.7)	34.9	(±3.2)	27.8	(±3.9)	22.2	(±5.3)	29.8	(±2.3)
Weight														
Overweight[d]	36.0	(±2.2)	27.8	(±2.2)	26.2	(±2.1)	41.0	(±2.9)	41.0	(±4.4)	38.1	(±7.7)	32.4	(±1.7)
Obesity[e]	10.3	(±1.3)	16.2	(±1.9)	5.8	(±1.0)	20.8	(±2.4)	25.0	(±4.0)	19.3	(±6.0)	12.8	(±1 .1)
Physical activity														
Any weekly vigorous[f]	38.9	(±2 4)	23.9	(±1.9)	35.8	(±2.5)	33.5	(±2.6)	22.3	(±3.5)	10.0	(±3.4)	31.6	(±1.7)
Any weekly activity[g]	56.9	(±2 6)	48.2	(±2.4)	57.7	(±2.4)	54.9	(±2.8)	43.8	(±3.9)	22.0	(±4.4)	52.6	(±1.7)
Ever checked														
Blood pressure	61.1	(±2.3)	73.9	(±2.0)	56.1	(±2.2)	78.7	(±2.4)	83.6	(±2.8)	81.9	(±5.0)	67.4	(±1.6)
Cholesterol	20.8	(±2.0)	16.1	(±1.8)	9.6	(±1.2)	26.0	(±3.0)	35.0	(±4.2)	28.0	(±5.4)	18.5	(±1.3)

[a] Confidence interval.

[b] Ever smoked ≥ 100 cigarettes during lifetime.

[c] Ever smoked ≥ 100 cigarettes during lifetime and currently smoke every day or some days.

[d] Body mass index (BMI) (i.e. ratio of weight in kilograms to height in meters squared (kg/m^2)) of 25.0–29.9.

[e] BMI ≥ 30.

[f] Vigorous activity (i.e. causing heavy sweating and large increases in breathing or heart rate for 20 minutes).

[g] Any moderate activity (i.e. causing light sweating and small increases in breathing or heart rate for 30 minutes) or vigorous activity.

Source: data from **Jordan Department of Statistics**. *Jordan in Figures*. Amman, Jordan: Jordan Department of Statistics, 2002, http://www.dos.gov.jo/dos_home_e/main/jorfig/2002/jor_f_e.htm, accessed 01 Aug. 2016.

Case study. Uncovering the hidden part of the US obesity epidemic

The epidemic of overweight and obesity in the United States has been long recognized and well documented. For public health purposes, however, reporting focuses on the prevalence of overweight or obesity (body mass index of 30 or greater) and the prevalence of clinically severe obesity (BMI of 40 or greater) is not generally reported. In 2003 Professor Roland Sturm reported that clinicians tended to believe that clinically severe obesity was a relatively rare pathological condition that would only affect a fixed proportion of the population and, crucially, would not increase as Americans, in general, became heavier.[17]

Sturm had, in fact, analysed data from the Centers for Disease Control and Prevention's long-running US Behavioural Risk Factor Surveillance Survey to explore this issue. His analyses of the BRFSS self-reported BMI data revealed that the prevalence of BMI of 40 or greater quadrupled—from about 1 in 200 adult Americans to 1 in 50—between 1986 and 2000.[18] The prevalence of BMI of 50 or greater increased by a factor of five, while standard obesity (BMI of 30 or greater) had only doubled over this time. Sturm concluded that the most dramatic part of the obesity epidemic has remained hidden and that clinically severe obesity is an integral part of the US population's weight distribution.

Sturm's conclusion that prevalence of clinically severe obesity would continue to increase has been borne out by more recent data. Following up on the research with an analysis of the BRFSS data between 2000 and 2010, Sturm and Hattori found the prevalence of BMI over 40 had increased by 70% and the prevalence of BMI over 50 had increased even faster. There was evidence, however, that the increase had been less rapid since 2005.[18]

There were major implications from this analysis of the surveillance data. As people in the USA got heavier, the heaviest categories would grow fastest. This underlined the urgent need for a population-based approach to prevent obesity, but also forewarned of the serious logistical challenges facing health services as extreme obesity increases. Services need to plan to ensure that they have appropriate resources and equipment available in order to be able to care for extremely obese patients—from larger blood pressure cuffs to appropriate wheelchairs, stretchers, and beds.[19] There are also issues around transport and the safety of care staff. The urgent need to plan for, and invest in, appropriate facilities and care arrangements underlines the importance of appropriate surveillance to be able to identify emerging problems.

Source: data from **Sturm R**. Increases in clinically severe obesity in the United States, 1986-2000. *Archives of Internal Medicine*, Volume 163, Issue 18, pp. 2146–48, Copyright © 2003 American Medical Association; **Sturm R** and **Hattori A**. Morbid obesity rates continue to rise rapidly in the US. *International Journal of Obesity*, Volume 37, Issue 6, pp. 889–91, Copyright © 2013 Macmillan Publishers Limited.

Acknowledgements

This chapter is largely drawn from presentations by Dr Nick Townsend, Dr Gauden Galea, and Dr Alexandra Krettek, with case study material from Dr Randa Hamadeh, Dr Rouham Yamout, and other sources cited.

References

1. **Wilson JMG, Jungner G.** Principles and practice of screening for disease. *WHO Chronicle* 1968; 22(11):473.
2. **Quinn M, Babb P, Jones J, Allen A** (on behalf of the United Kingdom Association of Cancer Registries). Effect of screening on incidence of and mortality from cancer of the cervix in England: evaluation based on routinely collected statistics. *BMJ* 1999; 318:904–8.
3. **Yamout R, Adib SM, Hamadeh R, Freidi A, Ammar W.** Screening for cardiovascular risk in asymptomatic users of the primary health care network in Lebanon, 2012-2013. *Preventing Chronic Disease* 2014; **11**:E120.
4. **Centers for Disease Control and Prevention.** *Behavioural Risk Factor Surveillance System.* Available at: http://www.cdc.gov/brfss/
5. **World Health Organization.** *Chronic Disease and Health Promotion—STEPS Manual.* Available at: http://www.who.int/chp/steps/manual/en/
6. **Centers for Disease Control and Prevention.** *Global Health Protection and Security—Field Epidemiology Training Program (FETP).* Available at: http://www.cdc.gov/globalhealth/fetp/
7. **World Health Organization.** *Global Status Report on Noncommunicable Diseases.* Geneva: WHO, 2010. Available at: http://www.who.int/nmh/publications/ncd_report2010/en/
8. **Aryal UR, Vaidya A, Shakya-Vaidya S, Petzold M, Krettek A.** Establishing a health demographic surveillance site in Bhaktapur district, Nepal: initial experiences and findings. *BMC Research Notes* 2012, *5*:489.
9. **Choulagai BP, Aryal UR, Shrestha B, Vaidya A, Onta S, Petzold M,** et al. Jhaukhel-Duwakot Health Demographic Surveillance Site, Nepal: 2012 follow-up survey and use of skilled birth attendants. *Global Health Action* 2015; **8**:29396.
10. **Vaidya A, Aryal UR, Krettek A.** Cardiovascular health knowledge, attitude, and practice/behavior in an urbanizing community of Nepal: a population-based cross-sectional study from Jhaukhel-Duwakot Health Demographic Surveillance Site. *BMJ Open* 2013; **3**:e002976.
11. **Oli N, Vaidya A, Subedi M, Krettek A.** Experiences and perceptions about cause and prevention of cardiovascular disease among people with cardiometabolic conditions: findings of in-depth interviews from a peri-urban Nepalese community. *Global Health Action* 2014; 7:24023.
12. **Oli N, Vaidya A, Subedi M, Eiben G, Krettek A.** Diet and physical activity for children's health: a qualitative study of Nepalese mothers' perceptions. *BMJ Open* 2015; 5:e008197.
13. **Al Hourani HM, Naffa S, Fardous T.** National commitment to action on social determinants of health in Jordan: Addressing obesity. Presentation to World Conference on Social Determinants of Health. Available at: http://www.who.int/sdhconference/resources/draft_background_paper18_jordan.pdf
14. **Nsubuga P, White ME, Thacker SB,** et al. Public health surveillance: a tool for targeting and monitoring interventions. In: **Jamison DT, Breman JG, Measham AR,** et al. (eds.), *Disease Control Priorities in Developing Countries*, 2nd edn. Washington, DC: World Bank; 2006. Available from: http://www.ncbi.nlm.nih.gov/books/NBK11770/

15. **Al-Nsour M, Zindah M, Belbeisi A, Hadaddin R, Brown DW, Walke H.** Prevalence of selected chronic, noncommunicable disease risk factors in Jordan: results of the 2007 Jordan Behavioral Risk Factor Surveillance Survey. *Preventing Chronic Disease* 2012; **9**:E25.

16. **Ministry of Health.** *The National Strategy and Plan of Action against Diabetes, Hypertension Dyslipidemia, and Obesity in Jordan.* Amman: Ministry of Health; 2011. Available from: https://www.mindbank.info/item/4967

17. **Sturm R.** Increases in clinically severe obesity in the United States, 1986-2000. *Archives of Internal Medicine* 2003; **163**(18):2146–48.

18. **Sturm R, Hattori A.** Morbid obesity rates continue to rise rapidly in the US. *International Journal of Obesity* 2013; **37**(6):889–91.

19. **US Department of Health and Human Services.** Planning considerations for the extremely obese. Public Health Emergency. Available at: http://www.phe.gov/Preparedness/planning/abc/Pages/obesity.aspx

Further reading

Wilson JMG, Jungner G. Principles and practice of screening for disease. Geneva: World Health Organization, 1968 (Public Health Papers No. 34).

Alwan A, Maclean DR, Riley LM, et al. Monitoring and surveillance of chronic non-communicable diseases: progress and capacity in high-burden countries. *Lancet* 2010; **376**:1861–68.

For more on WHO's STEPwise approach to surveillance see: http://www.who.int/chp/steps/en/

Part III

Solution generation

Chapter 8

Evidence for population-level approaches to the prevention of NCDs: Evaluating effectiveness and modelling

8.1 Effectiveness

In order to convince policy-makers to take action on non-communicable diseases (NCDs), and to persuade the general public that such action is justified, evidence is needed. Generating evidence on behavioural interventions to prevent NCDs poses a distinct set of challenges, compared with, for example, evidence on efficacy of a particular drug or treatment.

There is a vital role for public health research in generating evidence to guide policy and to stimulate change. There are a number of issues to consider to ensure that research is able to fulfil this role.

A solid evidence base alone is usually not enough to make policy change happen. A favourable environment in terms of public opinion and political will is also required. For example, evidence supporting the case for a ban on smoking in public places has existed for decades but such measures were generally not deemed to be politically acceptable until many years later. An 'implementation gap' exists—many interventions for which there is good evidence of effectiveness have not been put into practice. Conversely, some measures with weaker evidence—such as peer support, social marketing, stages of change or behaviour change models, and nudge theory—have been enthusiastically adopted.[1,2,3] To help address this gap, researchers who create public health evidence should also play a role in changing public opinion. Teams publishing findings on NCDs and, especially, on the efficacy or effectiveness of interventions should also prioritize issuing a press release and a policy brief at time of publication.

It is important to address some of the widespread assumptions that exist about evidence in relation to public health interventions (Box 8.1). For example, it has been argued that there is confusion about how public health interventions *should* work. Thinking about what causes disease—dominated by the pathogenic and predictive model of communicable disease whereby, within broad limits, a person develops a disease *because* they have been exposed to a pathogen—has become confused with thinking about how interventions work. In reality, things are often not so straightforward; models of disease prevention are probabilistic, involving predictions of outcomes that are much less secure than in the pathogenic model of disease aetiology. In the case of interventions for NCDs,

Box 8.1 Applying evidence-based medicine to public health interventions

Since 2005, the National Institute for Health and Care Excellence (NICE) in the UK has been working on methods for applying the principles of evidence-based medicine to public health. The key questions to be answered for any public health problem or intervention are:

- Do we know whether intervention *x* for public health problem *y* is effective?
- How do we know it is effective?
- How do we know whether it is more or less effective than intervention *z*?
- On what basis do we make that judgement of effectiveness?
- Do we know what it costs? And is it cost effective? If it is not cost effective, why is it still being used?
- What are the dangers posed to the public of interventions and actions about which we are scientifically uncertain?
- Are the interventions dangerous? Why are we using potentially dangerous or worthless interventions?

It is also important to recognize the problem of equipoise, in which it is finely balanced as to whether the evidence suggests whether something will work. This is a common scenario in public health.

Box 8.2 Research to influence public health policy: top-down or bottom-up?

Researchers involved in generating evidence on how NCDs can be prevented have, as described in section 8.1, an important role in guiding policy-makers. There are many different forms this dialogue between evidence producers and policy-makers can take. In a top-down project, for example, policy-makers might themselves commission research to address specific questions. The advantage for researchers of this approach is that results are likely to be taken up very readily by policy-makers. On the other hand, the research team may lose some control over the research details, and involvement of a wider group of stakeholders is often required. Alternatively, in a bottom-up project researchers may design a project with the intention of engaging policy-makers. In these cases, researchers retain more control over project design but it can be harder to feed the findings into the policy process and get the message through to the right decision-maker. As a result, take-up by policy-makers can be challenging.

predictions often concern human and organizational behaviour and relate to conditions with complex causal webs, so there is much less certainty about outcomes.

In order to overcome these challenges a dialogue between evidence producers and policy-makers is necessary. Such dialogue—which may be part of a 'top-down' or 'bottom-up' process—is rare (Box 8.2). The concerns of evidence producers—such as academic concerns about the integrity of the science or the need for more research to answer further scientific questions—are often different to those of policy-makers, who need brief explanations of complex ideas to address immediate policy needs. Story-based policy (as opposed to evidence-based) is very common and it is advisable for evidence producers to include stories and case examples, alongside research evidence, when talking to policy-makers, journalists, and the broader public.

Case study: Knowledge to action—fiscal policy in Europe

One area where the evidence is strong, but action lags far behind is fiscal policy—in other words, taxation on tobacco, alcohol, and unhealthy foods and/or subsidies on healthy foods. The evidence is so strong that the World Health Organization (WHO) classifies tobacco tax increases and increasing alcohol excise taxes as 'best buys' (WHO

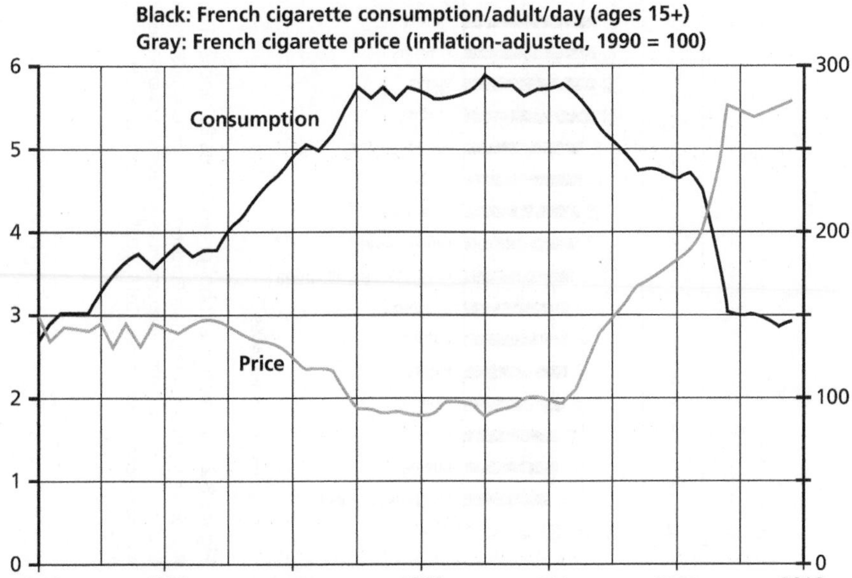

Figure 8.1 Tobacco control in France.

Reproduced by kind permission of Professor Catherine Hill, Copyright © 2016 Catherine Hill.

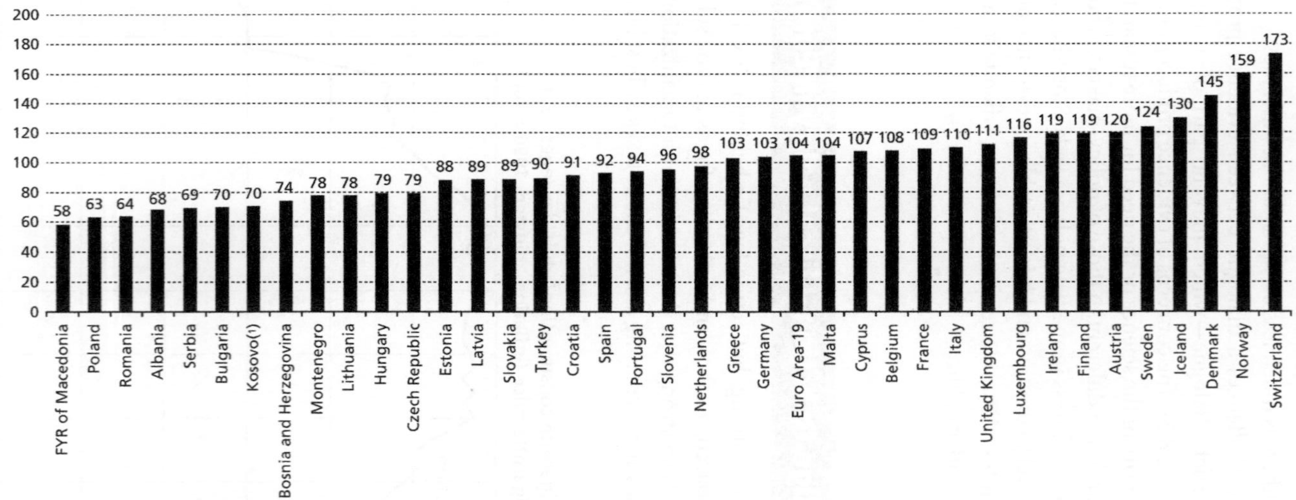

(1) Kosovo under UNSCR 1244/99

Figure 8.2 Variation in alcohol prices across Europe 2013.

Reproduced with permission from **Eurostat**. 'File:Price level index for food and non-alcoholic beverages, 2015, EU28 = 100 V2.png', http://ec.europa.eu/eurostat/statistics-explained/index.php/File:Price_level_index_for_food_and_non-alcoholic_beverages,_2015,_EU28%3D100_V2.png#filelinks, accessed 18 Aug. 2016, Copyright © 2016 European Union.

defines a best buy as an intervention that is not only highly cost-effective but also cheap, feasible, and culturally acceptable to implement).

Figure 8.1 illustrates this clearly, showing the effect of tobacco tax increases in France between 1990 and 2005. Over this period the cigarette price (adjusted for inflation) in France *tripled*, while consumption *halved* and government income (also adjusted for inflation, not shown) *doubled*.

Despite this strength of evidence, however, implementation lags behind. Figure 8.2 illustrates, for example, the challenges in implementing alcohol and tobacco taxes evenly across Europe. These variations in prices lead to problems with illicit marketing and cross-border sales, rendering tax increases less effective.

As with action on tobacco and alcohol, implementation of food taxes/subsidies lags behind the evidence. In the past few years, specific taxes have been introduced in, among others, Finland, Denmark, France, Hungary, and Mexico. Implementation is often in the face of fierce opposition from the food industry, despite growing evidence on the impact of these measures. The Danish tax on foods high in saturated fats, for example, appears to have led to about a 6% reduction in saturated fat consumption, but was repealed after only a year in force because industry mounted a national campaign to repeal the tax (see case studies in Chapter 4 and Chapter 14).

In addition to generating evidence for policy, in order to overcome the implementation gap—particularly for policies that threaten vested interests—policy-makers, researchers, and health advocates need to work together to change opinion, including influencing those responsible for approving new laws and policy initiatives (e.g. parliamentarians).

Case study: Restricting alcohol marketing in Lithuania—health advocates taking on vested interests

Recent experience with efforts to reduce harmful alcohol consumption in Lithuania illustrates how powerful vested interests can successfully undermine the best of policy intentions and also highlights the important role of non-governmental organizations (NGOs) and health advocates in fighting back.

In 2007–8, faced with one of the highest alcohol intakes in Europe (15.4 L of pure alcohol per capita per annum, compared to the 10.9 L average for the WHO European region) and a growing burden of alcohol-related harm, the Lithuanian parliament introduced a series of alcohol control measures. These included higher excise taxes, stricter penalties for drunk driving, a ban on the sales of alcoholic drinks between 10 p.m. and 8 a.m. (except in bars and restaurants), and time restrictions on advertising for alcoholic drinks on radio and television. At the same time, a total ban on advertising for alcoholic drinks—identified by WHO as one of the most cost-effective policy options available—was approved and would come into force in January 2012.

The alcohol industry campaigned vigorously against the pending advertising ban. Lobbying efforts by the drinks industry—combined with other vested interest groups—were successful in December 2011. The parliament voted to revoke the advertising ban and, rather than using her veto, the president of the republic signed the law onto the statute.

Figure 8.3 illustrates the incidence of one proxy measure of alcohol-related harm, alcohol-induced psychosis, against the evolution of different alcohol control policy measures over the past 25 years.

Paukšte and colleagues documented the campaign to overturn the advertising ban and many of the tactics reportedly employed were straight out of the tobacco industry playbook.[4] The anti-ban group included, amongst others, drinks industry bodies, commercial media, advertising and trade bodies, and sports bodies. The tactics reported include, for example:

Forming alliances with other vested interest groups—such as communication agencies, traders, media and advertising industry bodies and sporting bodies (spreading the message, for example, that basketball fixtures would no longer be broadcast if alcohol advertising were banned);

Lobbying of politicians—including sending joint letters to the speaker and, later,

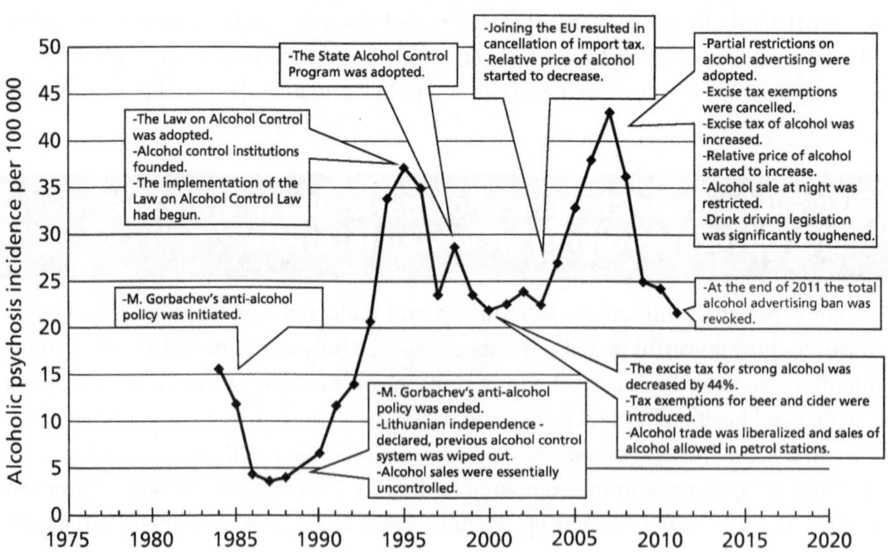

Figure 8.3 Incidence of alcoholic psychosis and alcohol control policy measures in Lithuania (1984–2011).

Reproduced with permission from **Paukštė E, Liutkutė V, Stelemėkas M, Goštautaitė Midttun N**, and **Veryga A**. Overturn of the proposed alcohol advertising ban in Lithuania. *Addiction*, Volume 109, Issue 5, pp. 711–9, Copyright © 2014 John Wiley and Sons.

detailed voting instructions to parliamentarians. Meetings between ministers and senior industry figures were also reported;

Financial incentives/gifts—four political parties received funding from an investment group with relevant interests; politicians were given free tickets to sporting events.

The anti-ban group benefited from positive publicity, while the NGOs and health groups advocating for the ban to be implemented were often portrayed, according to Paukšte and colleagues, as 'a handful or of radicals'. It appears, however, that the advocacy of these radicals did hinder the lobbying process of the vested interests. In June 2011, NGO Vilniaus Sajudis published an online photographic gallery with pictures of the MPs who voted to revoke the advertising ban. A group of NGOs met with representatives of the media industries and explored options that could compensate media organizations for the loss of sponsorship and allow them to get behind the ban (e.g. support for a tax exemption, different sources of sponsorship). Fifty NGOs sent an open letter to the president, prime minister, MPs, speaker of the parliament, and the Lithuanian people asking them to support the ban and challenging the industry arguments. The national tobacco and alcohol control coalition requested an official investigation of the potential conflicts of interest of ten MPs who supported overturning the ban. In 2012, a criminal investigation was opened into an allegedly corrupt relationship between one of the alcohol industry lobbyists and one of the parliamentarians behind the efforts to overturn the advertising ban. In December 2011, 256 NGOs signed a joint letter asking the president to veto the amendments overturning the ban.

Although their actions proved to be too little too late in this case, it is clear that health advocates did nonetheless manage to create obstacles and make the task of industry groups much more difficult. It is also evident that the voluntary sector has learned greatly from this experience, recognizing that a failure to monitor the process systematically *from the very beginning* had lead to damaging delays. Although there were grounds to challenge the legality of the processes involved to overturn the ban, for example, these findings emerged too late to influence the outcome. Nonetheless, those advocating for the ban did succeed in drawing public attention to the issue, increasing the pressure on decision-makers and laying the foundations for more public support for alcohol control measures proposed in the future.

Efforts to reduce alcohol consumption are continuing in the country—a specific goal to reduce per capita annual consumption down to the level of the European average was adopted in 2014 as part of the National Health Program. Yet there still appears to be ambivalence of politicians in power towards effective alcohol control measures in Lithuania, as evidenced by the newest attempt at the end of 2015 to overturn the ban on alcohol sale in petrol stations. Learning from previous experience of 2011, this latest attempt was anticipated by public health advocates. The process was counteracted with more effective resistance, focusing on early monitoring of the legal process and instant publication of events by creating a publicly available event chronology. That document mapped parliamentary processes, as well as the persons involved, and was followed attentively by the media. Success was a result of vigorous, time-consuming efforts by the public health lobby, combined with growing public support in response to some tragic and very public alcohol-related deaths. This restriction on alcohol availability has now been in force since January 2016 and has helped to eliminate nearly 600 points of alcohol sale.

It is worth noting that a total ban on advertising alcohol in Lithuania would have created an important precedent in Europe, with potential consequences for industry groups beyond the Lithuanian borders. Paukšte and colleagues—including some of those involved in advocating for maintenance of the advertising ban—conclude that, given the global nature of the alcoholic drinks industry, international regulation limiting the influence of vested interests on national law-making could be useful for protection of public health.

Source: data from **Paukštė E**, **Liutkutė V**, **Stelemėkas M**, **Goštautaitė Midttun N**, and **Veryga A**. Overturn of the proposed alcohol advertising ban in Lithuania. *Addiction*, Volume 109, Issue 5, pp. 711–9, Copyright © 2014 Society for the Study of Addiction.

8.2 **Modelling**

Modelling methods can play a role in improving public health decision-making. Modelling has been defined as 'a logical mathematical framework that permits the integration of facts and values to produce outcomes of interest to decision-makers and clinicians'.[5] In other words, in a simplified version of reality, researchers take an initial data set and apply a logical operation (sometimes mathematical) to that data to produce some findings. A model has to be built on a series of assumptions.

Modelling can be used, for example, to estimate the burden of disease associated with a particular risk factor, or to project how the disease patterns might change if policy measures are introduced to modify exposure to the risk factor.

Box 8.3 and Box 8.4 describe two examples of modelling with relevance to NCDs, including the extremely important global initiative to estimate the worldwide burden of disease and disability.

Modelling offers potential for public health decision-making when existing evidence is inadequate or incomplete and traditional research methods are unable to provide the solutions. In the case of complex, multifactorial conditions—such as the major NCDs under consideration in this book—it can be used to help explain trends and to explore future prevention policy options. Modelling can also show policy-makers where to invest to get the biggest gains, and illustrate how small reductions in risk factors could have big impacts on a population basis.

In addition to highlighting the significant potential of modelling, it is important to understand some of the limitations of these methods. Inevitably, modelling is based on a series of assumptions. Furthermore, faced with gaps in good quality data researchers are

Box 8.3 Estimating disease burden: understanding the Global Burden of Disease estimates

An extremely important piece of modelling work on global population health is the Global Burden of Diseases, Injuries and Risk Factors (GBD) project.[6] The GBD study uses the concept to disability-adjusted life years (DALYs) to show which conditions cause the greatest burden of death and health loss, by modelling partial, often incomplete data on disease progression (incidence, prevalence, duration, case fatality, and mortality) in different populations to estimate population attributable risks (PARs) for different disease–risk factor combinations. These PARs can be used to estimate the proportion of total disease burden in a specific population that is due to individual risk factors.

Definitions from the Global Burden of Disease studies[6]

Disability-adjusted life years

Disability-adjusted life years measure the state of a population's health. They are the sum of two components: years of life lost due to premature mortality and years lived with disability.

Years of life lost

Years of life lost (YLLs) are calculated by multiplying the number of deaths at each age x by a standard life expectancy at age x.

Years of life lived with disability

Years of life lived with disability (YLDs) are computed as the prevalence of different disease sequelae and injury sequelae multiplied by the disability weight for that sequela. Disability weights are selected on the basis of surveys of the general population about the loss of health associated with the health state related to the disease sequela. The GBD has identified 1150 sequelae of 291 diseases and injuries.

The GBD initiative is, and will continue to be, highly influential in debate and decision-making on global health priorities. Many countries have followed suit and used the GBD or similar methodology to produce national burden of disease studies. The authors of the 2010 GBD study concluded that 'quantifying health loss in terms of DALYs has led to increased attention to mental health problems and injuries, non-fatal health effects of neglected tropical diseases, and more generally non-communicable diseases'.[6]

It is useful to understand the GBD methods and their limitations. Broadly speaking, four sets of data are needed:

- Current burden of diseases in population;
- Relationships between diseases and risk factors;

- Current prevalence of risk factors in population; and
- Theoretical minimum risk distributions.

Figure 8.4 illustrates a highly simplified example of how to calculate one aspect of the burden of disease attributable to alcohol in the United Kingdom. For simplicity, the number of deaths attributed to alcohol are considered, but the same principles could be applied to DALYs or other health indices. A detailed exploration of the United Kingdom burden of disease, from the 2010 GBD study, was published by Murray and colleagues in the *Lancet* in 2013.[7]

This worked example is based on some simplifying assumptions. The relationship between alcohol and health is assumed to the same for everyone. Only three conditions are taken into consideration and possible short-term effects of alcohol, such as binge drinking and injuries, are ignored.

Figure 8.4a shows the current burden, in terms of number of deaths caused by liver cirrhosis, cancer, and cardiovascular disease (CVD).

Figure 8.4b plots the relationship between the diseases and the risk factor—the relative risk of each of these three conditions by amount of alcohol consumed. The risk of liver cirrhosis and cancer goes up with alcohol consumption, while small amounts of alcohol consumption lead to a reduced risk of CVD.

Figure 8.4c translates this information into mortality rates for the three conditions (see the J-shaped curve for CVD). The next important piece of the jigsaw is data on the current prevalence of the risk factor in the population.

Figure 8.4d shows the distribution of alcohol consumption.

Figure 8.4e illustrates how many people are dying at each level of alcohol consumption.

The next step is to agree the theoretical minimum risk distribution—in this example, this is assumed to be 100% non-drinkers (Figure 8.4f).

Figure 8.4g applies that new minimum risk distribution to the mortality curves, enabling calculation of the projected number of deaths if no one in the population was to drink alcohol.

In the final figure (Figure 8.4h) the red bars show the number of deaths if the population entirely abstained from alcohol. Because of the J-shaped relationship curve for alcohol and CVD, there would be a slight increase in CVD deaths to offset against the drop in cancer and cirrhosis deaths. In order to work out the total burden of disease attributed to alcohol, therefore, it is necessary to add the cirrhosis and cancer deaths that could be avoided if alcohol consumption were eliminated, and to subtract from this total the extra deaths due to CVD which would occur (a + b – c).

The number of deaths due to alcohol consumption is one way of expressing the burden of disease attributable to alcohol in the UK. To arrive at a more comprehensive estimate, it would be necessary to calculate the years of life lost to premature death, which would then need to be combined with calculations of the years of life lived with ill-health or disability caused by alcohol.

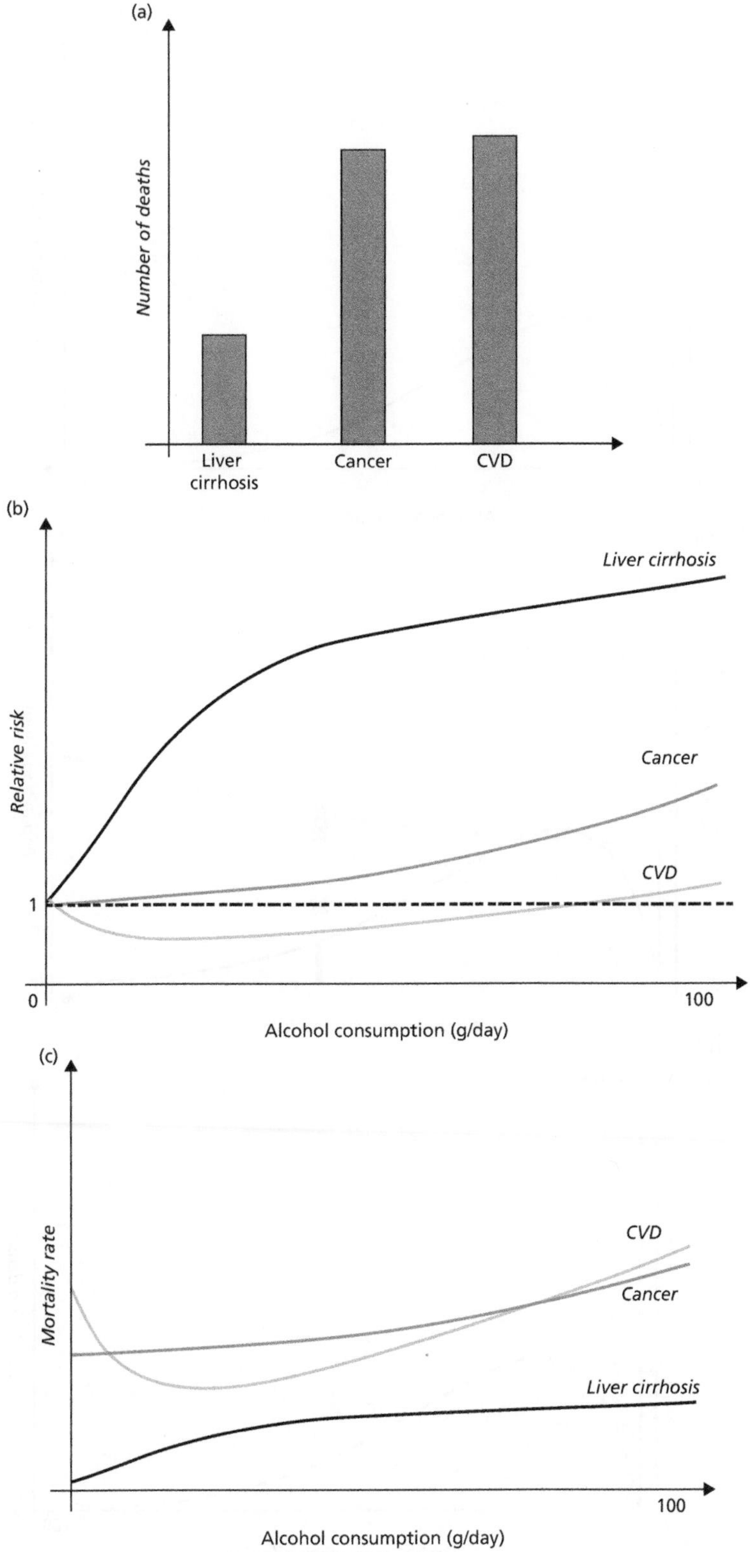

Figure 8.4 Simplified example of global burden of disease workings: alcohol consumption in the UK.

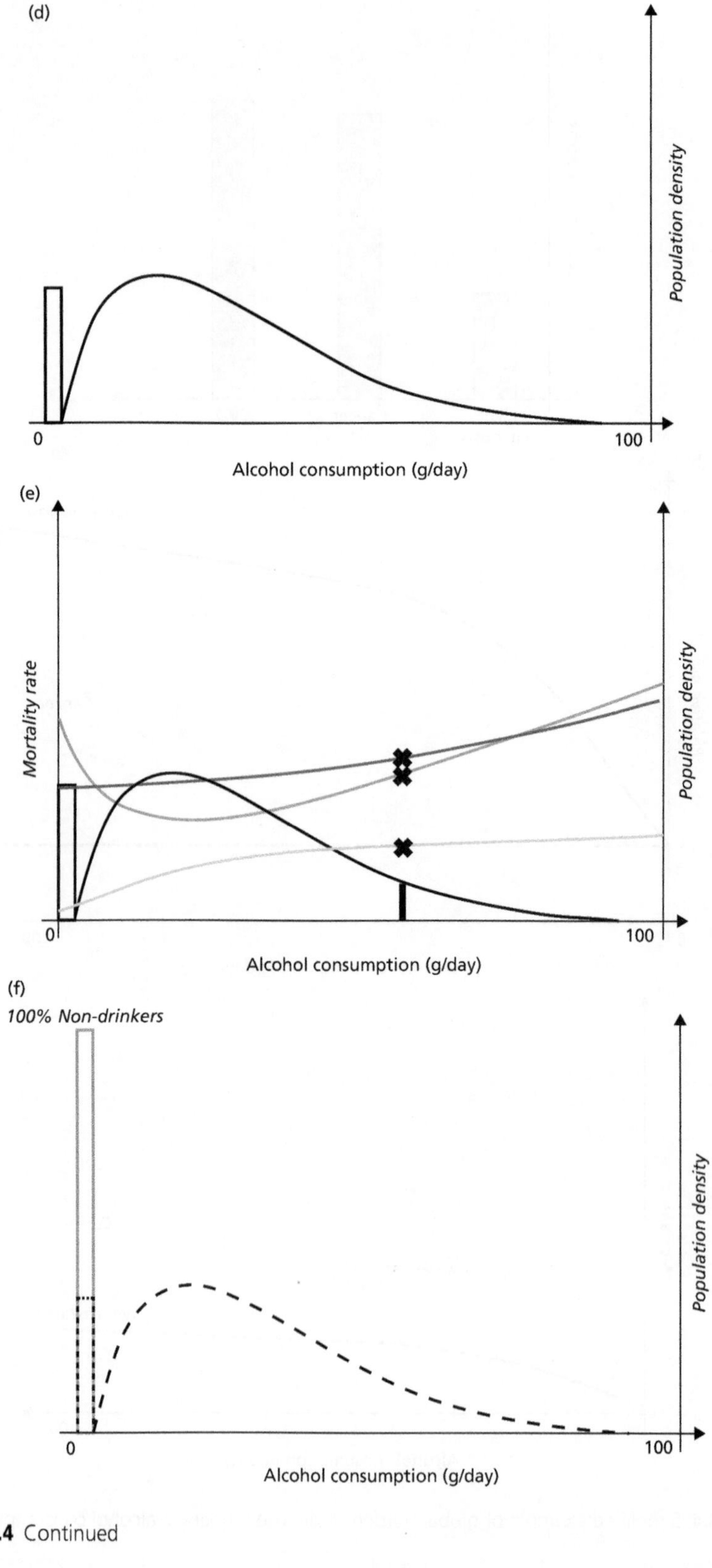

(d)
Population density
0
100
Alcohol consumption (g/day)
(e)
Mortality rate
Population density
0
100
Alcohol consumption (g/day)
(f)
100% Non-drinkers
Population density
0
100
Alcohol consumption (g/day)

Figure 8.4 Continued

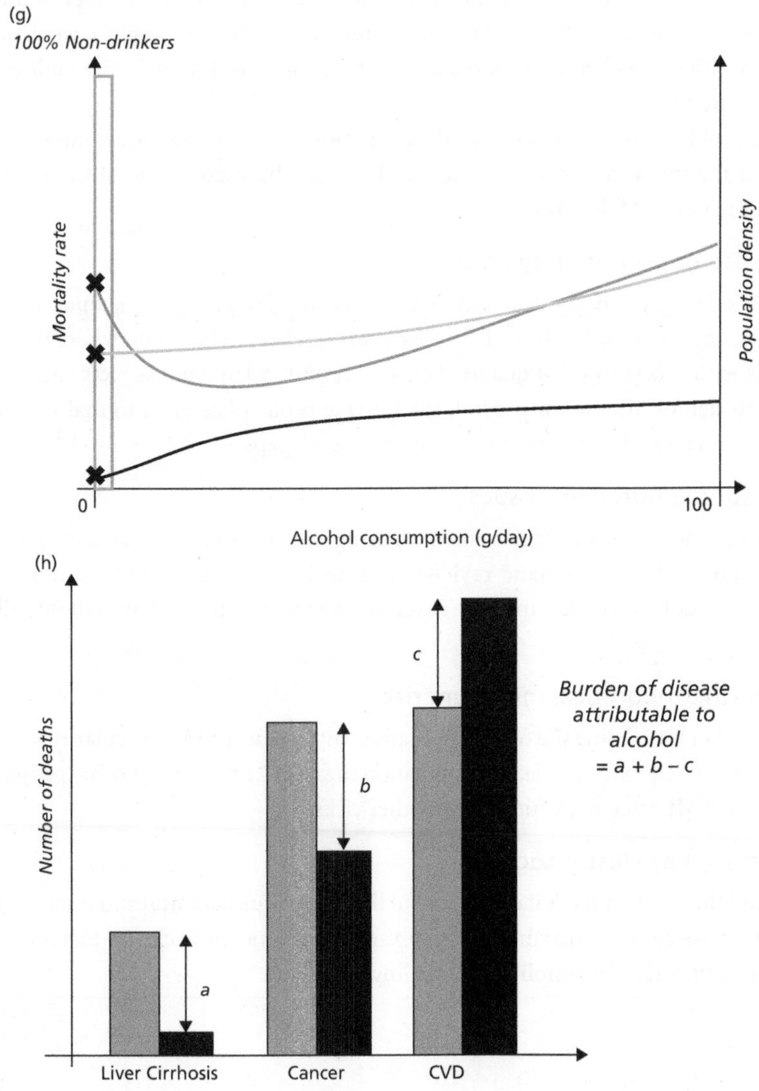

Figure 8.4 Continued

The GBD method has evolved since the initial work for the 1990 study. The respective strengths and weaknesses of the methodology have been discussed in the literature. In 2003, Christopher Murray and colleagues discussed many of the conceptual and methodological issues in their comparative risk assessment module of the GBD study in a paper in *Population Health Metrics*.[8] There has been debate about which risk factors for health burdens should be included. Some have argued that the high standard of evidence for causality (longitudinal and intervention studies) might have resulted in some health effects being overlooked and, thus, some health outcomes and/or risk factors omitted.[9]

It is helpful to understand some of the limitations of the GBD modelling methodology and the implications for how the findings can be used. Some of the issues to consider include the following.

Incomplete or poor quality data

There are often gaps in good quality data, especially for particular subpopulations. One of the key issues facing the GBD researchers has been what to do where there are problems with access to good quality data—even on fundamental aspects such as the current burden of disease. In general, the GBD approach has been to make the best possible estimate and extrapolate rather than to leave gaps.

Risk factor measurement issues

There are numerous challenges with measuring risk factors, such as diet, physical activity, and alcohol. Systematic reviews were widely used to compile estimates of exposure to risk factors, and, in some cases, observational studies have fed into those reviews.

Defining the theoretical minimum risk

It can be difficult to define the optimal situation with respect to a particular risk factor. In the case of BMI, for example, the population mean of 21 may mean some people fall into the low BMI category, which brings other risks.

Risk factors may cluster together

NCDs, and the risk factors that contribute to them, are multifactorial and inter-related. Risk factors like alcohol and smoking, for example, are known to cluster together. This can create difficulties for simplified modelling scenarios.

Box 8.4 Using the IMPACT model to understand disease trends

There is increasing interest in the use of modelling to help understand disease trends. One such example is the IMPACT epidemiological model which has been used to explain what has caused changes in coronary heart disease (CHD) death rates in several different countries including the UK, USA, Tunisia, and China.[10,11,12,13] These studies explored what proportion of the change in CHD deaths can be attributed to changes in different risk factors and also what proportion is due to advances in treatment or prevention.

The model incorporates evidence from meta-analyses (including meta-analyses of cohort studies) for all the major CHD risk factors and also evidence from meta-analyses of the effectiveness of available treatments to calculate the causes of the deaths postponed or prevented. (See References for full description of the model.)

Findings of the IMPACT model studies suggest that 25–50% of the fall in CHD mortality in countries like the UK and USA is due to improvements in treatment, while between 50 and 75% can be attributed to changes in risk factors.[11] Figure 8.5 illustrates, by way of example, the findings from the study on the fall in CHD mortality in the USA between 1980 and 2000.

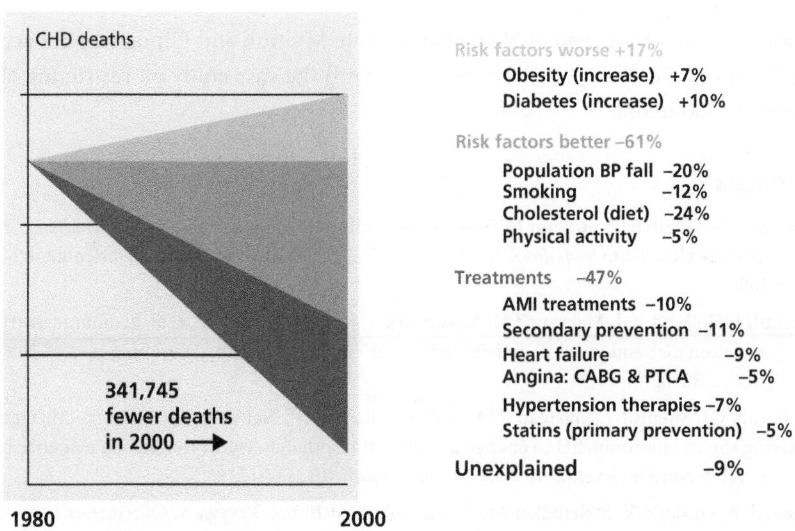

Figure 8.5 IMPACT study explanation of fall in CHD deaths in the US, 1980–2000.

Reproduced from **Capewell S**. *Studying mortality trends: The IMPACT CHD policy model*, 14th January 2008, https://www.actuaries.org.uk/documents/studying-mortality-trends-impact-chd-policy-model, accessed 10 Aug. 2016, by kind permission of Professor Simon Capewell.

Source: data from **Ford ES**, **Ajani UA**, **Croft JB**, **Critchley JA**, **Labarthe DR**, **Kottke TE**, **Giles WH**, and **Capewell S**. Explaining the decrease in US deaths from coronary disease, 1980-2000. *New England Journal of Medicine*, Volume 356, pp. 2388–98, Copyright © 2007 Massachusetts Medical Society.

The IMPACT model can be extended to a number of other uses:

- Replication in other populations (including in different socioeconomic groups);
- Estimating the impact of increasing treatment or reducing risk factors still further in a population;
- Calculating life-years to be gained by particular policies or interventions; and
- Calculations on cost effectiveness of interventions.

It is important to understand the limitations of the model. For one thing, the model assumes that efficacy in a randomized controlled trial (RCT) is equivalent to effectiveness. Another limitation is that data remain patchy—a factor which must be borne in mind when considering its potential application in LMICs.

often required to make judgement calls about how best to proceed. The precise limitations will, of course, vary from one model to another.

Acknowledgements

This chapter is drawn from presentations by Professor Mike Kelly, Dr Peter Scarborough, Colin Mitchell, Professor Richard Peto, Dr Gauden Galea, Dr Oliver Mytton, and Professor Simon Capewell.

We are grateful for the help of Nijole Gostautaite Midttun and Lithuanian Tobacco and Alcohol Control Coalition for their assistance with the case study on restricting alcohol marketing in Lithuania.

References

1. **Marteau TM, Ogilvie D, Roland M, Suhrcke M, Kelly MP.** Judging nudging: can 'nudging' improve population health? *British Medical Journal* 2011; **342:** d228. http://www.bmj.com/content/342/bmj.d228.full
2. **Shemilt I, Hollands GJ, Marteau TM, Nakamura R, Jebb SA, Kelly MP,** et al. Economic instruments for population diet and physical activity behaviour change: a systematic scoping review. *PLOS One* 2013; **8**(9):e75070.
3. **Hollands GJ, Shemilt I, Marteau TM, Jebb SA, Kelly MP, Nakamura R, Suhrcke M, Ogilvie D.** Altering micro-environments to change population health behaviour: towards an evidence base for choice architecture interventions. *BMC Public Health* 2013; **13**:1218.
4. **Paukštė E, Liutkutė V, Stelemėkas M, Goštautaitė Midttun N, Veryga A.** Overturn of the proposed alcohol advertising ban in Lithuania. *Addiction* 2014; **109**(5):711–19.
5. **Weinstein MC, O'Brien B, Hornberger J, Jackson J, Johannesson M, McCabe C,** et al. Principles of good practice for decision analytic modeling in health-care evaluation: report of the ISPOR Task Force on Good Research Practices—Modeling Studies. *Value Health* 2003; **6**(1):9–17.
6. **Murray CJ, Vos T, Lozano R, Maghavi M, Flaxman AD, Michaud C,** et al. Disability-adjusted life years (DALYs) for 291 diseases and injuries in 21 regions, 1990-2010: a systematic analysis for the Global Burden of Disease Study 2010. *Lancet* 2012; **380**:2197–23.

7. **Murray CJL, Richards MA, Newton JN, Fenton KA, Anderson HR, Atkinson C**, et al. UK health performance: findings of the Global Burden of Disease Study 2010. *Lancet* 2013; **381**:997–1020.

8. **Murray CJ, Ezzati M, Lopez AD, Rodgers A, Vander Hoorn S.** Comparative quantification of health risks: Conceptual framework and methodological issues. *Popular Health Metrics* 2003; **1**:1.

9. **Watts C, Cairncross S.** Should the GBD risk factor rankings be used to guide policy? *Lancet* 2012; **380**:2060–1.

10. **Saidi O, Ben Mansour N, O'Flaherty M, Capewell S, Critchley JA**, et al. Analyzing recent coronary heart disease mortality trends in Tunisia between 1997 and 2009. *PLoS ONE* 2013; **8**(5):e63202.

11. **Ford ES, Ajani UA, Croft JB, Critchley JA, Labarthe DR**, et al. Explaining the decrease in US deaths from coronary disease, 1980-2000. *New England Journal of Medicine* 2007; **356**:2388–98.

12. **Bajekal M, Scholes S, Love H, Hawkins N, O'Flaherty M**, et al. Analysing recent socioeconomic trends in coronary heart disease mortality in England, 2000-2007: A population modeling study. *PLoS Medicine* 2012; **9**(6):e1001237.

13. **Cheng J, Zhao D, Zeng Z, Critchley JA, Liu J, Wang W**, et al. The impact of demographic and risk factor changes on coronary heart disease deaths in Beijing, 1999-2010. *BMC Public Health* 2009; **9**:30.

Chapter 9

Evidence for population-level approaches to the prevention of NCDs: Economic evaluation

9.1 Introduction

Against a backdrop of scarce resources and costs that are continually increasing—driven by ageing populations, developments of new and expensive medical technology, and increasing consumer awareness—health economics and economic appraisal of health programmes play an important role in providing evidence on value for money. Governments and other funders are increasingly demanding evidence for safety, efficacy, and cost-effectiveness.

It is clear that no health-care system can afford to fund *all* the health services that could, in theory, be provided. Priority setting is essential, therefore, for good stewardship in health system management and for making the most efficient use of scarce resources. Policy-makers should seek to get the 'biggest bang for the health-care buck'. This is true for population-based prevention approaches, just as it is for treatment and health service provision.

This is where health economics can be useful. Health economics applies economic theories—on the supply and demand for scarce resources—to the supply of and demand for health.

9.2 Health economics

According to health economics, a market for health care is created from a demand for health. The market facilitates the buying and selling of health care, and in a 'perfectly competitive' market, efficient allocation of resources will occur. Health and health care, however, are not ordinary economic commodities that can be exchanged in a market. There are many instances where the allocation of health care related goods and services is not efficient. These instances, sometimes described as 'market failures', are caused by a number of factors:

- Consumption of health care does not necessarily lead to production of health or improved well-being for the individual;
- Uncertainties (e.g. in the efficacy of treatments) lead to irrational decisions;

- Notion of risk also leads to health insurance, which can create perverse incentives to over-consume health (e.g. there is no financial benefit from taking measures to reduce demand);
- The buyer (patient) and seller (doctor) do not have equal access to information on the patient's health and their health care options ('informational asymmetries'); this leads to a potentially conflicting role for the doctor as the patient's advisor and supplier of the health care ('supplier-induced demand'); and
- There are barriers to market entry, brought about by the need for licensing of doctors and restrictions on the number of training places in medical schools and hospitals. This is usually done in the interests of maintaining quality, but it acts to restrict supply and therefore increase the costs of healthcare.

When market failures occur, non-market institutions (e.g. government) can step in to encourage efficient allocation of resources. Economic evaluation can help in this process.

9.3 **Economic evaluation**

Economic evaluation is 'the comparative analysis of alternative courses of action in terms of both their costs and consequences'.[1]

In order to complete an economic evaluation, information is required on costs. This could comprise direct costs for diagnosis, treatment, rehabilitation, and prevention costs. Direct costs include, for example, GP, hospital, and pharmaceutical costs. It could also cover indirect costs—including lost production due to less days worked or less productivity per hour—and intangible costs—for example, a monetary value attributed to the pain, grief, and suffering of the patient and family.

Any decision on which of these costs are relevant depends on the perspective—that is, whether the aim is to assess the costs to the health-care sector, to patients, or to society at large. The costs of key interest are the opportunity costs. In other words, it is what society *gives up* in order to pay for a particular health intervention.

The scarcity of health resources forces choices to be made and choices imply a sacrifice or foregone opportunity. Opportunity cost is the value of the best alternative that is foregone. It reflects the fact it is not possible to do everything or that finances over time are limited. Spending health resources on one service, such as, for example, dialysis for renal disease, means that those resources cannot be spent for another purpose, such as childhood vaccination.

Economic evaluation also requires information on the consequences, or effects, of interventions. Examples include:

- Change in body mass index;
- Change in life years (LY) lived; and
- Change in disability-adjusted life years (DALYs) or quality-adjusted life years (QALYs).

The key criteria for a full economic evaluation are:

- Comparison of at least two alternatives; and
- Examination of both costs and consequences of the alternatives.

Table 9.1 Types of economic evaluation

Type of economic analysis	Measure of costs	Measure of consequences	Example result
Cost-effectiveness analysis	Monetary units	Natural units	Cost per LY saved Cost per kg lost
Cost–utility analysis	Monetary units	Utility measure	Cost per DALY averted Cost per QALY gained
Cost–benefit analysis	Monetary units	Monetary units	Net $ (net present value)

Evaluations that examine only consequences are efficacy or effectiveness evaluations. Those that only examine costs are cost analyses. Those which examine the costs and consequences, but only of one alternative, are cost–outcome descriptions.

The types of economic evaluation include cost-effectiveness analysis, cost–utility analysis, and cost–benefit analysis (see Table 9.1).

9.3.1 Cost–benefit analysis

Cost–benefit analysis aims to determine whether the social and private benefits of a health project exceed its costs. Since cost–benefit analysis assigns monetary values to health outcomes it is useful for comparing health with other programmes (e.g. education) and for assessing whether a health programme pays for itself. The challenge, however, is to assign money values to life, health, and other outcomes of health projects.

9.3.2 Cost-effectiveness analysis

For cost-effectiveness analyses, outcomes are measured in units relevant to the intervention. For cancer screening interventions, for example, the outcome could be the number of cases detected. This approach is useful for the decision-maker who is working within a given budget and/or is considering options within a certain field (e.g. cancer prevention).

Cost-effectiveness analysis is not, however, useful for comparison of different types of interventions (e.g. weight reduction and cancer screening).

9.3.3 Cost–utility analysis

In cost–utility analyses the outcomes are measured in units that are relevant across many health interventions. These can include QALYs, DALYs, and similar measures, which combine impact on quantity and quality into a single measure, by including a measure of change in mortality and a change in morbidity or quality of life. Cost–utility analysis is useful for decisions on how best to allocate an existing budget ('priority setting'). There are different opinions, however, on how best to measure quality of life (e.g. ability to see, read, walk; feelings of anxiety, pain, discomfort, etc.) or how to weigh disability.

9.3.4 What type of economic evaluation should you choose?

Many economists favour cost–benefit analysis because it can establish net benefit (i.e. worth) of a programme, and options can be ranked and a budget allocated accordingly. Governments and other funders, however, are increasingly demanding cost-effectiveness analyses or cost–utility analyses. The National Institute for Health and Clinical Excellence (NICE) in the UK, the Pharmaceutical Benefits Advisory Committee (PBAC) in Australia and the Pharmaceutical Management Agency (PHARMAC) in New Zealand, all require estimates of clinical effectiveness and cost-effectiveness in making decisions about funding pharmaceuticals.

9.4 Cost-effectiveness analysis

Two approaches to cost-effectiveness analysis can be distinguished—one based on *observed* data, usually as part of a clinical trial, and one involving *modelling* of costs and expected benefits based on best available evidence (e.g. a clinical trial or meta-analysis of outcomes from many trials). Cost-effective analysis of observed data is usually easier, but it will only capture events over the length of the trial, while benefits (and costs) may continue over the lifetime, and it will only determine cost-effectiveness under trial conditions, rather than in the real world.

9.4.1 Calculating cost-effectiveness

In a situation when A is the intervention being evaluated and B is the comparator, an equation can be applied to calculate the cost-effectiveness ratio (CER):

$$\text{CER} = \frac{\Delta\text{Costs}}{\Delta\text{Effects}} = \frac{\text{Cost}_A - \text{Cost}_B}{\text{Effects}_A - \text{Effects}_B}$$

For example, compared to usual care (**B**), the cost-effectiveness of giving dietary advice to reduce salt intake to everyone with a systolic blood pressure > 140 mmHg (**A**) is $160,000/DALY.

Interventions can be plotted according to their effectiveness and their cost, with those which are more effective and less costly preferable (Figure 9.1).

9.4.2 When is an intervention 'cost-effective'?

Having calculated the cost-effectiveness ratio ($ per DALY), this can feed into decisions about whether an intervention is 'cost-effective'. To be able to make such a decision, thresholds need to be set—such that everything below a particular threshold can be classified as 'cost-effective' or 'highly cost-effective'.

The Commission on Macroeconomics in Health, for example, suggests the following thresholds:

- Highly cost-effective is < 1 × GDP per capita per DALY averted;
- Cost-effective is < 3 × GDP per capita per DALY averted; and
- Cost-ineffective is > 3 × GDP per capita per DALY averted.

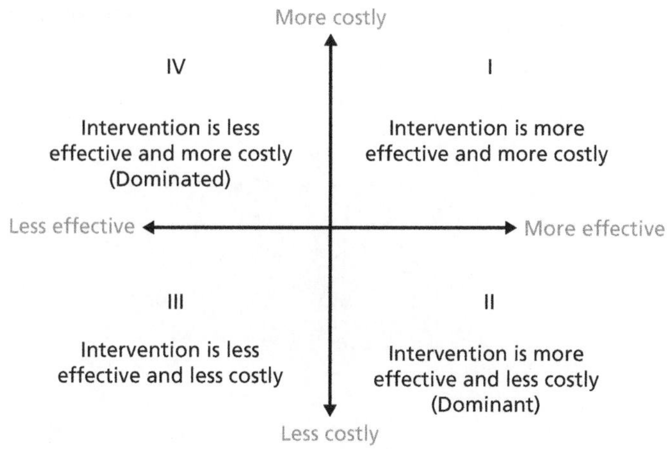

Figure 9.1 Plotting cost-effectiveness.

Adapted from **Black WC**, The cost-effectiveness plane: a graphic representation of cost-effectiveness, *Medical Decision Making*, Volume 10, Number 3, pp. 212–15, Copyright © 1990 by Society for Medical Decision Making. Reprinted by permission of SAGE publications.

In relation to assessing the public funding of drugs, for example, authorities may use thresholds to appraise drugs. Authorities are usually reluctant to state threshold levels. Cost-effectiveness is not the only factor to be taken into account, and where thresholds are given they are accompanied by a number of qualifying statements. NICE in England, however, has stated that when the cost per QALY gained is above £20,000 (around US$26,000) per QALY, judgements will have to be taken about the acceptability of the technology as an effective use of National Health Service resources, taking into account a number of factors. If every QALY gained cost is estimated to cost more than £30,000 (around US$40,000), then NICE's Committee 'will need to identify **an increasingly stronger case** for supporting the technology as an effective use of NHS resources', taking into account a number of other specified factors.[2] It has been reported that the threshold above which drugs were regarded as not providing good value for money by the Australian Pharmaceutical Benefit System between 1991 and 1996 was around 76,000 Australian dollars (US$56,000) per life year gained and 42,000 Australian dollars (US$31,000) per QALY gained.[3]

An example of how cost-effectiveness could be plotted and used to determine whether an intervention is below or above the threshold is shown in Figure 9.2.

9.4.3 Assessing health system performance

Cost-effectiveness analysis can also be used to assess health system performance. It can help to determine how much is currently being spent on interventions and to identify the associated health outcome(s), then to compare this against the ideal package of

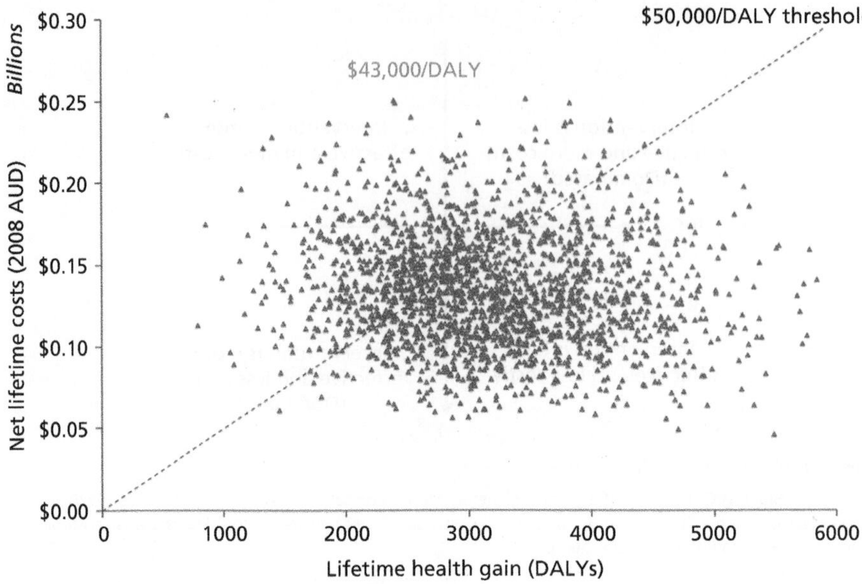

Figure 9.2 Example of cost-effectiveness threshold use.

Reproduced with permission from **Cobiac LJ** and **Vos T**. Cost-effectiveness of extending the coverage of water supply fluoridation for the prevention of dental caries in Australia. *Community Dentistry and Oral Epidemiology*. Volume 40, Issue 4, pp. 369–76, Copyright © 2012 John Wiley and Sons.

interventions ('expansion pathway'). In this way, it is possible to have a measure of efficiency of a current health system (Box 9.1).

Cost-effectiveness analysis can be used for large-scale priority setting, in other words to help determine priorities for allocating health care resources at a global or national scale.

The WHO-CHOICE (CHOosing Interventions that are Cost-Effective) initiative provided national policy-makers with information on cost-effectiveness, costs, and strategic planning. It also reported the costs and effects of a wide range of health interventions in the 14 WHO subregions using standardized methods that can be applied to all interventions in different settings. Results are grouped into a database and costs and effectiveness of a wide range of interventions at the subregion level are available for download.

9.5 Key steps in conducting an economic evaluation

There are a number of key steps involved in doing an economic evaluation. These include:

Decide upon the study question.

Make statement of alternatives to be appraised.

Assess costs and benefits of alternatives.

- List the appropriate costs and benefits to include in the appraisal.
- Measure resources, used and saved by the programme alternatives, and the outcomes produced by each.
- Value resources used (and saved) and outcomes produced in appropriate units for comparison.

Box 9.1 Cost-effectiveness of interventions for reducing blood pressure and cholesterol in Australia

Researchers evaluating the optimal mix of lifestyle, pharmaceutical, and population-wide measures to prevent cardiovascular disease in Australia evaluated the cost-effectiveness of a number of interventions on blood pressure and cholesterol (Figure 9.3).[4]

The interventions included in the evaluation were a community heart health programme; mandatory reduction of salt in bread, margarines, and cereals; six pharmaceutical interventions targeting high-risk individuals; and three behaviour change interventions for those at high risk. For comparison, current practice in Australia—comprising voluntary salt reductions, dietary advice from a general practitioner, and blood pressure- and cholesterol-lowering drug therapy—was also modelled.

Current practice on reducing blood pressure and cholesterol in Australia is shown above the curve. The vertical dotted line shows the point on the curve where the same level of health could be achieved with lower expenditure. The horizontal line shows where greater health could be achieved at the same level of expenditure.

The study found that mandatory salt reductions were easily the most effective and cost-effective strategy for primary cardiovascular disease (CVD) prevention. Lowering blood pressure with diuretics, calcium channel blockers, and

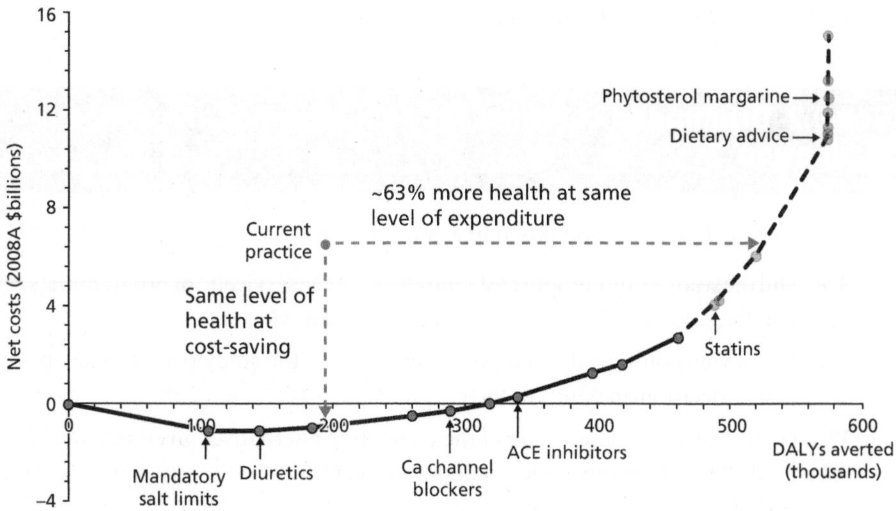

Figure 9.3 Cost effective of interventions for reducing blood pressure and cholesterol in Australia.

Adapted with permission from **Cobiac LJ**, **Magnus A**, **Lim S**, **Barendregt JJ**, **Carter R**, and **Vos T**. Which interventions offer best value for money in primary prevention of cardiovascular disease? *PLoS ONE*, Volume 7, Issue 7, Article e41842, Copyright © 2012 L Cobiac et al.

angiotensin-converting-enzyme inhibitors was also cost-effective. The authors concluded that implementing a package of mandatory salt limits in processed foods and provision of diuretic, calcium channel blocker, angiotensin-converting-enzyme inhibitor, and low-cost statin drugs for everyone with at least a 5% five-year risk of CVD could achieve a threefold improvement in population health and reduce lifetime health-care expenditure by 4.2 billion Australian dollars.

Adjust for timing.

- Discounting

Adjust for risk

- Modelling and sensitivity analysis

Make a decision.

Calculate and use decision rules:

- Net present value of programme
- Comparison of cost-effectiveness ratios

9.5.1 Critical appraisal of an economic evaluation

A ten-point checklist for evaluating an economic evaluation was developed by Drummond (Box 9.2). This sets out ten key questions—and some more specific questions under each of these—to be able to evaluate an economic evaluation.

Box 9.2 Drummond checklist for evaluation of an economic evaluation

1. Was a well-defined question posed in answerable form?
   - 1.1. Did the study examine both costs and effects of the service(s) or programme(s)?
   - 1.2. Did the study involve a comparison of alternatives?
   - 1.3. Was a viewpoint for the analysis stated and was the study placed in any particular decision-making context?
2. Was a comprehensive description of the competing alternatives given (i.e. can you tell who did what to whom, where, and how often)?
   - 2.1. Were there any important alternatives omitted?
   - 2.2. Was (should) a do-nothing alternative be considered?
3. Was the effectiveness of the programmes or services established?
   - 3.1. Was this done through a randomized, controlled clinical trial? If so, did the trial protocol reflect what would happen in regular practice?

3.2. Was effectiveness established through an overview of clinical studies?

3.3. Were observational data or assumptions used to establish effectiveness? If so, what are the potential biases in results?

4. Were all the important and relevant costs and consequences for each alternative identified?

4.1. Was the range wide enough for the research question at hand?

4.2. Did it cover all relevant viewpoints? (Possible viewpoints include the community or social viewpoint, and those of patients and third-party payers. Other viewpoints may also be relevant depending upon the particular analysis.)

4.3. Were the capital costs, as well as operating costs, included?

5. Were costs and consequences measured accurately in appropriate physical units (e.g. number of physician visits, lost work-days, gained life-years)?

5.1. Were any of the identified items omitted from measurement? If so, does this mean that they carried no weight in the subsequent analysis?

5.2. Were there any special circumstances (e.g., joint use of resources) that made measurement difficult? Were these circumstances handled appropriately?

6. Were costs and consequences valued credibly?

6.1. Were the sources of all values clearly identified? (Possible sources include market values, patient or client preferences and views, policy-makers' views, and health professionals' judgements.)

6.2. Were market values employed for changes involving resources gained or depleted?

6.3. Where market values were absent (e.g. volunteer labour) or did not reflect actual values (such as clinic space donated at a reduced rate), were adjustments made to approximate market values?

6.4. Was the valuation of consequences appropriate for the question posed (i.e. has the appropriate type or types of analysis—cost-effectiveness, cost–benefit, cost–utility—been selected)?

7. Were costs and consequences adjusted for differential timing?

7.1. Were costs and consequences that occur in the future 'discounted' to their present values?

7.2. Was there any justification given for the discount rate used?

8. Was an incremental analysis of costs and consequences of alternatives performed?

8.1. Were the additional (incremental) costs generated by one alternative over another compared to the additional effects, benefits, or utilities generated?

9. Was allowance made for uncertainty in the estimates of costs and consequences?

9.1. If data on costs and consequences were stochastic (randomly determined sequence of observations), were appropriate statistical analyses performed?

9.2. If a sensitivity analysis was employed, was justification provided for the range of values (or for key study parameters)?

9.3. Were the study results sensitive to changes in the values (within the assumed range for sensitivity analysis, or within the confidence interval around the ratio of costs to consequences)?

10. Did the presentation and discussion of study results include all issues of concern to users?

10.1. Were the conclusions of the analysis based on some overall index or ratio of costs to consequences (e.g. cost-effectiveness ratio)? If so, was the index interpreted intelligently or in a mechanistic fashion?

10.2. Were the results compared with those of others who have investigated the same question? If so, were allowances made for potential differences in study methodology?

10.3. Did the study discuss the generalizability of the results to other settings and patient/client groups?

10.4. Did the study allude to, or take account of, other important factors in the choice or decision under consideration (e.g. distribution of costs and consequences, or relevant ethical issues)?

10.5. Did the study discuss issues of implementation, such as the feasibility of adopting the 'preferred' programme given existing financial or other constraints, and whether any freed resources could be redeployed to other worthwhile programmes?

9.6 **Summary and conclusions**

When considering the role of cost-effectiveness analyses in the decision-making process, the formulaic use of cost-effective analysis results is not recommended. There can be good justification in particular circumstances for policy-makers to implement less cost-effective interventions or to not implement more cost-effective interventions. There may be practical constraints such as, for example, a shortage of persons qualified to deliver a particular intervention.

Policy decisions should, however, be made with information on the opportunities to improve population health that are foregone elsewhere.

A variety of criteria may be taken into account in decisions on public spending. Economic efficiency, for example, could include cost-effectiveness, public goods (something for which there is no market), externalities (e.g. herd immunity from vaccination), and catastrophic costs (e.g. costly healthcare that could send non-poor into poverty if it is not publicly funded). Ethical reasons could take into account poverty, equity, and the 'rule of rescue', whereby the cost-effectiveness of an intervention may be given lower priority if the only alternative for an individual is death. Other criteria may relate to political considerations, such as the respective demands of the population, providers, or suppliers.

In summary, economic evaluation provides a method for assessing the efficiency of interventions in improving health and can be used to, among other things, guide resource allocation decisions and to measure the efficiency of the health system. It remains a challenge to engage policy-makers and advocates in the use and generation of cost-effectiveness while considering impacts on other decision-making criteria. In this way, priority-setting in health policy will be more explicit and will also be evidence-based.

Case study: ACE-Prevention—assessing cost-effectiveness of preventive interventions

The five-year ACE-Prevention study, funded by the National Health and Medical Research Council and led by the University of Queensland and Deakin University, evaluated preventive interventions in Australia to identify those that would prevent the most illness and those that are best value for money.[5]

With a view to providing a comprehensive analysis of the comparative cost-effectiveness of NCD prevention intervention options, with a specific focus on Indigenous Australians, the study assessed 123 prevention measures and, for comparison, 27 treatment interventions. Around 130 top health experts were involved and a standard protocol was developed to ensure comparability of results. To ensure valid comparisons between results:

- Each intervention was modelled to apply to the relevant people in the 2003 Australian population and the costs and health outcomes were measured for as long as they occur, often over a lifetime;
- All results were expressed as a cost per disability-adjusted life year (DALY) averted, where:
  - The DALY is a measure of the difference in healthy time lived comparing an intervention scenario with 'current practice' or 'do nothing'; the disability adjustment reflects the severity of disease or disability. More DALYs 'saved' means a longer life, a life with less disability, or a combination of these;
- Costs take into account the expenditure required to implement each health intervention as well as the downstream consequences for disease treatment;
- Best available evidence on effectiveness was derived from the international literature, preferably using estimates that are pooled across all available studies;

- Costs and outcomes were modelled based on realistic expectations of how interventions would be implemented under routine health service conditions in Australia;
- Uncertainty was explicitly quantified and presented around all results; and
- Stakeholders from government, health non-governmental organizations (NGOs), academia, and service providers provided guidance to the researchers and helped to formulate conclusions taking the technical results into consideration, together with other policy relevant considerations such as acceptability, feasibility, and equity.

The categories used to classify interventions according to cost-effectiveness ratio, health impact, intervention cost, strength of evidence, and other issues are set out in Table 9.2.

Table 9.2 Categories used in ACE Prevention project to classify interventions according to various aspects

Aspect	Categories		
Cost-effectiveness ratio	◆ *Dominant*: interventions that improve health and save money; ◆ *Very cost-effective*: interventions that improve health at a cost of less than $10,000 per DALY; ◆ *Cost-effective*: interventions that improve health at a cost of between $10,000 and $50,000 per DALY; ◆ *Not cost-effective*: interventions that improve health at a cost of more than $50,000 per DALY; and ◆ *Dominated*: interventions with worse health outcomes at a cost; or more cost-effective alternatives are available that 'replace' the dominated intervention.		
Health impact (lifetime)	+	++	+++
	Small	Medium	Large
	0–10,000 DALYs	10,000–100,000 DALYs	>1,00,000 DALYs
Intervention cost (annual)	+	++	+++
	Small	Medium	Large
	<$10 million	$10-100 million	>$100 million
Strength of evidence (Table 9.3)	Comparative evidence: ◆ sufficient; ◆ limited; or ◆ inconclusive;	No comparative evidence: ◆ likely; ◆ maybe; or ◆ no evidence	
Other issues	No pre-defined categories		

Reproduced with permission from **Vos T**, **Carter R**, **Barendregt J**, **Mihalopoulos C**, **Veerman JL**, **Magnus A**, et al. *Assessing Cost-Effectiveness in Prevention (ACE–Prevention): Final Report, September 2010*. Brisbane, Australia: University of Queensland, and Melbourne, Australia: Deakin University, https://public-health.uq.edu.au/filething/get/1836/ACE-Prevention_final_report.pdf, accessed 20 Jul. 2016.

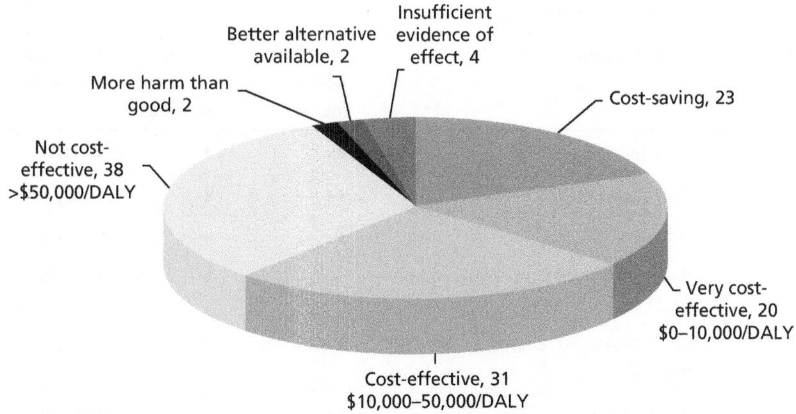

Figure 9.4 Cost-effectiveness of the 123 preventive interventions.

Source: data from **Vos T, Carter R, Barendregt J, Mihalopoulos C, Veerman JL, Magnus A**, et al. *Assessing Cost-Effectiveness in Prevention (ACE–Prevention): Final Report, September 2010*. Brisbane, Australia: University of Queensland, and Melbourne, Australia: Deakin University, https://public-health.uq.edu.au/filething/get/1836/ACE-Prevention_final_report.pdf, accessed 20 Jul. 2016.

A summary of the results is shown in Figure 9.4, with 31 interventions assessed as being cost-effective, 20 considered as being very cost-effective, and 23 as cost saving (dominant).

Twenty-three cost-saving (dominant) prevention interventions were identified. Of these, 12 aim to reduce exposure to harmful risk factors by taxation (of alcohol, tobacco, and unhealthy food) or regulation (alcohol advertising bans, raising minimum age of drinking, limiting salt in processed food, and fluoridation of drinking water). There were four health promotion interventions and seven screening interventions to identify, and treat, those who are at high risk (Table 9.3).

In the 'very cost-effective' category—with a cost-effectiveness ratio less than $10,000 per DALY—there were 20 interventions, of which 15 involved screening (in primary care or schools) followed by a drug, psychological, health promotion, or surgical intervention. Two regulatory interventions were also classified as highly cost-effective—namely, licensing controls on alcohol retailing and responsible media reporting of suicide. Two health education interventions, targeting physical activity or fruit and vegetable intakes, and a universal infant vaccination programme also met the criteria for very cost-effective.

The taxation and regulatory initiatives are the least costly to implement for health systems and can lead to substantial health gains. The ACE-Prevention study report concludes that 'from a public health point of view there are no hesitations to advocate the implementation of these interventions', although it also recognizes that implementation of such measures is highly dependent on political will.

Table 9.3 Preventive interventions for non-communicable disease assessed as cost saving (dominant) by the ACE–Prevention project

Topic area	Intervention	Lifetime health impact*	Annual intervention cost*	Strength of evidence
Alcohol	Volumetric tax	++	+	Likely
	Tax increase 30%	+++	+	Likely
	Advertising bans	+	+	Limited
	Raise minimum legal drinking age to 21	+	+	Limited
Tobacco	Tax increase 30% (with or without indexation)	+++	+	Likely
Physical activity	Pedometers	++	++	Sufficient
	Mass media	++	++	Inconclusive
Nutrition	Community fruit and vegetable intake promotion	+	++	May be effective
	Voluntary salt limits	+	+	Likely
	Mandatory salt limits	+++	+	Likely
Body mass	10% tax on unhealthy food	+++	+	May be effective
Blood pressure and cholesterol	Community heart health program	++	+	May be effective
	Polypill $200 for >5% CVD risk	+++	+++	Likely
Osteoporosis	Screen women aged 70+ and alendronate	++	++	Sufficient
Hepatitis B	Vaccine and immunoglobulin to infants born to carrier or high-risk mothers	+	+	Sufficient
	High-risk infant vaccination	+	+	Sufficient
	Selective vaccination of infants with mothers from highly endemic countries	+	+	Sufficient
Kidney disease	Proteinuria screen and angiotensin-converting enzyme inhibitors for diabetics	++	+	Sufficient
Mental disorders	Problem-solving post-suicide attempt	+	+	Sufficient
	Treatment for individuals at ultra-high risk for psychosis	+	+	Likely
Oral health	Fluoridation drinking water, non remote	+	+	Limited

CVD, cardiovascular disease.

Note: Some infectious disease interventions and treatment interventions were included in the study as a benchmark.

Reproduced with permission from **Vos T, Carter R, Barendregt J, Mihalopoulos C, Veerman JL, Magnus A**, et al. *Assessing Cost-Effectiveness in Prevention (ACE–Prevention): Final Report, September 2010*. Brisbane, Australia: University of Queensland, and Melbourne, Australia: Deakin University, https://public-health.uq.edu.au/filething/get/1836/ACE-Prevention_final_report.pdf, accessed 20 Jul. 2016.

Case study: Cost-effectiveness of interventions to tackle unhealthy diets, physical inactivity, and obesity in six low- and middle-income countries

WHO and the Organisation for Economic Cooperation and Development (OECD) created a chronic disease prevention model based on a causal web of inter-related lifestyle risk factors for selected chronic diseases (Figure 9.5). This model uses a microsimulation approach, which is able to answer complex questions that it would take a very long time—given that results may be realized over whole lifetimes—and considerable resources to address with empirical research.

In a 2015 study, the researchers applied this model to assess a number of public health strategies designed to tackle obesity, unhealthy diet, and physical inactivity in Brazil, China, India, Mexico, Russia, and South Africa. One high-income country, England, was included for comparative purposes. The six low- and middle-income countries were selected because they have a high burden of NCDs, they are relatively large and prominent in their regions, and they had more data available than other countries.

A number of interventions, for which evidence of effectiveness was available, were assessed:

- School-based health promotion interventions;
- Worksite health promotion interventions;
- Mass media health promotion campaigns;
- Counselling of individuals at risk in primary care;
- Fiscal measures affecting the prices of fruit and vegetables and foods high in fat;
- Regulation of food advertising to children; and
- Compulsory food labelling.

Country-specific information was used to establish potential population coverage and to adapt effectiveness to the local population distribution of risk factors. Interventions were then implemented in the model by applying the effects on risk factors to the relevant target age groups, taking into account the likely coverage of those age groups. The costs of interventions were calculated using a standardized methodology and included any costs relating to individuals using health services and the costs associated with implementing the programme, such as administration, training, communication costs, or any other activities.

Limitations of the model include, among others, its reliance on the availability of national or subnational data for many parameters, its inability to take into account some potential confounding effects and possible interactions between risk factors, and relatively limited data on the intervention effects, particularly in the long term. Key strengths of the model, however, include its capacity to handle a combination

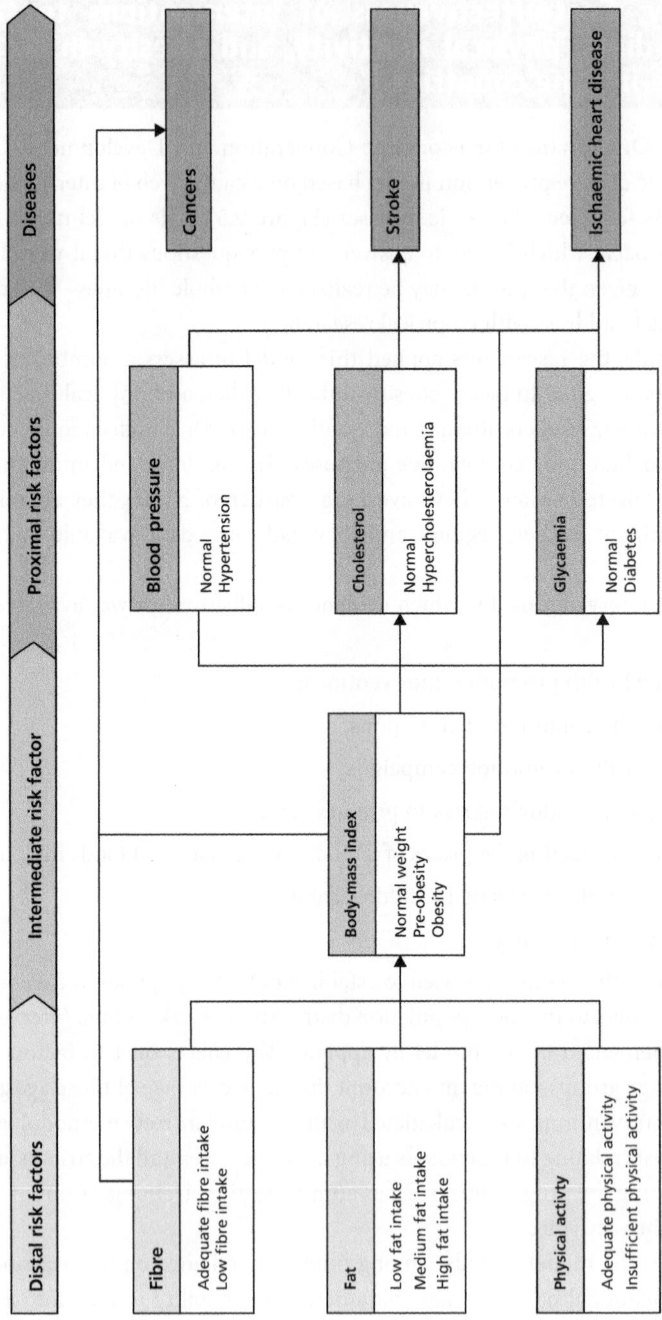

Figure 9.5 Causal web for risk factors and disease events implemented in the chronic disease prevention model.

Reprinted from *The Lancet*, Volume 376, Issue 9754, **Cecchini M**, **Sassi F**, **Lauer JA**, **Lee YY**, **Guajardo-Barron V**, and **Chisholm D**. Tackling of unhealthy diets, physical inactivity, and obesity: health effects and cost-effectiveness, pp. 1775–84, Copyright © 2010, with permission from Elsevier.

Table 9.4 Effectiveness and cost-effectiveness of interventions after 20 years and 50 years

	Brazil		China		England		India		Mexico		Russia		South Africa	
	DALYs	**CE***	**DALYs**	**CE***	**DALYs**	**CE***	**DALYs**	**CE***	**DALYs**	**CE***	**DALYs**	**CE***	**DALYs**	**CE***
20 years														
School-based interventions	4	†	10	704863	0	†	8	†	3	†	12	830177	3	†
Worksite interventions	1187	8270	399	7785	1725	45630	405	6151	644	37912	1759	6187	254	25409
Mass media campaigns	627	5074	688	7188	1361	25897	246	15552	533	6858	811	12911	421	23221
Fiscal measures	1642	CS	1027	CS	1496	CS	139	CS	509	CS	1696	CS	528	CS
Physician counselling	2805	8503	864	9390	5562	25284	523	6155	2796	23811	6988	5982	719	23841
Food advertising regulation	38	CS	145	556	245	25672	49	3186	**112**	11151	288	918	89	13241
Food labelling	1030	9962	779	71	1134	12577	495	952	358	3974	1176	396	389	7953
50 years														
School-based interventions	170	93350	337	35174	245	152 989	232	59665	83	235957	696	26114	152	153233
Worksite interventions	3323	3541	1383	3393	6078	20506	939	4491	2175	16932	5929	2926	739	14561
Mass media campaigns	1803	1994	2500	3177	4025	13796	670	8575	1530	2778	2914	5822	1047	15211
Fiscal measures	5483	CS	3909	CS	6049	CS	355	CS	1978	CS	5898	CS	1725	CS
Physician counselling	7163	5156	2306	5718	14776	15731	1045	5553	7477	15108	16644	4331	1739	16591
Food advertising regulation	988	CS	1314	CS	2179	4278	752	332	658	3415	5823	552	610	3352
Food labelling	3259	CS	2805	CS	4019	5268	1089	776	1304	CS	4099	CS	1157	3927
Cost-effectiveness threshold (US$/DALY)‡		15000		5000		50000t		2500		20000		15000		15000

DALYs, disability-adjusted life-years saved per million population. CE, cost-effectiveness. CS, cost-saving.

* Cost-effectivenes ratios are expressed in US$ per DALY averted, and represent the net cost of gaining 1 additional year of healthy life, relative to a no-prevention or treatrnent-ony scenario.

† Cost-effectivenes ratio is higher than US$1,000,000 per DALY.

‡ For countries other than England, the guideline amount of three times gross domestic product per head (US$2005) is used as a cost-effectiveness threshold. In England, US$50,000 DALY is a threshold commonly adopted by the UK's National Institute for Health and Clinical Excellence to denote that an intervention is cost effective.

of multiple and heterogeneous sources of data, along with the possibility to test the consistency of input data and the robustness of results. A specific analysis to examine the uncertainty in relation to both costs and effectiveness (a 'probabilistic uncertainty analysis') found that substantial variation did exist but, despite such variation, confirmed the cost-effectiveness of the most efficient interventions.

The model produced results for effectiveness, measured as DALYs saved per million population, and cost-effectiveness ratios, expressed as US$ per DALY averted (Table 9.4). The study found that, when compared to a scenario where there is only treatment and no prevention, fiscal measures are consistently cost saving in all six settings after both 20 and 50 years. Regulation of food advertising to children and mass media health promotion campaigns also both have very favourable cost-effectiveness ratios, and after 50 years, regulation of food advertising is cost saving in several countries. The health effects of advertising restrictions and school-based health promotion interventions remain small within the 50-year modelling period, but this to be expected because the real benefits of interventions targeted at children will probably only start to accrue after 40–50 years, even though the overall benefits may be as large over the longer term. The returns for worksite health-promotion initiatives are quicker, and these also have favourable cost-effectiveness. Primary care counselling of high-risk individuals is one of the most effective interventions, but it depends on widespread access to primary health care.

In addition, a multi-intervention strategy that combined a mass media campaign, fiscal measures, food advertising regulation, and food labelling was assessed. Such a strategy would achieve substantially larger health gains than would individual interventions, often with even better cost-effectiveness, and would be cost saving in about half the countries examined.

The authors concluded that 'several population-based prevention policies can be expected to generate much needed health gains while entirely or very largely paying for themselves through their reduction of future healthcare costs'.[6] These policies include health information and communication strategies, fiscal measures, and regulatory measures to improve nutritional information or restrict the marketing of unhealthy foods. The authors point out that these highly cost-effective (or cost-saving) interventions are different from the more targeted strategies that were also considered (namely, those that were school-based, work-based, or specifically targeted at higher-risk individuals) because they covered a greater proportion of the population and were relatively inexpensive to implement. They concluded that 'a package of measures for the prevention of chronic diseases would deliver substantial health gains, with a very favourable cost-effectiveness profile'.[6]

Source: data from *The Lancet*, Volume 376, Issue 9754, **Cecchini M**, **Sassi F**, **Lauer JA**, **Lee YY**, **Guajardo-Barron V**, and **Chisholm D**. Tackling of unhealthy diets, physical inactivity, and obesity: health effects and cost-effectiveness, pp. 1775–84, Copyright © 2010 Elsevier.

Acknowledgement

This chapter is based on a presentation by Dr Linda Cobiac, which is based on her PhD thesis (Cobiac LJ. 2010. Cost-effectiveness of interventions to prevent lifestyle-related disease and injury in Australia. PhD Thesis, School of Population Health, University of Queensland. Available from: http://espace.library.uq.edu.au/view/UQ:213020) and the case study sources cited.

References

1. **Drummond MF, Sculpher MJ, Claxton K, Stoddart GL, Torrance GW.** *Methods for the Economic Evaluation of Health Care Programmes*. 2005.
2. **National Institute for Clinical Health and Excellence.** *Guide to the methods of technology appraisal 2013*. 4 April 2013. Available from: https://www.nice.org.uk/process/pmg9/chapter/1-foreword
3. **George B, Harris A, Mitchell A.** Cost-effectiveness analysis and the consistency of decision making: evidence from pharmaceutical reimbursement in Australia (1991 to 1996). *Pharmacoeconomics* 2001; **19**(11):1103–9.
4. **Cobiac LJ, Magnus A, Lim S, Barendregt JJ, Carter R, Vos T.** Which interventions offer best value for money in primary prevention of cardiovascular disease? *PLoS ONE* 2012; 7(7):e41842.
5. **Vos T, Carter R, Barendregt J, Mihalopoulos C, Veerman JL, Magnus A, et al., ACE–Prevention Team.** *Assessing Cost-Effectiveness in Prevention (ACE–Prevention): Final Report*. Melbourne: University of Queensland, Brisbane and Deakin University, 2010.
6. **Cecchini M, Sassi F, Lauer JA, Lee YY, Guajardo-Barron V, Chisholm D.** Tackling of unhealthy diets, physical inactivity, and obesity: health effects and cost-effectiveness. *The Lancet* 2010; **376**(9754):1775–84.

Chapter 10

Developing a prevention strategy

10.1 Building a prevention strategy

Equipped with knowledge about the issues around non-communicable diseases (NCDs) in the current global context and armed with an understanding of prevention and a population-based approach, the next step is to explore how to build a strategy.

In general terms, a strategy can be defined as a plan of action designed to achieve a vision. In public health policy, there are five elements that all strategies have, whether or not these are explicitly expressed. These are aims, context, philosophy, logic/evidence, and values.

It is obviously important that any strategy should have explicit aims and these need to be clear and transparent. Some strategies go further and crystallize their aims into a series of targets. Such targets should aim at being SMART—that is, specific, measurable, attainable, realistic, and time-specific.

The context in which the strategy will operate should also be taken into consideration. Strategies may operate at different levels—such as local, national, or global—or may be for different groups of actors such as governments, commercial organizations, and non-governmental organizations (NGOs).

All strategies will be underpinned by a particular philosophy. As described earlier (see section 1.3, Key Concepts) the underlying philosophy or a prevention strategy could be, for example, a population-based approach, a high-risk approach, or a combination of the two.

A strategy also needs to be informed by logic and/or evidence, which means that a certain degree of understanding of the causal pathways is required. Although strong evidence of causality is obviously ideal, it is also possible to progress with a good logic model. This is where the causal webs highlighted in Chapter 3 may be particularly useful.

In drawing up a strategy it can also be useful to use a systematic process to organize elements such as possible interventions. This framework may inform the process of prioritizing actions (see section 10.3).

Finally, all NCD prevention strategies are driven by values, regardless of whether these are explicitly acknowledged. An example of a list of values behind an NCD prevention strategy is the list of overarching principles found at the beginning of the World Health Organization (WHO) Global NCD Action Plan (Box 10.1).

It is often difficult to know what expression of these values means in practice for the development of a strategy. Are they just normative assumptions that are being made? It is generally assumed, for example, that multisectoral action is more effective than unilateral

Box 10.1 Examples of values driving a prevention strategy—the overarching principles behind the Global NCD Action Plan

Life course approach
Empowerment of people and communities
Evidence-based strategies
Universal health coverage
Management of real, perceived of potential conflicts of interest
Human rights approach
Equity-based approach
National action and international action and solidarity
Multisectoral action

action. Are they simply aspirational goals setting out ideals to aim for? Some degree of equity in health outcomes, for example, is often a goal of public health strategy. Or can they be meaningfully translated into clear features of a strategy? Table 10.1 sets out some common aspirational values for strategies and shows how these can be translated into normative values, which can be clearly applied to a strategy.

All strategies have the five elements described at the start of this section—whether or not these are explicit. In addition, every strategy needs the following in order to be successful:

Time—there is no such thing as a 'short-term' NCD plan;

Resources (money and people) for implementation;

Evidence for effectiveness of interventions and/or understanding of causality;

Buy-in from stakeholders; and

Leadership and teamwork.

Table 10.1 Common aspirational and normative values for prevention strategies

Normative	Aspirational
Has clear purpose (aims) Is appropriate for that purpose Operationalizes that purpose	Efficiency
Is evidence based Is rational and logical	Effectiveness/efficacy
Is concerned with all population groups	Equity
Is published Process of development is documented	Transparency
Involves all stakeholders, including the least powerful	Cooperativity/autonomy

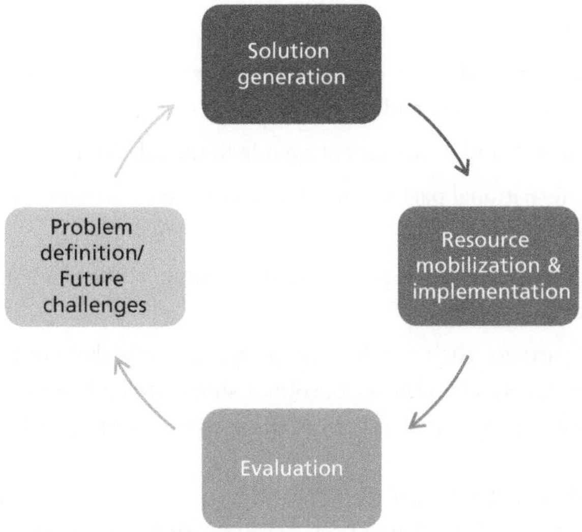

Figure 10.1 The strategy/policy-making cycle.

10.2 **Stages in developing a strategy**

When drawing up a strategy, the problem must initially be described and consideration then given to the time available and resource constraints, before identifying key stakeholders and designing a monitoring system. As the problem is being described possible solutions should be identified and considered. However, given limited resources, it is important to maximize resources that may already be available. Then the plan can be implemented and evaluation should take place throughout the cycle of planning and implementation. Figure 10.1 summarizes this cycle in a simple manner.

In order to help national policy-makers to build a prevention strategy, the Global Action Plan for the Prevention and Control of NCD's 2013–2020 (see Chapter 5) provides a menu of policy options and cost-effective interventions (Box 10.2).

Box 10.2 WHO Global NCD Action Plan—Menu of Policy Options

Policy options for countries, international partners, and WHO are set out under each of the Action Plan's six objectives:

1. *To raise the priority accorded to the prevention and control of non-communicable disease in global, regional, and national agenda and internationally agreed development goals—through strengthened international cooperation and advocacy.*

Policy options for countries:

- Gather evidence and advocate on the effectiveness of NCD interventions and policies, thereby raising public and political awareness.
- Broaden the health and development agenda to include NCDs.
- Strengthen international partnerships for resource mobilization, capacity building, and exchange of best practices.
- Mobilize civil society and the private sector to support the implementation of the action plan at all levels.
- International partners, such as other UN organizations, global health initiatives, and financial institutions and private sector entities, should strengthen the capacity of member states and advance the political commitment to reduce the global NCD burden.

2. *To strengthen national capacity, leadership, governance, multisectoral action, and partnerships to accelerate a country's response for the prevention and control of NCDs.*

Policy options for countries:

- Develop and implement a national multisectoral policy and plan.
- Increase domestic budgetary allocations for NCD control and universal health coverage
- Improve efficiency of resource utilization through integrated and shared planning across sectors.
- Conduct periodic epidemiological assessments of health impacts of policies in sectors beyond health.
- Set up high-level commission, agency, or task force for multisectoral NCD action.
- Provide training and educational programming to health, social services, and community workforces.
- Empower communities and individuals to facilitate social mobilization, engaging and empowering a broad range of actors.
- International partners should support national authorities in implementing evidence-based multisectoral action to address functional gaps in the response to NCDs.

3. *To reduce modifiable risk factors and underlying social determinants through health promotion activities.*

Policy options on tobacco control for countries:

- Accelerate full implementation of the WHO Framework Convention on Tobacco Control.
- Protect tobacco control policies from the tobacco industry.
- Legislate 100% tobacco-free environments in all indoor public places.
- Warn people of the dangers of tobacco smoke through effective health warnings.

- Ban tobacco advertising, promotion, and sponsorship.
- Offer assistance programming to people who want to stop using tobacco.

Policy options on promoting healthy diets for countries:

- Develop new policies or strengthen existing policies pertaining to national food and nutrition programming and infant and young child feeding.
- Promote and support exclusive breastfeeding for the first six months.
- Implement WHO's set of recommendations on the marketing of foods and non-alcoholic beverages to children.

Policy options for increasing physical activity for countries:

- Implement the WHO Global Strategy on Diet, Physical Activity, and Health.
- Promote the ancillary benefits from increasing population levels of physical activity.
- Develop appropriate partnerships and engage all stakeholders in actively implementing programmes aimed at increasing physical activity across all ages.
- Develop national and regional urban planning initiatives that improve infrastructure for walking and cycling.
- Improve quality of physical education in school settings.
- Create and preserve recreational and national environments which support physical activities in institutions and communities.

Policy options for reducing harmful use of alcohol for countries:

- Strengthen awareness of alcohol-attributable burden.
- Provide prevention and treatment interventions for those at risk of or affected by alcohol disorders.
- Implement effective drink-driving policies and countermeasures.
- Regulate commercial and public availability of alcohol.
- Restrict or ban alcohol advertising and promotions.
- Use pricing policies such as excise taxes on alcoholic beverages.
- International partners should support the policies developed and implemented by member states.

4. *To enhance and orient health systems to prevent and control NCDs through people-centred primary health care and universal health coverage.*

Policy options for countries:

Expand quality services coverage

- Harness the potential of all providers to address NCDs' equitably and meet the needs for long-term care of chronic NCD patients.
- Empower people to seek early detection and encourage self-management.

Strengthen human resources

- Provide incentives for health workers to service underserved areas.
- Develop career tracks for health workers through strengthening postgraduate training in various professional disciplines.
- Optimize the role of nurses and allied health professions.

Improve equitable access to prevention programmes

- Include relevant medicines in national essentials medicines list.
- Facilitate access to preventive measures for occupational NCDs.
- Promote access to affordable, safe, and quality medicines, life-saving technologies, and diagnostic tools.
- International partners should support these policy efforts by mobilizing sustained financial resources for orienting health systems to provide universal coverage and improving access to quality medicines through trade-related aspects of intellectual property rights.

5. *To strengthen national capacity for high-quality research for the prevention and control of non-communicable diseases.*

Policy options for countries:

- Develop and implement a national policy and plan on NCD-related research.
- Increase investment in research to fill in gaps around NCD interventions.
- Enhance research competency by building on skills to conduct quality research.
- Incentivize innovation and encourage the establishment of national reference centres and networks to conduct policy relevant research.
- Track the domestic and international resource flows for national research output and the information applicable to the prevention and control of NCDs.
    - International partners should support member states and in addition:
        - Strengthen institutional capacity through the creation of fellowships and scholarships for NCD research.
        - Promote the use of information and communications technology to improve programme implementation, health outcomes, health promotion, and surveillance systems.

6. *To monitor trends and determinants of NCDs and evaluate progress in their prevention and control.*

Policy options for countries:

- Increase and prioritize budgetary allocations for surveillance and monitoring systems.
- Strengthen vital registration and cause of death registration systems.

- Integrate monitoring systems to include prevalence of key interventions, risk factors, determinants of risk exposure, and dimensions into national health information systems.
- Develop, maintain, and strengthen disease registries.
- Disseminate results by reporting on trends with respect to morbidity, mortality by cause, risk factors, and other determinants, providing information to the WHO.
- International partners should support the policies developed and implemented by member states

The Global Action Plan and this menu of policy options provide a roadmap for the development and implementation of regional and national NCD action plans. WHO is charged with providing support to countries in all six areas and a number of tools to help with implementation are available at http://www.who.int/ncds/prevention/en/.

Adapted with permission from: **World Health Organization**. *Global action plan for the prevention and control of noncommunicable diseases 2013-2030*. Geneva: WHO, Copyright © 2013 World Health Organization.

10.3 Tools for priority setting

Having identified the problem and analysed the needs, the next steps are to assess potential solutions and then effectively to identify priority areas for action. This prioritization should involve working with stakeholders throughout the process and should be guided by evidence.

One tool to guide the prioritization process has been developed specifically in relation to obesity. The ANGELO process uses the analysis grid for elements linked to obesity (ANGELO) to help communities analyse the environmental influences affecting their physical activity and eating patterns and then to work out which factors they can more readily alter (see Case study: Community prioritization of action on childhood obesity in Geelong, Victoria, Australia).[1]

WHO has issued guidance on determining and identifying priority areas for action on childhood obesity.[2] This document presents a set of tools, including the ANGELO framework, and gives practical advice on how to use such tools.

Case study: Community prioritization of action on childhood obesity in Geelong, Victoria, Australia

A team from Deakin University supported the community of Geelong (population 200,000) in Victoria, Australia to work through the ANGELO process.[1] Geelong is in Barwon South-West region. Crucially, the community itself conducted the process, over a period of two days, with the academic team providing information and evidence to feed into the process and advising on the process itself.

Originally developed by Swinburn and colleagues, the ANGELO framework categorized obesogenic environments by components into two environment sizes (i.e. micro and macro) and into four types of environments (sociocultural, policy, physical, and economic).[3] Since then, the framework has been used as a tool to assess environmental determinants of obesity or potential interventions. It is a practical tool for identifying and prioritizing potential behaviours, knowledge/skills, and environments for interventions and for guiding the process of creating community action plans. The key priority setting criteria in the ANGELO process are changeability and importance (relevance and impact). The intended outcome of the ANGELO process is to have a community action plan with agreed objectives and strategies. The process, which engages a wide range of stakeholders, follows the steps shown in Figure 10.2.

In Geelong the first step was a process of stakeholder engagement, with initial discussions with relevant people in schools, health and education departments, churches, local government, and other key local organizations or influential people. Through these discussions, priorities were identified.

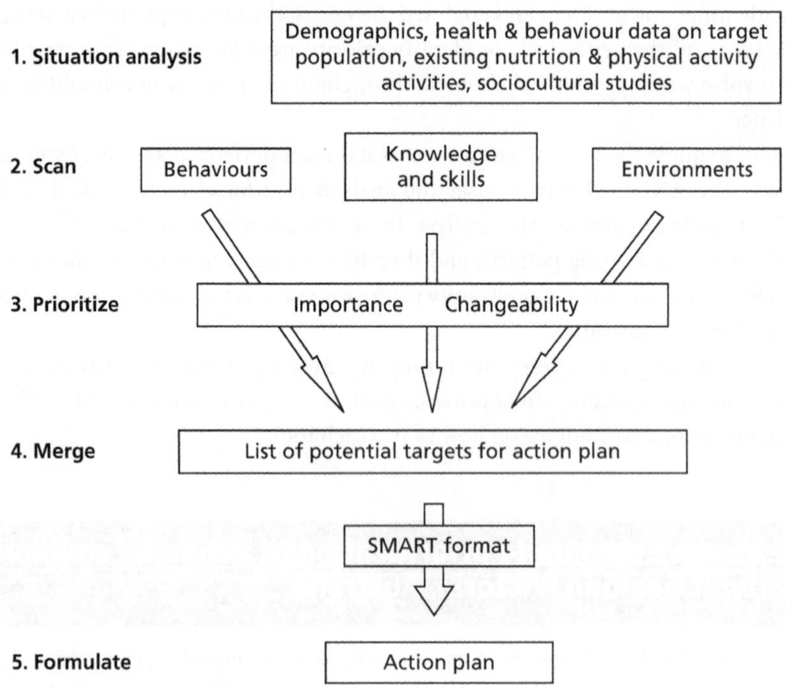

Figure 10.2 The ANGELO process.

Reproduced with permission from Simmons A, Mavoa HM, Bell AC, De Courten M, Schaaf D, Schultz J, and Swinburn BA. Creating community action plans for obesity prevention using the ANGELO (Analysis Grid for Elements Linked to Obesity) Framework. *Health Promotion international*, Volume 24, Issue 4, pp. 311–24, Copyright © 2009 Oxford University Press.

The next step was a two-day stakeholder workshop to come up with a draft action plan. To start the workshop researchers presented data from technical assessments and community consultations and other aspects of the situation. The workshop then moved on to discuss key behaviours to target, knowledge and skill gaps, and environmental barriers. Participants then scored each element for importance and changeability and the elements were ranked according to those scores. The workshop was able to reach a consensus on goals and priorities and these were pulled together to form a structured action plan for community-level obesity prevention.

As a result of this process, three projects were initiated over the following three years—the *Romp n Chomp* project in under 5s, the *Be Active, Eat Well* project in primary schools, and the *It's Your Move* project with adolescents. All three reported a positive impact, in terms of anthropometric changes.[4,5,6] A positive impact on community capacity measures, such as community readiness to change, was also reported.

Case study: The NOURISHING policy framework for promoting healthy diets and reducing obesity

Another tool that exists for helping policy-makers to take action on NCDs and their risk factors is the NOURISHING policy framework. This tool, developed by World Cancer Research Fund International, is designed to help policy-makers, researchers, and civil society organizations worldwide take action to tackle unhealthy diets.

NOURISHING sets out a comprehensive package of policies to promote healthy diets and reduce overweight/obesity and NCDs. Each letter in the word NOURISHING represents one of ten areas where governments need to take action (Figure 10.3).

The ten areas take place across three domains: food environment, food system, and behaviour change communication. Each domain is important in influencing what people eat. The rationale for inclusion of these three areas was set out clearly when the policy framework was first developed.[7] Food environments have a significant influence on dietary patterns. Different aspects of food environments—whether it is a mix of shops and food outlets in a neighbourhood or the array of products produced and promoted by food companies—influence what is available and affordable. This, in turn, influences what people eat. Policy areas in relation to food environments address issues such as nutrition labelling, nutrition standards for food in public institutions, economic tools such as taxes/subsidies on unhealthy or healthy foods, restricting food advertising, changing the nutritional content of food products, and policies to create a healthier food retail and catering environment. The second domain in the framework is the food system, which exerts influence on food availability, affordability, and acceptability through, for example, agriculture, trade, and other upstream policies

NOURIS		H	ING
FOOD ENVIRONMENT		FOOD SYSTEM	BEHAVIOUR CHANGE
	POLICY AREA		
N	Nutrition label standards and regulations on the use of claims and implied claims on foods		
O	Offer healthy foods and set standards in public institutions and other specific settings		
U	Use economic tools to address food affordability and purchase incentives		
R	Restrict food advertising and other forms of commercial promotion		
I	Improve nutritional quality of the whole food supply		
S	Set incentives and rules to create a healthy retail and food service environment		
H	Harness supply chain and actions across sectors to ensure coherence with health		
I	Inform people about food and nutrition through public awareness		
N	Nutrition advice and counselling in health care settings		
G	Give nutrition education and skills		

Figure 10.3 The NOURISHING Framework.

Reproduced with permission from **World Cancer Research Fund International**. 'NOURISHING framework', http://www.wcrf.org/int/policy/nourishing-framework, accessed 20 Jul. 2016, Copyright © 2015 World Cancer Research Fund International.

such as supply chain logistics. The third aspect is behaviour change communication, relating to the provision of information, education, literacy, and skills to encourage behaviour change, complementary to action of food environments and food systems.

The NOURISHING policy database was initially developed on the basis of experience in 11 countries, but now includes more than 260 implemented government policy actions across over 100 countries (as of April 2016). The database is updated quarterly. World Cancer Research Fund International has a two-stage process for populating and updating the database. The first stage involves a structured approach to sourcing and reviewing policy actions intended to promote healthy diets and reduce overweight/obesity. The second stage is to verify the details of the policy actions with in-country or regional representatives to ensure the policy action has actually been implemented. The methods for updating and populating the database, including the verification process, will be made publicly available in 2016.

NOURISHING is intended to help policy-makers, civil society, and researchers. It aims to help policy-makers to identify where action is needed, select and tailor options, and, importantly, see what other countries are doing. It is also intended to be a tool for civil society to monitor what governments are doing, benchmark progress, and hold governments to account. For researchers, the database will enable them to identify the available evidence, identify research gaps, and use that for policy monitoring and evaluation.

Source: **Hawkes C**, **Jewell J**, and **Allen K**. A food policy package for healthy diets and the prevention of obesity and diet-related non-communicable diseases: the NOURISHING framework. *Obesity Reviews*, Volume 14, Issue S2, pp. 159–168, Copyright © 2013 C Hawkes et al.

Acknowledgements

This chapter draws on presentations by Professor Mike Rayner and Professor Steven Allender and incorporates material supplied by Simone Bösch, World Cancer Research Fund International.

References

1. **Simmons A, Mavoa HM, Bell AC, De Courten A, Schaff D, Schultz J, Swinburn BA.** Creating community action plans for obesity prevention using the ANGELO (Analysis Grid for Elements Linked to Obesity) Framework. *Health Promotion International.* 2009: **24**(4): 311–24
2. **World Health Organization.** *Prioritizing areas for action in the field of population-based prevention of childhood obesity: A set of tools for Member States to determine and identify priority areas for action.* Geneva: World Health Organization, 2012.
3. **Swinburn B, Gill T, Kumanyika S.** Obesity prevention: a proposed framework for translating evidence into action. *Obesity Reviews.* 2005; **6**:23–33.
4. **De Silva-Sanigorski AM, Bell AC, Kremer P, Nichols M, Crellin M, Smith M, Sharp S, de Groot F, Carpenter L, Boak R, Robertson N, Swinburn BA.** Reducing obesity in early childhood: results from Romp & Chomp, an Australian community-wide intervention program. *Am J Clin Nutrition.* 2010 Apr;**91**(4):831–40.
5. **Sanigorski AM, Bell AC, Kremer PJ, Cuttler R, Swinburn BA.** Reducing unhealthy weight gain in children through community capacity-building: results of a quasi-experimental intervention program, Be Active Eat Well. *Int J Obes (Lond)*, 2008 Jul;**32**(7):1060–7.
6. **Millar L**, et al. Reduction in overweight and obesity from a 3-year community-based intervention in Australia: the 'It's Your Move! project'. *Obesity Reviews* **12**.s2 (2011): 20–28.
7. **Hawkes C, Jewell J, Allen K** (2013). A food policy package for healthy diets and the prevention of obesity and diet-related non-communicable diseases: the NOURISHING framework. *Obesity Reviews* **14** (Suppl. 2), 159–68. Accessible free of charge on Wiley Online Library (http://bit.ly/23uqaxY).

Further reading

On strategy and priority setting:

Swinburn B, Gill T, Kumanyika S. Obesity prevention: a proposed framework for translating evidence into action. *Obesity Reviews* 2005; **6**:23–33.

World Health Organization. *Prioritizing Areas for Action in the Field of Population-Based Prevention of Childhood Obesity: A Set of Tools for Member States to Determine and Identify Priority Areas for Action.* Geneva: World Health Organization, 2012.

Rose G. *Rose's Strategy of Preventive Medicine.* Revised edition with commentary from Kay-Tee Khaw and Michael Marmot. Oxford: Oxford University Press, 2008.

For more information on NOURISHING see www.wcrf.org/nourishing

Part IV

Resource mobilization and implementation

Chapter 11

Capacity building

11.1 Capacity building

Capacity building emerged as a key concept in international development in the 1990s, with an emphasis on supporting people and communities to be able to solve their own problems. The 1986 Ottawa Charter for Health Promotion was important in the development of capacity building as a key concept for health, in that it acknowledged that people are the principal resource for health.

Community capacity building, also known as capacity development, is defined as 'a conceptual approach to development that focuses on the understanding of obstacles that inhibit people, governments, international organizations, and non-governmental organizations from achieving their development goals while enhancing their ability to achieve measurable and sustainable results'.[1]

As the definition suggests, although it is important to build the capacity of individuals, capacity building should be seen as a much wider concept which also incorporates change to communities, systems, and environments. The United Nations Development Programme (UNDP) sets out three levels of capacity that are required for 'individuals, institutions and societies to perform functions, solve problems, and achieve objectives in a sustainable manner':

- Enabling environment (social system, laws, policies, power relations);
- Organization/structure (internal structure, policies, and procedures); and
- Individual (skills, experience, knowledge).[2]

Many potential responses are available to build capacity at each level. Clearly different solutions are needed when it comes to building knowledge and skills of individuals than are needed to generate change in the enabling environment. UNDP has identified four core issues—institutional arrangements, leadership, knowledge, and accountability—all of which need to be underpinned by information and knowledge. The essential five steps in the capacity building process are shown in Figure 11.1.

In addition to building institutional capacity, building the capacity of young professionals and health advocates needs to be part of a long-term strategy. Examples of three different attempts to achieve this are shown in the three case studies in this chapter.

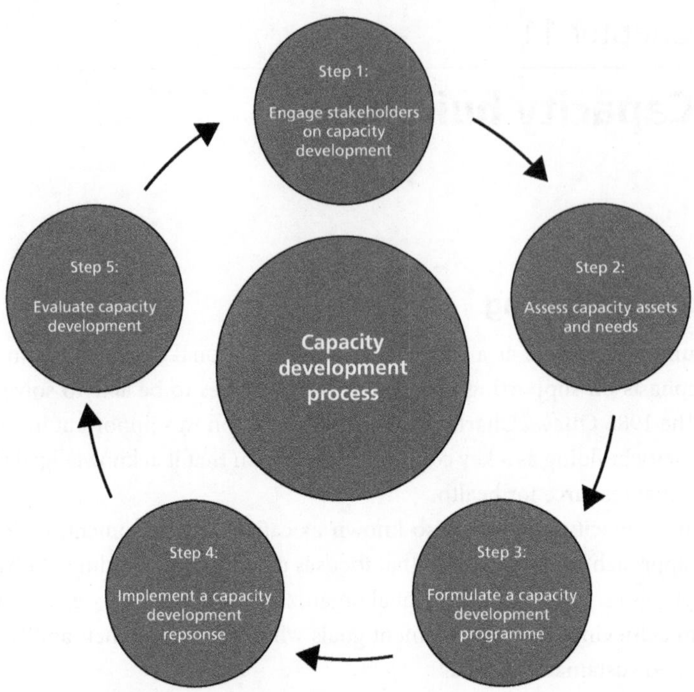

Figure 11.1 A process for capacity building.

Case study: The Young Professionals–Chronic Disease Network (YP-CDN)

The Young Professionals–Chronic Disease Network (YP-CDN) is a civil society organization whose mission is to mobilize a global community of young leaders to take action against the social injustice driving non-communicable diseases (NCDs).

Its members—over 6,000—are young-minded professionals from around the globe in over 150 nations working in diverse fields (within and outside of health care), who are dedicated to policy analysis, advocacy, and social change. YP-CDN unifies these professionals and gives them the tools, resources, and powerful connections needed to confront and change the social injustices that contribute to making NCDs the leading cause of death worldwide.

YP-CDN believes that every person—regardless of income or geographic location—has the right to preventive measures (such as a healthy environment or healthy foods), as well as to medicines, vaccines, and technologies for treating NCDs. The global community has advanced the NCD agenda in some ways; yet, we still have a long way to go to prevent and treat NCDs adequately and more equitably across and within countries.

In particular, YP-CDN equips the next generation with the knowledge, technical skills, networks, and experiences they will need to impact policies and changes within their own communities and countries. This is achieved through trainings and advocacy campaigns through local chapters in places such as Boston (USA), Mexico City (Mexico), Lucknow (India), Lagos (Nigeria), Kampala (Uganda), Kigali (Rwanda), Addis Ababa (Ethiopia), and Nairobi, Eldoret, and Thika (all in Kenya).

The organization has invested in the preparation of future leaders through a Next Generational Leaders programme that will equip emerging leaders in the East African region with the tools to lead advocacy and action on NCDs, while providing the technical knowledge and evidence needed to lead lasting improvements in policy for health. In particular, it aims to prepare cohorts of young people to help governments hit the 80% essential medicines availability target described in the WHO NCD Action Plan and advance the implementation of NCD plans and strategies in East Africa.

For more information see http://ypchronic.org/.

Case study: The NCDFREE crowd-funded, crowd-sourced global social movement for a world free from preventable noncommunicable diseases

In 2013 brothers Sandro and Guiseppe Demaio successfully raised funds through an online Indiegogo crowdfunding campaign to launch NCDFREE at the University of Melbourne's Festival of Ideas. Concerned by the pressing need for action to tackle the leading global cause of death and motivated to raise awareness and address widespread misunderstandings about NCDs, the doctor and designer sibling team launched NCDFREE to change the way society perceives NCDs and inspire a new generation of young, community-level change-makers.

NCDFREE is a global social movement, in partnership with design agency Local Peoples, the Harvard Global Equity Initiative, the University of Melbourne, and the Copenhagen School of Global Health. Combining Global Health and medical know-how with designed-to-inspire communication techniques—and with support from global health and communication professionals—NCDFREE proposes a variety of innovative solutions.

Bootcamps are organized to bring young professionals and students together to address NCDs through a lens of global health, sustainability, and community action. By 2016, such advocacy, innovation, and leadership bootcamps had been held in Melbourne, Sydney, Brisbane, London, Ottawa, Cairo, and Copenhagen. The camps are designed to create links between the next generation of change-makers and community leaders from a wide range of sectors and to build capacity in advocacy, innovative thinking, and leadership. Additionally, the bootcamps are a means for NCDFREE to crowdsource new solutions and ideas from camp participants—in other words, NCDFREE gets camp participants to do some work. Bootcamp activities include 'Ted talk'-inspired presentations from emerging local leaders, panel discussions, group exercises, and 60-minute incubation sessions—where the ideas of bootcampers from all backgrounds converge, co-create, and come alive.

At the first camp in Melbourne, for example, the 50 participants were split into working groups and asked to come up with a pitch for a campaign to mobilize the millennial generation to bring about social change. The various pitches were judged by an expert panel and the winning pitch was for a humorous campaign 'Breaking up with Alcohol' intended to provoke discussion about young people's relationship with alcohol. NCDFREE then offered the winning team financial and practical support in order to turn the pitch into a real campaign.

Another idea for bringing young professionals and students together is the 'long lunch'. NCDFREE organizes these gatherings in order for young change-makers to share an afternoon meal and to hear about and discuss important NCD issues. After the initial launch in Melbourne, the event progressed to Sydney, Copenhagen, and Giessen focusing on topics such as community medicine, mental health, and diabetes.

On social media, NCDFREE launched the #theface campaign in October 2014 to 'put a face to the world's biggest global health challenge'.[3] This crowdsourced campaign invited people to share their photos and stories of how their lives had been touched by NCDs. In one month the campaign reached over a million people in more than 50 countries and hundreds of stories were shared. In its 2016 campaign NCDFREE aims to use food to bring people together to engage in NCDs on a global scale.

With an important social media presence, NCDFREE has over 12,000 followers on social media with over 1.5 million organic impressions on Twitter and Facebook between January 2015 and May 2016. Creation of infographics, blogging, production of a fortnightly newsletter, and promotion of live events through Instagram and Periscope are other communication tools NCDFREE uses to spread latest news and key messages about NCDs.

NCDFREE also communicates through the medium of short film. Advocacy films—aimed at sharing the personal narratives of inspiring young people in countries such as Peru, Mongolia, Sri Lanka, USA, Mexico, and Ghana—have been produced, tackling issues such as migrant health, sugar taxes, and indigenous population health. In the first 18 months of NCDFREE ten short films were produced, and more than 2.5 million people were reached.

For more information see http://ncdfree.org/.

Case study: Engaging medical students in prevention and control of NCDs in the Emirate of Sharjah

In order to foster understanding of NCDs among future doctors, and to build their capacity for prevention and control, the University of Sharjah, in the United Arab Emirates, has designed two programmes to engage medical students.

First-year students are introduced to a variety of prevention health services in the Emirate of Sharjah and surrounding areas through Health Awareness Week and World Health Day events. Through participation in a range of activities, students develop a greater awareness of prevention health services, communities, and practices. These experiences help the students to develop an understanding of the mechanisms and issues involved in providing prevention health services to various populations as well as identifying areas in need of improvement.

During this week, students celebrate World Health Day through a wide variety of activities. These actives are observe and practice under supervision at selected prevention health-care organizations, and attend presentations on different prevention health services in the UAE, such as health services (in general), maternal and child health services including immunization, health education and promotion, and preventive services. During the last two days of this week, students are divided into groups and subgroups that are assigned to prepare presentations, posters, and an educational videos on various aspects related to the week's activities.

The university has also designed a community health programme (CHP) for third-year medical students, in order to enhance and strengthen their understanding of

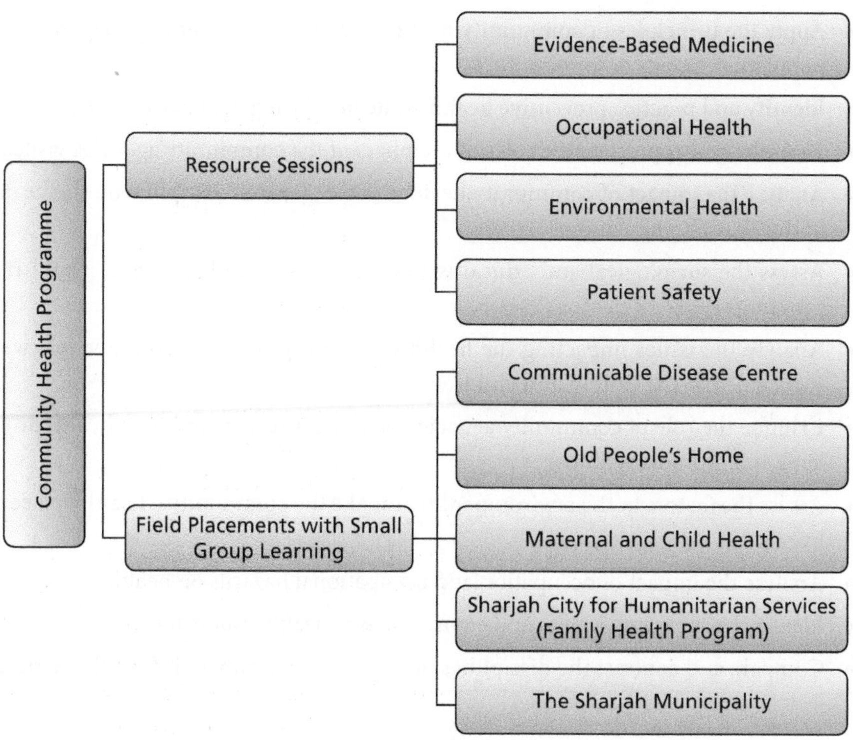

Figure 11.2 Community health programme for third-year medical students.

prevention concepts (to which they had been introduced in their first year). The programme aims to provide the students with essential knowledge, skills, and attitudes to community health through field activities, classroom sessions, and self-directed assignments.

The scope of the programme is depicted in Figure 11.2. These activities examine the scope and potential impact of community health as an organized health-care intervention and discipline, encompassing theory and practice. The focus of attention is on common preventive activities to address the needs of vulnerable populations, i.e. people with special needs, those living with chronic and disabling disease states, elderly people, maternal and child health, and socioeconomically disadvantaged groups. Students also explore ethical issues associated with health and health risk prevention, as well as issues impacting these community groups, and contributing environmental and occupational factors and problems. The role of community health agencies and programmes related to all levels of prevention and health promotion is also examined.

By the end of the CHP in year 3, students are expected to:

- Appreciate the role of community health in clinical medical practice;
- Identify the main concepts, principles, components, and strategies of community health;
- Apply the principles of community health assessment (community diagnosis) on population groups or families;
- Identify and practice preventive health strategies during field placements;
- Describe and appreciate the roles of members of the community agencies visited;
- Analyse the impact of community health as an organized discipline on the health of the Sharjah population;
- Assess the sociological and ethical issues associated with health and health risk prevention;
- Analyse the issues impacting the health of special groups including people with special needs, the elderly, and children;
- Critique the role of community agencies to assess, prevent, and treat health problems and promote wellness;
- Assess the factors in the environment that make the community a healthy place to live in;
- Analyse the impact of occupation and occupational hazards on health;
- Identify major occupational and environmental health issues; and
- Compare and contrast the disciplines of community health and clinical practice.

11.2 **A systems approach**

It is important to acknowledge that the problem of NCDs exists within a highly complex system. This means that the responses in turn need to be complex. Each intervention needs to be considered as one piece of the solution, rather than viewed as the entire solution. This perspective, which recognizes the complexity of the problem and required solutions, is called a systems approach. When considering efforts to improve public health, there are five different levels where interventions can be made (see Box 11.1). Most commonly interventions tend to tackle the structural elements of level 1—focusing, for example, on particular operational elements, such as smoking cessation and access to affordable food. Changing the paradigm (level 5), in contrast, means completely changing the way we understand a problem, and how to respond to it. An example of this type of change would be the transformation in understanding of the issue of exposure to second-hand tobacco smoke and the way in which this change in understanding enabled the acceptance and introduction of more effective responses.

A systems approach recognizes the interconnectedness of different elements and stresses the importance of different relationships, links, feedback loops, and other interactions. A systems-thinking perspective can be useful because it allows a better understanding of the system as a whole, rather than focusing on any specific detail, and of how things change over time. This approach was initially developed to enable a more nuanced understanding of highly complex issues such as climate change. As shown previously with the causal webs in Chapter 3, the development of NCDs is also highly complex and thus amenable to a systems approach.

To help understand exactly what systems thinking means in practice, the Waters Foundation has compiled some resources for schools, including a list of habits of a systems thinker and useful questions to consider.[4]

To illustrate the complexity of solutions required, Figure 11.3 shows the milestones in reducing prevalence of tobacco smoking in Australians aged 14 years or older between 1991 and 2013. This suggests that no one element—pricing, advertising bans, changing attitudes, or stronger epidemiological evidence—can be picked out as being the sole driver of declining smoking rates. Australia's response to reducing smoking has been complex and involved many different elements.

Box 11.1 Levels for public health interventions

- **Structural elements**: individual variables, actors and subsystems.
- **Feedback and delays:** reinforcing and balancing feedback loops.
- **Structure of the system as a whole:** variables, connections and networks.
- **Goals:** What the system is trying to achieve.
- **Paradigm:** Changes in the way we understand the problem, leading to a complex systems approach and appropriate solutions for such complex problems.

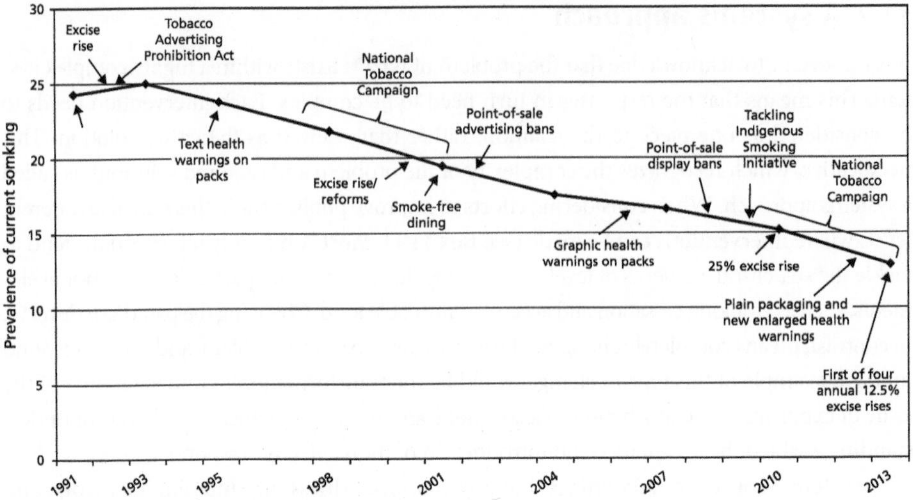

Figure 11.3 Milestones in reducing smoking in Australia 1990–2014.

Reproduced with permission from Appendix 1.6 'Smoking prevalence and tobacco control in Australia'. In: **Scollo MM** and **Winstanley MH** (eds.), *Tobacco in Australia Facts and Issues. History of tobacco in Australia*, Melbourne: Cancer Cancer Victoria, Copyright © 2016 Cancer Council Victoria, http://www.tobaccoinaustralia.org.au/appendix-1/a1-6-history-of-tobacco-in-australia/a1-6-prevalence-and-tobacco-control.html, accessed 16 Nov. 2016.

11.3 **Translating strategies that work into low- or middle-income settings**

It is clear that differences between cultures, settings, and populations—coupled with rapid epidemiological transitions—mean that a one-size approach will not fit all when it comes to translating NCD interventions from one setting to another. This means that interventions that have been shown to be effective in, for example, a high-income setting must be feasible for 'real world implementation' in a resource-poor context. This is the challenge of translation to a low- or middle-income (LMIC) setting. An influential paper on the lessons for LMICs from high-income countries' experience in implementing NCD programmes identified a number of key issues (Box 11.2).[5]

When interventions are adopted in a new context, they need to be culturally tailored so that they are appropriate (see example of a programme translated from Finland to Kerala in Box 11.3). Failure to ensure that programmes are culturally attuned can seriously hamper the effectiveness of the intervention.

Acknowledgements

This chapter draws on presentations by Professor Harry Rutter, Professor David Matthews, and Professor Brian Oldenburg with case study material provided by Dr Alessandro de Maio, Dr Sandeep Kishore, and Professor Nabil Sulaiman.

Box 11.2 Recommendations for NCD prevention programmes

- **Community diagnosis**—work with the community to combine the epidemiological data with risk factor profiles and a study of what the community needs to establish a diagnosis.
- **Multicomponent strategies**—strategies should combine a broad range of activities.
- **Dose**—An effective quantity or administration level of the intervention is needed.
- **Multilevel**—individual, environmental, and policy changes are important.
- **Monitoring and evaluation**—good and reliable monitoring and evaluation system are essential.
- **Dissemination and upscale**—use effective interventions as demonstration programmes to achieve impact on a wider scale.
- **Collaboration and networks**—sharing through international collaboration and other networks is valuable.

Source: data from **Nissinen A**, **Berrios X**, and **Puska P**. Community-based noncommunicable disease interventions: lessons from developed countries for developing ones. *Bulletin of the World Health Organization*, Volume 79, Issue 10, pp. 963–970, Copyright © 2001 World Health Organization.

Box 11.3 Preventing diabetes in Kerala, India

Prevalence of type 2 diabetes is a major public health challenge in the state of Kerala, India. A community-based diabetes prevention programme (the K-DPP programme), incorporating group-based peer support, is being implemented.[6] The programme is modelled on a diabetes prevention programme initially developed in Finland, then scaled up in Finland and Australia, and draws on other programmes in China and the United States.

Analysis of the Indian and Kerala contexts and community meetings during the piloting phase informed the process of adapting the programme to the specific situation.[7] The team realized, for example, that the group they had hoped to interest in the intervention (at-risk individuals) considered themselves to be healthy and were not interested in participating. The high prevalence of diabetes, however, meant that nearly everyone had a family member affected by the disease. As a result, the programme was adapted to offer women the opportunity to learn more about the condition, to help other family members manage the condition, and to learn about prevention. Another key difference is that the programme was designed not to be dependent on people coming into health services. Instead, methods of taking services to the population were developed, and mobile clinics have proved popular.

References

1. **Capacity building**. In *Wikipedia, The Free Encyclopedia*. Available at: http://en.wikipedia.org/wiki/Capacity_building. Accessed 5 October 2016.
2. **United Nations Development Programme**. *Capacity Development: A UNDP Primer*. New York: United Nations, 2009.
3. The face of NCDS. N.p., 2016. Available at: http://www.thefaceofncds.org. Accessed 29 October 2016.
4. **Waters Foundation**. Habits of a systems thinker. N.p., 2016. Available at: http://watersfoundation.org/systems-thinking/habits-of-a-systems-thinker/. Accessed 29 October 2016.
5. **Nissinen A, Berrios X, Puska P.** Community-based Noncommunicable disease interventions: lessons from developed countries for developing ones. *Bulletin of the World Health Organization* 2001; 79:963–70.
6. Based on presentation by Professor Brian Oldenburg, Monash University, Australia.
7. **Daviadanam M, Absetz P, Satish T, Thankappan KR, Fisher EB, Philip NE** et al. Lifestyle change in Kerala, India: needs assessment and planning for a community-based diabetes prevention trial. *BMC Public Health* 2013; 13:95.

Chapter 12

Implementation of an NCD prevention strategy

12.1 Defining implementation

Implementation can be defined as a specified set of activities designed to put into practice an intervention or policy of known dimensions. According to this definition, implementation processes are purposeful and are described in sufficient detail such that independent observers can detect the presence of the 'specific set of activities' related to implementation. Another element is that the intervention or policy being implemented is described in sufficient detail for independent observers to be able to detect its presence and strength.[1]

There are different ways of thinking about the purposes and outcomes of implementation. Some may pursue 'paper implementation', focusing on new policies and procedures, and a paper trail, which is helpful for monitoring but may not result in putting innovation into practice. Others may focus on 'process implementation', with an emphasis on putting new operating procedures into place—this means that the planned activities are happening, but these may not all be functionally related to the new policy or intervention. Changing health service structures and systems, for example, might not of itself result in a change of culture and practice that enhances the focus on prevention. Implementation that produces actual benefits and results (performance implementation) needs more a more careful, thoughtful approach.[1]

A relatively new field of science and research has emerged to help investigate and improve the implementation process—by, for example, developing strategies and tools or by studying how interventions are implemented in practice. This field also studies how the process of translating evidence-based interventions into policy and practice can be accelerated, taking into account realities on the ground. Implementation science aims to identify the factors, processes, and methods that facilitate successful implementation of evidence-based interventions into policy and practice to improve population health.[2]

This type of research (implementation research) is important for a number of reasons. When implementation of a policy or intervention fails, for example, it is key to be able to understand why. It is important to be able to judge whether the intervention failed because it was not effective in the particular context in question (intervention failure) or because it was not deployed properly (implementation failure).

A number of frameworks and theories have emerged from this research, and through the learning from decades of experience of trying to implement evidence-based policies or interventions. These can be useful in guiding the planning and organization of implementation.

One such framework, the Consolidated Framework for Implementation Research (CFIR) developed by Damschroder and colleagues, identifies five main domains that are critical to successful implementation, and a number of constructs within each of these domains.[3] The CIFR provides a useful list of factors to consider when considering how to implement a plan or policy.

The domains and constructs of the CIFR:

- Intervention characteristics (e.g. where the intervention comes from; strength and quality of evidence; perceived relative advantage compared to alternatives; adaptability to local needs; trialability—ability to test on a small scale and to undo implementation if needed; design quality and packaging; cost);
- The outer setting (patient needs and resources; networking with other organizations; peer pressure; external policy; and incentives such as regulations, guidelines, or recommendations);
- The inner setting (structural characteristics; networks and communications; culture; implementation climate; and readiness for implementation including leadership engagement, available resources, and access to knowledge/information);
- The characteristics of the individuals involved (knowledge; self-efficacy (self belief); stage of change; identification with organization; and other personal attributes); and
- The process of implementation (planning; engaging (opinion leaders, implementation leaders, champions, and external change agents); executing; reflecting; and evaluating).

There is often a need for guidance to fill the information gap between research that shows interventions work and understanding of how to put them into practice. Guidelines are often needed to help with implementation—how to translate theory into reality in policy and/or practice on the ground. Sometimes problems with implementation are not related to a lack of information, rather they are self-evident but there can also be a 'knowing-doing gap', a failure to translate knowledge into action.

The World Health Organization is producing a practical guide to implementation which gives pragmatic advice for those seeking to implement policies or interventions.

12.2 Strengthening health systems for NCD prevention and control

National health systems have an important role to play in the response to non-communicable diseases (NCDs). One of the objectives of the Global NCD Action Plan is to 'strengthen and orient health systems to address the prevention and control of NCDs and the underlying social determinants through people-centred primary health care and universal health coverage.'[4] The action plan goes on to specify that this means improved prevention, early detection, treatment, and sustained management of people with, or at high risk of, NCDs.

Health systems will be required to contribute to many different aspects of national strategies, but have an especially key role in attainment of three in particular of the Global NCD Action Plan's voluntary targets:

- At least 50% of all eligible people receive drug therapy and counselling (including glycaemic control) to prevent heart attack and strokes;
- An 80% availability of the affordable basic technologies and essential medicines, including generics, required to treat major NCDs in both public and private facilities; and
- A 25% relative reduction in the prevalence of raised blood pressure or containment of the prevalence of raised blood pressure, according to national circumstances.

12.3 What do we mean by health systems?

The World Health Organization (WHO) puts forward two definitions for a health system:

- All the activities whose primary purpose is to promote, restore, and/or maintain health; and
- The people, institutions, and resources, arranged together in accordance with established policies, to improve the health of the population they serve, while responding to people's legitimate expectations and protecting them against the cost of ill-health through a variety of activities whose primary intent is to improve health.[5]

The multiple roles of health systems include treating illness, preventing illness, promoting health, rehabilitation and care for people with disabilities, monitoring illness, monitoring or evaluating treatment and prevention, and finding effective and practical solutions. In many countries, however, the vision of the role of health systems has traditionally been much narrower—focusing on the hospital-based curative aspects, principally designed to treat communicable disease and trauma. Where prevention was considered at all, this was most likely to have been in relation to maternal and child health and infectious diseases.

Case study: Cardiovascular risk assessment among refugees in Jordan

Since the outbreak of the civil war in Syria, nearly one million official refugees have settled in Jordan, most of whom live outside of refugee camps in urban and rural areas. A cross-sectional survey of Syrian refugees (2014) estimated that more than half of Syrian refugee households in Jordan had at least one member with an NCD and although care seeking was high, cost was identified as the main barrier to seeking healthcare.[6] Since the burden of NCDs amongst refugees, and the associated cost for care, was so high, *Médecins Sans Frontières* (MSF) opened two outpatient primary health-care clinics in the Irbid Governorate of Jordan specifically targeting urban refugees and vulnerable Jordanians with NCDs.

Chronic disease care in humanitarian settings is largely unprecedented; as such, MSF developed its own NCD guidance for use in these clinics with a focus on CVD, diabetes, hypertension, chronic obstructive pulmonary disease, and asthma. Many aspects of MSF's guidance were based on the World Health Organization's (WHO) Package of Essential NCD Interventions for Primary Health Care in Low-Resource Settings (WHO PEN),[7] most notably from Protocol One for the prevention and management of CVD.[8] This protocol includes total cardiovascular risk assessment charts developed by the WHO and the International Society of Hypertension (WHO/ISH), and guidance for their use.[8,9]

WHO PEN provides a suite of tools and clinical protocols for the integrated management of NCDs in primary care, and for many low- and middle-income countries (LMICs) offers the only available standard of practice tailored for low-resource settings. As WHO PEN standards—and NCD control strategies in low-resource settings in general—are continually evolving, it is important to generate evidence of their effectiveness in new contexts.

In order to evaluate and improve MSF's NCD guidance, a mixed methods clinical audit of MSF's NCD mission in Jordan was carried out. A collaboration between the Centre for Evidence Based Medicine (Oxford), MSF (Operational Centre Amsterdam and Jordanian Country Management Team), and the Jordanian Ministry of Health was developed to ensure key stakeholders were engaged with a vision towards coordinated guideline development at a national or regional level. Given the unprecedented nature of NCD prevention in humanitarian settings, the audit focused on service development and consisted of both quantitative and qualitative strands. The quantitative analysis used routinely collected clinical data to determine the adoption and adherence to total cardiovascular risk assessment, which is a key component of integrated CVD prevention. Semi-structured interviews of clinical staff to explore reasons for discordance from guidance and to help inform the update of clinical guidance were conducted.

The most immediate beneficiaries of this work are the patients of the clinics which were audited, as results are being used to improve the quality of care in these settings. This work is relevant to a larger audience given the scale of the Syrian refugee community, the growing provision of NCD health care in humanitarian settings, and the increasing use of WHO/ISH CVD risk charts in the Eastern Mediterranean.

When complete, the audit will result in published recommendations for the use of total cardiovascular risk assessment for the prevention of CVD in humanitarian settings. Knowledge translation will occur through academic publications, lay summaries, presentations to key stakeholder groups, and at academic conferences.

This work will help to inform national, regional, and humanitarian guidelines for NCD prevention in low-resource settings. Given that NCD prevention and control in low-resource settings, not least humanitarian settings, is an area with limited evidence, this project will help generate evidence that is directly relevant to the humanitarian sector, and national and regional organizations in the Eastern Mediterranean.

12.4 Building health systems to face the NCD challenge

Health systems need to adapt and evolve to respond effectively to the growing challenge of NCDs. There are many challenges facing health systems trying to adapt in this way. These include, but are not limited to:

- Shortage of skilled human resources (new health worker roles may be needed);
- Inadequate infrastructure;
- Lack of tools;
- Resistance to change within the health system; and
- Funding and resources gap.

The previous case study from Jordan and the experience in Anhui Province, China (Box 12.1) highlight two examples of national health systems seeking to adapt to the NCD challenge. A number of important elements in the process have been identified.

Box 12.1 Community-based peer support to improving diabetes self-management in Anhui Province, China

In Anhui Province, China, a community-based programme to improve diabetes self-management supplements primary care services with peer support from people living with diabetes within the community. In the communities selected for the programme the aim was to establish a primary health services team, with very simple facilities and providing a limited range of services, in every building. Their remit includes health education and the management of NCDs. To supplement the activities of these teams, over 700 diabetic patients were recruited to give peer support. By leading or co-leading group activities (sometimes bringing several buildings together), organizing meetings and linking group members with the community health centre the peer supporters help people to manage their conditions, provide social and emotional support, and help people access primary care services.

12.4.1 Equipping the health workforce

Equipping the health workforce to tackle NCDs will be an important element of health system adaptation. Health professionals may need a new set of skills. The Global NCD Action Plan highlights a number of policy options in relation to human resources:

- Identifying the competencies required and investing in improving the knowledge, skills, and motivation of existing health workers to address NCDs;
- Incorporating the prevention and control of NCDs in all health worker training, with an emphasis on primary care, and developing specialist post-graduate NCD training;
- Providing adequate compensation and incentives for health workers to provide services in underserved areas;
- Ensure adequate deployment of a skilled health workforce, by promoting the production, training, and retention of health workers in line with the WHO Global Code of Practice on the International Recruitment of Health Personnel; and
- Optimizing the role of nurses and allied health professionals in prevention and control of NCDs.

12.4.2 Health financing

Strong and sustainable health systems require a solid funding base. The Global NCD Action Plan outlines some policy options for financing health systems. These promote a shift from reliance on charging patients (user fees) to systems based on pooled contributions and prepayments (e.g. health insurance, tax funding, cash transfers, and health savings schemes). Such systems should include preventive, curative, and palliative services at all levels of the health system, and should cover NCDs.

12.4.3 Organization of quality services

In terms of improving the efficiency, equity, and coverage of quality health services, the Global NCD Action Plan highlights a number of policy options:

- Organize services around close-to-user and people-centred primary health care, which is fully integrated with secondary and tertiary care systems;
- Enable all providers (including non-governmental organizations (NGOs) and private and non-profit providers) to address NCDs and harness potential of wide array of other services to deal with these conditions;
- Improve efficiency of service delivery to increase coverage of NCD interventions, linking NCD services with other disease-specific programmes;
- Develop innovative, effective, and integrated models of long-term care for people with NCDs, connecting community-based services with primary care and other health services;
- Establish quality assurance and improvement for NCD prevention and management (e.g. use of evidence-based guidelines, treatment protocols, management tools);

- Provide incentives and tools for self-care and self-management of NCDs;
- Review existing programmes (e.g. on nutrition, HIV, tuberculosis, sexual and reproductive health, maternal and child health, mental health) and, where possible, integrate NCD prevention and control services.

Health services clearly have a key role to play, yet it is important to recognize that strong health systems alone will not be able to tackle NCDs. Community engagement and mobilization are also vital. People need to be involved in the development of appropriate services, and be supportive of changes, for strategies to be successful. Innovative ways to involve communities in programmes are needed, such as involvement of peer educators or peer support workers. Multisectoral action, which extends beyond the health sector, is also of fundamental importance (see Chapter 13).

12.5 Tackling inequalities

Previous sections have highlighted the widespread social inequalities in health and the broad range of social, economic, cultural, and environmental determinants contributing

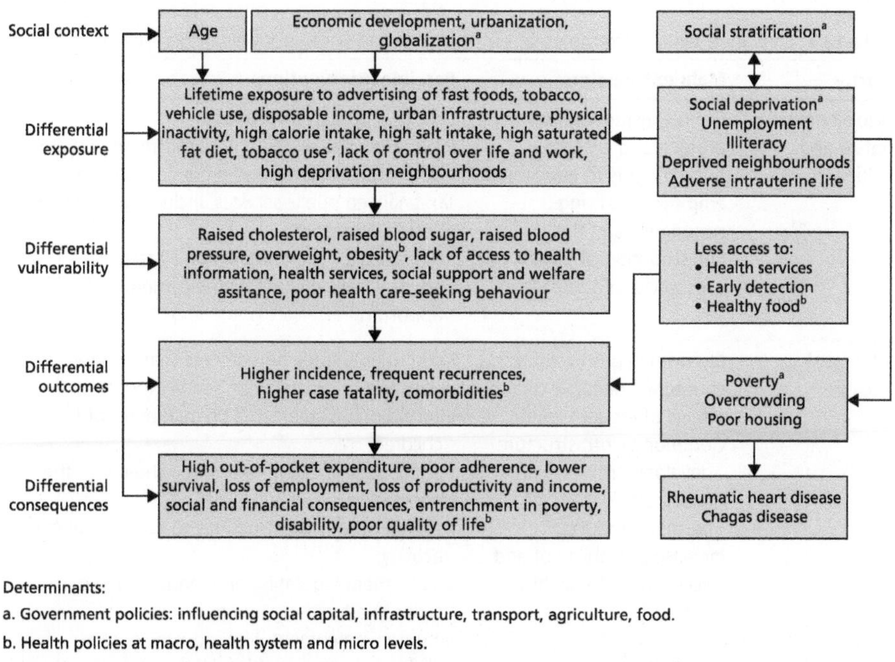

Figure 12.1 Conceptual framework for understanding health inequalities, pathways, and entry-points.

Reproduced with permission from Mendis S and Banerjee A. Cardiovascular disease: equity and social determinants. In: Blas E and Kurup AS (Eds.), *Equity, social determinants and public health programmes*. Geneva: WHO, http://apps.who.int/iris/bitstream/10665/44289/1/9789241563970_eng.pdf, accessed 20 Jul. 2016, Copyright © 2010 World Health Organization.

to these inequalities. The fact that many inequities are socially produced gives grounds for optimism that they can also be prevented.

As outlined previously, the Commission on the Social Determinants of Health made three overarching recommendations:

- Improve daily living conditions;
- Tackle the inequitable distribution of power, money, and resources; and
- Measure and understand the problem and assess the impact of action.

The very broad scope of these recommendations highlights the importance of a multisectoral, whole-government approach to reducing health inequalities. A conceptual framework for inequalities in relation to cardiovascular disease is shown in Figure 12.1.

More concrete ideas for action can be found in a 2010 WHO report identifying a number of entry points for tackling health inequalities and possible interventions (Table 12.1). Both the table and the framework relate specifically to CVD, but many of the points may be equally applicable to other NCDs.

Table 12.1 CVD inequalities: Examples of entry points and some possible interventions

Priority	Main entry points	Possible interventions
Socioeconomic context and position	Define, institutionalize, protect, and enforce human rights to education, employment, living conditions, and health; Redistribution of power and resources in populations.	Universal primary education; Programmes to alleviate undernutrition in women of childbearing age and pregnant women; Tax-financed public services, including education and health; Multifaceted poverty reduction strategies at country level, including employment opportunities.
Differential exposure	Strengthen positive and counteract negative health effects of modernization; Community infrastructure development; Reduce affordability of harmful products; Increase availability of and accessibility to healthy food.	International trade agreements that promote availability and affordability of healthy foods; International agreements on marketing of food to children; Use tobacco tax for promotion of health of the population; Develop urban infrastructures to facilitate physical activity; Government legislation and regulation, e.g. tobacco advertising and pricing; Voluntary agreement with industry, e.g. trans fats and salt in processed food; User-friendly food labelling to help customers to make healthy food choices.

(continued)

Table 12.1 Continued

Priority	Main entry points	Possible interventions
Differential vulnerability	Subsidize healthy items to make healthy choices easy choices; Compensate for lack of opportunities; Empower people.	Provide healthy meals free or subsidized to schoolchildren; Subsidize fruits and vegetables in worksite canteens and restaurants; Facilitate a price structure of food commodities to promote health, e.g. lower price for low-fat milk; Improve early case detection of individuals with diabetes and hypertension by targeting vulnerable groups, e.g. deprived neighbourhoods, slum dwellers; Improve population access to health promotion by targeting vulnerable groups in health education programmes; Combine poverty reduction strategies with incentives for utilization of preventive services, e.g. conditional cash transfers, vouchers; Provide social insurance and fee exemptions for basic preventive and curative health interventions; Education and employment opportunities for women.
Differential health-care outcomes	Medical procedures; Provider practices: compensate for differential outcomes.	Increase awareness among providers of ethical norms and patient rights; Provide universal access to a package of essential CVD interventions through a primary health-care approach; Provide incentives within public and private health systems to increase equity in outcome, e.g. fees and bonuses for disadvantaged groups; Provide dedicated services for particular groups, e.g. smoking cessation programmes for people in deprived neighbourhoods.
Differential consequences	Social and physical access	Policies and environments in worksites to reduce differential consequences; Increase access of services for people with specific health conditions, e.g. cardiac rehabilitation; Improve referral links to social welfare and health education services.

12.6 Disadvantaged groups as key stakeholders

Discussion on social inequalities often focuses on groups with lower income, low educational status, or some other wealth-related measure. In fact, there are many more reasons that particular groups may be disadvantaged or excluded. Box 12.2 lists some, but not necessarily all, of the groups that can be considered to be particularly vulnerable. All of these groups have one thing in common—they are often socially marginalized or excluded from mainstream processes.

Box 12.2 Examples of disadvantaged subgroups of the population

- People experiencing mental health problems/personality disorder
- Brain-injured individuals
- Children
- Children in care
- Carers
- People with a learning difficulty
- Ethnic minorities
- Asylum seekers, refugees, and other migrants
- Travellers
- Homeless people
- Frail, older persons
- Older persons in general
- Those experiencing forms of dementia
- People for whom speech and/or hearing is not their principle means of communication
- Visually impaired people
- People suffering from a life-limiting illness
- Disabled people
- People who use drugs
- Single parents
- People who cannot read or write
- People in poverty
- People who need, but are not receiving, health or social care services
- People in receipt of forensic mental health services
- Prisoners

Many of these groups are considerable in size. There are, for example, an estimated 214 million migrants globally, including around 43 million who have been forcibly displaced.[10] An estimated 10 million people are currently incarcerated in prisons.[11]

Some of the groups, such as prisoners and migrants, tend to be relatively young, and thus could be expected to be relatively healthy. However, they are not necessarily low risk for NCDs because they may have greater exposure to NCD risk factors and their determinants.

An important principle in global and national strategies to prevent and control NCDs should be the empowerment and engagement of communities. It is important that this approach of involving people in defining problems and identifying solutions should extend to disadvantaged groups. Disadvantaged populations often suffer from further exclusion as they are marginalized from health strategies. These people deserve a much greater voice.

Chapter 10 described the ANGELO process for priority setting. This process trusts communities as a whole to come together and to be able to articulate the problems they face, in terms of NCDs, and to identify possible solutions. A similar level of trust should be accorded to disadvantaged groups. Box 12.3 describes an example where poor rural

Box 12.3 Understanding of childhood obesity, its causes, and possible solutions among poor communities in Peru

> *"All that junk, you see more of it now. The children want fried chicken, fried potatoes. This is their diet … It is not like before when our diets were a little bit healthier here." Mother, Chachapoyas*

This quote from one of 27 mothers interviewed in a study on obesity in Peru illustrates a clear understanding of some of the factors contributing to the obesity epidemic in the country. Focus groups with 70 children and 27 mothers took place in four sites—some rural, some urban—along with 28 interviews with teachers (20) and primary care givers (8) as part of the Young Lives international study of childhood poverty.[12]

> *"Children now live more sedentary lives. Before, to go from one district to another meant walking or going on horse, mule. There was not the mobility that there is now. Now we have combis, trici-taxis, moto-taxis. Camana has changed a lot from that it was." Mother, Camana*

The participants identified the increasing problem of childhood obesity, despite the coexistence of over- and undernutrition within this population. They also identified key factors responsible for the adverse changes (greater access to junk food and decreased opportunities for physical activity).

> *"We had proposed to not have mobile vendors outside of the school but the Municipality did not do anything to help us." Mother, Camana*

As the quote above illustrates, mothers also identified appropriate interventions at the local and national level.

and urban groups in Peru successfully described the factors associated with the growing problem of obesity and identifying issues to be tackled. As this example neatly illustrates, neither money nor higher educational levels are prerequisites for capacity to understand NCDs and their impact on communities.

Case study: Brazil's Bolsa Família—cash transfers to break the intergenerational cycle of poverty

It is clear that reducing health inequalities means thinking outside the 'health box'. WHO's Commission on the Social Determinants of Health powerfully argued that action to tackle the inequitable distribution of power, money, and resources is needed. One approach to tackling such inequitable distribution, which emerged in Latin America in the 1990s, and has since been widely copied, is the provision of regular, predictable payments—known as cash transfers—directly to people living in poverty. Some types of cash transfers—known as conditional cash transfers—are only paid if recipients comply with certain conditions, such as ensuring children attend school or take up preventive health services.

Brazil's *Bolsa Família* (family grant) programme is the largest conditional cash transfer programme in the world and is said to have played a substantial role in the drop in inequality recorded in the country. Launched by then President Lula in 2003 as part of the *Fome Zero* (Zero Hunger) strategy, the programme initially covered 3.6 million families and now reaches around 14 million families, (one quarter of all Brazilian households) living in poverty or extreme poverty. Eligibility criteria are simple—households with per capita income below the programme threshold are eligible to join. In order to stay in the programme, families are obliged to ensure that school-age children and adolescents attend school (85% attendance or higher) and to ensure that young children are immunized and have regular growth monitoring and health checks. Pregnant women are obliged to attend prenatal health services and meet certain nutritional care requirements.

Total inequality in Brazil fell by about 5% from the mid-1990s to the mid-2000s, and *Bolsa Família* was a key contributor, estimated to be responsible for 21% of the 2.7 percentage point fall in the country's Gini index (a measure of inequality).[13] More generally, cash transfer programmes are effective instruments for tackling extreme poverty. The UK Department for International Development (DfID) concluded that there is very consistent evidence that cash transfers can raise living standards, reduce the severity of poverty, and reduce the gap between the rich and poor.[14] Figure 12.2 illustrates the mutually reinforcing improvements to household welfare that may be possible with cash transfers.

In relation to health outcomes, *Bolsa Família* is associated with better outcomes—a community-based study found significantly better health outcomes, including improved health-care utilization (increased attendance at appointments for child

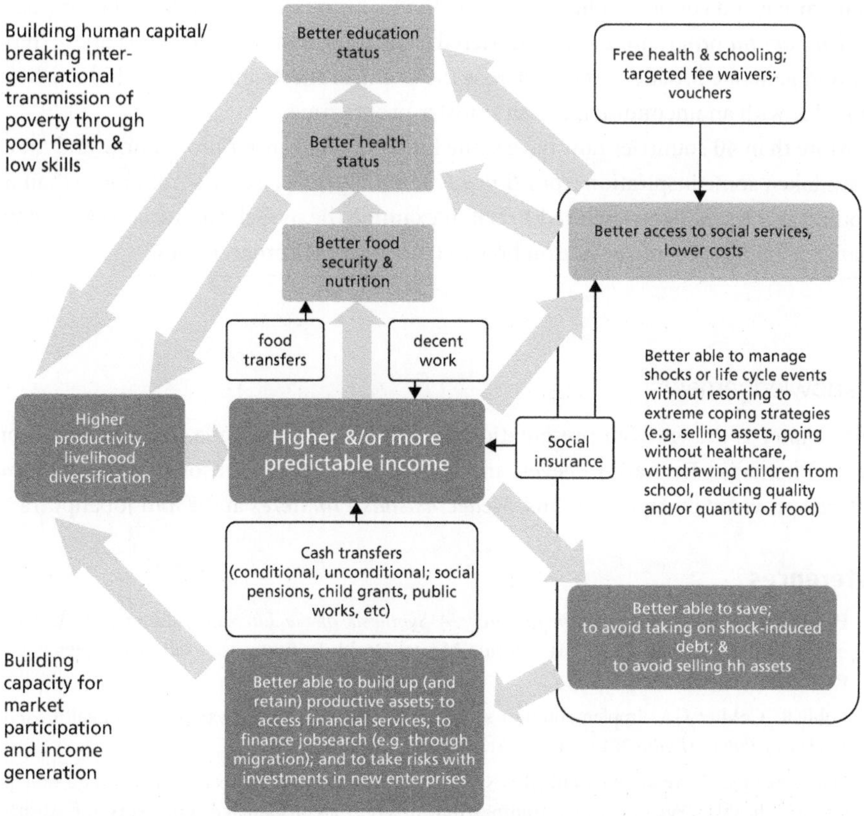

Figure 12.2 Causal pathways by which cash transfers can improve household welfare.

Reproduced from UK Department for International Development, Policy Division. *Cash Transfers: Evidence paper 2011*, http://webarchive.nationalarchives.gov.uk/+/http:/www.dfid.gov.uk/Documents/publications1/cash-transfers-evidence-paper.pdf, accessed 10 Aug. 2016, Copyright © 2011 Crown Copyright.

growth monitoring, immunization, and health checks) and improved psychosocial health.[15] A 2009 Cochrane review of six conditional cash transfer interventions found strong evidence of a positive impact on the use of health services, nutritional status, and other health outcomes, including improving access to preventive services.[16] While many of the improved outcomes in children—such as nutritional status—may have consequences for later trajectories of NCDs, very few interventions have focused directly on adult health outcomes or NCDs specifically.

Where conditional cash transfers are designed to incentivize people to access health services it is obvious that there need to be good quality public services for them to access. In Brazil, despite the *Bolsa Família* and other social protection measures, there were mass protests in 2015 to call for better public service provision.

Some research suggests that it is not necessary to attach conditions to cash transfers for them to be effective, and there have been criticisms that the setting of conditions is intrusive and condescending. In Brazil, the inclusion of conditions in the proposed *Bolsa Família* programme was considered to be important to be able to achieve 'buy-in' and generate broader support across the political spectrum than would have been possible with an unconditional cash transfer programme.

More than 40 countries now have some kind of cash transfer programme and many have taken some inspiration from *Bolsa Família*. By 2016, experts from more than 60 countries are said to have visited Brazil to examine the model, and twice-yearly seminars are held to provide advice on how to launch similar programmes.[17]

Acknowledgements

This chapter is drawn from presentations by Dr Prasad Katalunda, Dr Xuefeng Zhong, Prachi Bhatnagar, Dr Aaron Reeves, and Dr Emma Plugge, with some of the case study material provided by Dylan Collins, *Médecins sans Frontières* and Kiran Jobanputra.

References

1. **Fixsen DL**, et al. *Implementation research: A Synthesis of the Literature*. Tampa, FL: University of South Florida, Louis de la Parte Florida Mental Health Institute, The National Implementation Research Network, 2005.
2. **Lobb R, Colditz GA.** Implementation science and its application to population health. *Annual Review of Public Health* 2013; **34**:235–51.
3. **Damschroder LJ, Aron DC, Keith RE, Kirsh AR, Alexander JA, Lowery JC.** Fostering implementation of health services research findings into practice: a consolidated framework for advancing implementation science. *Implementation Science* 2009; **4**:50.
4. **World Health Organization.** *Global Action Plan for the Prevention and Control of Noncommunicable Diseases, 2013-2020*. Geneva: World Health Organization, 2013.
5. **World Health Organization.** *Health Systems Strengthening Glossary*. Available at: http://www.who.int/healthsystems/hss_glossary/en/index5.html
6. **Doocy S, Lyles E, Roberton T**, et al. Prevalence and care-seeking for chronic diseases among Syrian refugees in Jordan. *BMC Public Health* 2015; **15**:1097.
7. **World Health Organization.** *Package of Essential Noncommunicable (PEN) Disease Interventions for Primary Health Care in Low-Resource Settings*. Geneva: World Health Organization, 2010. http://apps.who.int/iris/handle/10665/44260. Accessed 27 October 2014.
8. **World Health Organization.** *Implementation tools for the Package of Essential Noncommunicable (PEN) Disease Interventions for Primary Health Care in Low-Resource Settings*. Geneva: World Health Organization, 2013. Available at: http://apps.who.int/iris/bitstream/10665/133525/1/9789241506557_eng.pdf?ua=1&ua=1
9. **International Society of Hypertension.** WHO/ISH Risk prediction charts for 14 WHO epidemiological sub-regions. 2007. http://ish-world.com/downloads/activities/colour_charts_24_Aug_07.pdf
10. **International Organization of Migration.** *Facts and figures infographic*. Available at: http://www.iom.int/files/live/sites/iom/files/infographics/iom_infographics.jpg

11. **Institute for Criminal Policy Research.** *World Prison Brief.* Available at: http://www.prisonstudies.org/

12. **Young Lives.** Department of International Development, University of Oxford. Available at: http://www.younglives.org.uk

13. **Soares S, Osorio RG, Soares FV, Medeiros M, Zepeda E.** Brazil, *Chile and Mexico: Impacts upon Inequality.* International Poverty Centre. UNDP, 2007.

14. **Arnold C, Conway T, Greenslade M.** *Cash Transfers—Literature Review.* UK Department for International Development Policy Division, 2011. http://r4d.dfid.gov.uk/PDF/Articles/cash-transfers-literature-review.pdf

15. **Shei A, Costa F, Reis MG, Ko AI.** The impact of Brazil's Bolsa Família conditional cash transfer program on children's health care utilization and health outcomes. *BMC International Health and Human Rights* 2014; **14**:10.

16. **Lagarde M, Haines A, Palmer N.** The impact of conditional cash transfers on health outcomes and use of health services in low andmiddle income countries. *Cochrane Database of Systematic Reviews* 2009, (4): CD008137.

17. **Tepperman J.** Brazil's antipoverty breakthrough. *Foreign Affairs* January/February 2016. Available at: https://www.foreignaffairs.com/articles/brazil/2015-12-14/brazils-antipoverty-breakthrough

Further reading:

On tackling inequalities:

Commission on the Social Determinants of Health. *Closing the Gap in a Generation: Health Equity through Action on thee Social Determinants of Health. Final Report of the Commission on Social Determinants of Health.* Geneva: World Health Organization, 2008.

Blas E, Kurup AS (Eds). *Equity, Social Determinants and Public Health Programmes.* Geneva: World Health Organization, 2010.

Chapter 13

Implementation: Beyond the health sector

13.1 Beyond the health sector: multisectoral action

Given the many varied determinants contributing to the development of non-communicable diseases (NCDs), it is clear that the health sector alone is unable to tackle all the issues needed for prevention to be effective. A multisectoral approach involving other sectors—ranging from agriculture to youth affairs—is essential to bring about changes to the environmental and social factors involved in NCD development.

The importance of this approach is highlighted by the Global NCD Action Plan, which specifies that multisectoral action is one of its overarching principles. This calls for 'coordinated multistakeholder engagement for health both at the government level and at the level of a wide range of actors'. A multisectoral approach, involving different levels of government, can be referred to as a health-in-all-policies or a whole-of-government approach.

A health-in-all-policies approach can be defined as an approach 'to public policies across sectors that systematically takes into account the health implications of decisions, seeks synergies and avoids harmful health impacts in order to improve population health and health equity'.[1] Health authorities at national, regional, and local levels have a key role in promoting a health-in-all-policies approach.

Table 13.1 lists some of the other sectors which the health sector will have to work with in order to establish a cross-sectoral government approach and multisectoral action.

It is important to recognize that, in practice, such a multisectoral approach can be extremely challenging. Sectors outside health may need to be convinced of their role.

The Adelaide Statement on Health in All Policies, from a 2010 international meeting in South Australia, specifies that health in all policies works best when the following conditions are met:

- 'a clear mandate makes joined-up government an imperative;
- systematic processes take account of interactions across sectors;
- mediation occurs across interests;
- accountability, transparency and participatory processes are present;

- engagement occurs with stakeholders outside of government;
- practical cross-sector initiatives build partnership and trust'.[2]

The statement also identified an array of tools and instruments that can help to ensure a health-in-all-policies approach. These include:

- Interministerial and interdepartmental committees;
- Cross-sector action teams;
- Integrated budgets and accounting;
- Cross-cutting information and evaluation systems;
- Joined-up workforce development;
- Community consultations and Citizens' Juries;
- Partnership platforms;
- Health lens analysis;
- Impact assessments; and
- Legislative frameworks.

In January 2014, the World Health Organization (WHO) issued a framework document to serve as a 'starter kit' for countries to apply health in all policies to decision-making and implementation.[1]

This document states that a national multisectoral action plan should include:

- **Making the national investment case for addressing NCDs:** Given the immense burden NCDs pose on countries' economies, it is important to quantify the costs of the management of NCDs and interventions to prevent and control NCDs, their returns, and the costs of inaction.
- **Enhancing national coordination beyond the health sector**: National governance and regulatory frameworks need to strengthen multistakeholder partnerships that will contribute to the implementation of national NCD responses.

Table 13.1 Multisectoral action: examples of sectors to be involved

Agriculture	Health	Transport
Communication	Housing	Urban planning
Education	Justice/security	Youth affairs
Employment	Legislature	
Energy	Social welfare	
Environment	Socio-economic development	
Finance	Sports	
Food/catering	Tax and revenue	
Foreign Affairs	Trade and industry	

Source: data from WHO. *Global Action Plan for the Prevention and Control of Noncommincable Diseases*, Geneva: World Health Organization, pp. 77–78, Copyright © 2013 World Health Organization, http://apps.who.int/iris/bitstream/10665/94384/1/9789241506236_eng.pdf?ua=1, accessed 20 Jul. 2016.

- **Strengthening municipal engagement on NCDs:** Unmanaged rapid urbanization is one of the underlying drivers for the NCD epidemic, alongside poverty, population ageing, and the globalization of marketing and trade in the absence of regulatory, statutory, and policy frameworks.

13.2 Multisectoral coordination mechanisms

Coordination of multisectoral activity presents another challenge. A variety of different mechanisms exists for countries to coordinate multisectoral action (see Box 13.1 for some examples from three Pacific countries).

Box 13.1 Multisectoral mechanisms for tackling NCDs in Pacific countries

Examination of some of the mechanisms adopted in Pacific countries to coordinate multisectoral action on NCDs illustrates the characteristics that increase the likelihood of such arrangements being effective.

Parliamentary advocacy in Samoa

Samoa set up a high-level multisectoral structure in the form of a parliamentary group. The Samoan Parliamentary Advocacy Group on Healthy Lifestyles (SPAGHL) comprises six members of parliament, including cabinet ministers, and four government chief executive officers. It advocates for NCD prevention at various different levels, from parliamentary discussions to village-based events. This advocacy provides the oversight and coordination of NCD action and, because it is based in parliament rather than a specific ministry, ensures buy-in across different sectors. There is no specific funding for NCD action attached to SPAGHL.

With the Minister of Health sitting as a member of the group—which is chaired by the Speaker of the House—this group provides very high-level political leadership. This is highlighted by the participation of the Prime Minister as a champion of physical activity in a popular promotional video.

State of health emergency in Palau

In May 2011, concerned that at least 55% of the country's health budget was being spent on managing NCDs, the government of Palau declared a state of health emergency on NCDs.[3] By adopting this crisis status—comparable to those created by a natural disaster—the President was able to order the Minister of Health (MOH) to utilize the MOH Incidence Command System to coordinate activities to manage the NCD crisis. The President also ordered, among other things, all ministers and heads of national government agencies to assist the Minister of Health when called upon.

The Minister of Health was able convene regular meetings, request action, demand frequent reports on progress, and mobilize public funds.

The momentum behind this approach faltered when there was a change of government, and change in Minister of Health, following an election two years after the crisis was declared. Initial signs, however, were that this approach is extremely powerful.

Palau also championed this issue at the Pacific Island Forum Leaders meeting in September 2011, and the leaders adopted a statement declaring NCDs as a 'human, social and economic crisis requiring an urgent and comprehensive response' and expressing 'alarm that 75 per cent of all adult deaths in the Pacific are due to NCDs and the majority of whom are in the economically active age bracket'.[4]

Cabinet committee in Tonga

In Tonga a subcommittee on NCD prevention was established at cabinet level, involving a number of government ministers and other cabinet members, and chaired by the Minister of Health. Under the umbrella committee on NCD prevention further specific subcommittees were established on tobacco and alcohol, diet, and physical activity. Each of the subcommittees is chaired by the relevant minister for the sector concerned.

Crucially, this high-level mechanism is bolstered in its work by the establishment of a Health Promotion Foundation (see the longer case study on the Tonga Health Promotion Foundation in this chapter), at the initiative of the cabinet subcommittee. This foundation has a high degree of operational autonomy from government, but is allocated its funding from central government.

This arrangement involving a coordination mechanism at a very high political level—with a solid mandate and considerable political clout—coupled with a semi-autonomous funding body, has enabled leverage of funds for NCD prevention.

Key characteristics for efficacy

A number of key characteristics for effective institutional coordination mechanisms can be identified through these and other examples:

- High profile leadership from a senior politician to chair or a high-level institution;
- A legislative or statutory basis for the mechanism—giving a strong institutional mandate; and
- The authority and means to mobilize resources.

13.3 Developing and implementing a multisectoral action plan

WHO has developed a number of tools—including practical tools and various templates—to assist with the development, implementation, and monitoring of a national multisectoral action plan for NCD prevention and control.[5] Box 13.2 sets out the key steps for policy-makers to follow.

Box 13.2 Key steps for developing, implementing, monitoring a National Multisectoral Action Plan for NCD Prevention and Control

Step 1: **Conduct a comprehensive situation assessment**

It is vital to fully comprehend a country's NCD burden and the current status of practices to effectively address the problems, the needs, discrepancies, and capacity for NCD prevention and control within the population. Performing the following activities lends insight into the specifics of the NCD burden.

Activity 1: **Collect background sociodemographic and economic information**—population and health indicators, economic and health expenditure, social determinants including income, education, gender, etc.

Activity 2: **Review of data on magnitude and trends of NCDs and their determinants**—leading causes of death, burden of NCDs, risk and protective factors.

Activity 3: **Review of international evidence-based interventions**—experience and best practices for NCD prevention and control, focusing on those most relevant to country.

Activity 4: **Examination of the existing strategies, policies, plans, and programmes relevant to development, health, and NCDs**—national NCD strategies, policies, programmes, and plans, assessment of capacity of health-care/health system for NCD prevention and control, review of national policies, analysis of gaps related to policy, implementation and research for NCD prevention and control, discussion of potential for improvement/up-scaling/expansion/integration.

Activity 5: **Stakeholder mapping**—identification of the roles and responsibilities of relevant non-health stakeholders for NCD prevention and control.

Step 2: **Engagement of all stakeholders**

Only advocacy and partnerships together can be used to create a national dialogue on NCD prevention and control. Advocacy campaigns call upon the situation assessment from step 1 to garner popular support, influence decision makers in the policy sphere, and inform the potential for intersectoral partnerships.

Activity 6: **Establish an engagement strategy:** optimize strategies to engage with diverse stakeholders and maintain participation and motivation for NCD prevention and control programmes.

Activity 7: **Initiate a proposal for developing multisectoral action plan** on NCDs—establish a national NCD structure/coordination mechanism.

Activity 8: **Develop a strategy to involve relevant sectors to foster partnership**—develop engagement plan, use a framework to foster common understanding between sectors, identify need for multisectoral action, and assess capacity of non-health sectors.

Step 3: **Development of a national multisectoral action plan (MSAP)**

The development of the national MSAP sets the foundation for implementation and requires the convening of stakeholders to draft an outline of recommended actions. The action plan must be considered from an economic perspective, as it should be both economically feasible and socioculturally relevant for the population.

Activity 9: **Multisectoral process and estimation of the potential health and economic impact of the MSAP**—NCD core team to brainstorm on key challenges and a proposed outline of recommended action.

Activity 10: **Draft a multisectoral action plan on NCDs**—develop a strategy to involve relevant sectors to foster partnerships.

Activity 11: **Broad consultation**—bring together all stakeholders to discuss the draft MSAP within their respective area.

Activity 12: **Costing of the multisectoral action plan:** derive an estimate for the cost of each intervention and subsequent logistical activities; assess and maximize existing resources and mobilize additional necessary tools.

Step 4: **Validation and implementation of the MSAP**

The highest level of authority should approve the national MSAP in order to improve and ensure sound implementation. Successful implementation of MSAP relies on gaining and maintaining political and public support, generating stakeholder participation, capacity building, and scaling up existing programmes or establishing pilot projects.

Activity 13: **Implementation of MSAP**—Gain and maintain political and public support, generate appropriate stakeholder participation, and scale up existing programmes or establish pilot projects.

Step 5: **Monitoring and evaluation of progress**

Monitoring and evaluation of the NCD epidemic are fundamental to its prevention and control and need to be seen as essential components of national public health infrastructure. By establishing monitoring and evaluation alongside the establishment of new policies, plans, and programmes, appropriate changes can be made when needed and the effectiveness of new interventions can be evaluated.

Box 13.3 Multisectoral NCD control and prevention in China

In China, where prevalence of NCDs in adults over 40 is predicted to double over the next 20 years, the government responded to the NCD epidemic by introducing a National Plan for NCD Prevention and Control 2012–15.[14] The national plan was issued jointly by 15 ministries and commissions. It sets out three principles, eight goals, 24 indicators, seven strategies, and five guarantee measures. A number of measures are being, or have been, implemented, including interventions targeted at the whole population as well as measures for high-risk groups and patient management. This national plan on NCDs has been implemented alongside major measures to reform the national health system (to ensure access to basic primary care for the whole population, with integrated NCD care), efforts to expand coverage of health insurance and investment in public health services. It is also accompanied by nationwide initiatives on tobacco control, salt reduction and healthy lifestyles. NCD prevention and control rests on three pillars of the Chinese Centre for Disease Control and Prevention system: centre for disease control system (surveillance and prevention), community health centres (delivering essential public health services, early diagnosis and treatment, and management of NCDs and palliative care), and hospitals (involved in treatment, education, and research) (Figure 13.1). Figure 13.2 illustrates how this division of responsibility works out in practice.

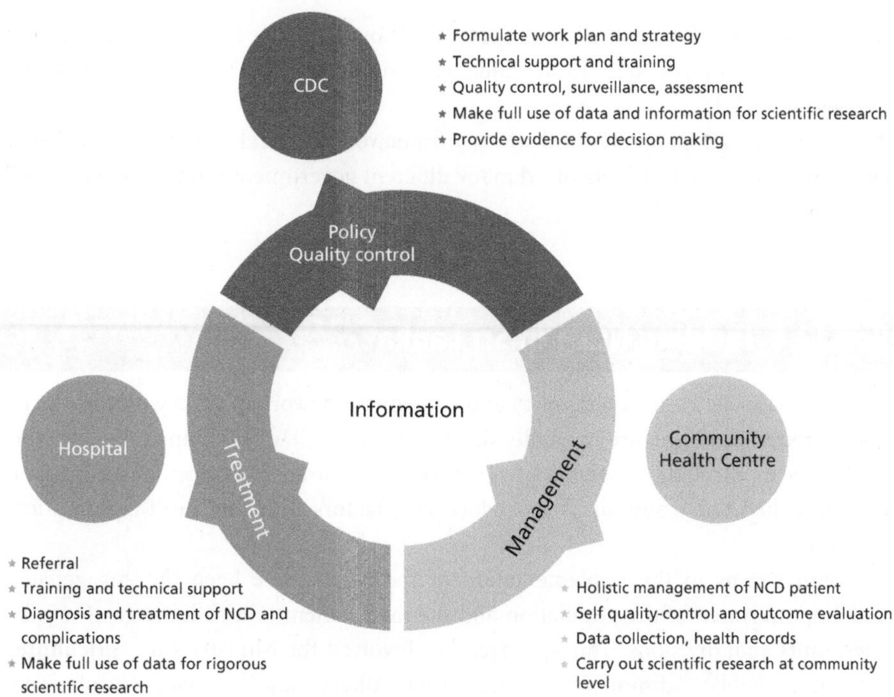

Figure 13.1 Division of responsibilities for NCD control and prevention in China.
Reproduced by kind permission of Dr Xuefeng Zhong.

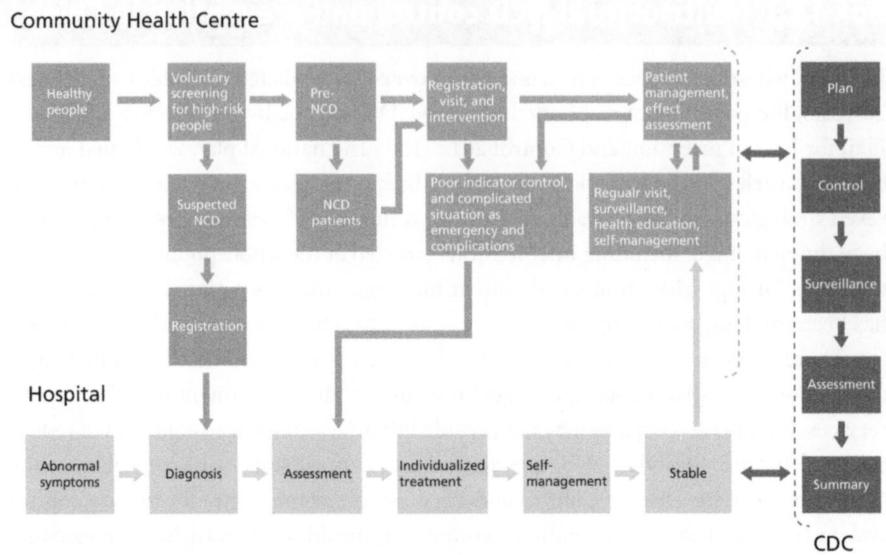

Figure 13.2 Organization of NCD prevention and control in China.
Reproduced by kind permission of Dr Xuefeng Zhong.

In one example of a national multisectoral action plan, the National Plan for NCD Prevention and Control 2012–15 in China was issued jointly by 15 ministries and commissions (Box 13.3).

Similarly, the national policy and strategy framework for tackling NCDs in Sri Lanka, to give another example, has involved many different government ministries and coordinating bodies (Box 13.4).

Box 13.4 Tackling NCDs in Sri Lanka

Sri Lanka launched a national policy and strategy framework in 2009 with the objective of 'reducing premature mortality due to chronic NCDs by 2% annually over the next 10 years through expansion of evidence-based curative services, and empower the individual and community to reduce risk factors by using health promotion measures'.[15]

Essential steps in the implementation of the policy have been the engagement and empowerment of the population and the involvement of a wide range of ministries, units and, divisions. This approach has involved the Ministries of Agriculture, Education, Public Administration and Home Affairs, Social Services, Trade, and Media and Mass Communication.

Implementation of the programme has been supported by a raft of coordinating bodies—from the Ministry of Health at country level to NCD units at the provincial level and down to NCD cells and other institutions at district level. Around 300 healthy lifestyle centres were established in districts to provide health guidance to people aged between 35 and 65 years (with no previous diagnosis of NCDs). Outreach clinics were established to provide support to people living in remote areas. A community awareness programme organized activities in the community to raise awareness of NCD prevention and healthy lifestyles. There was also a focus on promoting healthy lifestyles in the workplace. Media activities to help mobilize the population used the participation of popular figures, such as the First Lady, to generate interest and support.

In addition to involving the full range of different sectors within government, for truly effective action a whole-of-society approach is needed. Such an approach requires many different stakeholders, outside of government, to be involved. Examples include civil society and non-governmental organizations, academia, industry, and professional bodies. One example of an intervention that mobilized a wide range of stakeholders, beyond government, is the introduction of *ciclovia* days to reduce air pollution in Bogota, Colombia (Box 13.5).

Box 13.5 *Ciclovia* days in Bogota, Colombia: reducing air pollution and promoting physical activity

One example of how different elements of society can play a valuable role in creating healthier environments can be found in Bogota, Colombia.[16] The city has *ciclovia* days on Sundays and holidays when certain streets and main avenues are closed to cars. First introduced in 1974, *ciclovia* days gradually grew in popularity so that by 2005 10% of the population cycles as part of *ciclovia* every Sunday. The city now has a *ciclortura* transport system comprising 300 km of cycle paths that provide access to workplaces, schools, colleges, and recreational facilities. These cycle paths also connect to other public transport. The city has also extended traffic restrictions, such as occasional days when it is totally car free between 6.30 am and 7.30 pm and restrictions on certain days of the week according to vehicle license plate numbers.

This programme came about because of a combination of, among other things, community mobilization and political leadership. In the 1970s there were mass protests by cyclists calling for some road closures. Although some *ciclovia* days were introduced there was not a great deal of institutional commitment to the idea. In the 1990s, however, the city's then mayor did a great deal to promote *ciclovia* and to increase the network of cycle paths. The next mayor shared the enthusiasm for *ciclovia* and continued to introduce improvements. Street theatre was used to disseminate messages about sensible vehicle use and the benefits of traffic restrictions. Commute time, pollution, and congestion are all reported to have been reduced.

The involvement of such a wide range of stakeholders, although essential, also poses potential questions about conflicts of interest, particularly where private sector stakeholders are involved. It is clear that real or perceived conflicts of interest should be explicitly acknowledged and need to be managed.

Just as multisectoral action can present difficulties at the national level, it is challenging for international partners. WHO has established a framework for monitoring implementation of the action plan and has established a global coordination mechanism for NCDs (see Chapter 5). It is also hoped that this global coordination mechanism will help to bring different sectors together at the national level.

Case study: Tonga Health Promotion Foundation—A multisector approach to tackle noncommunicable diseases

What is the problem that is being addressed?

In the Pacific kingdom of Tonga the burden of NCDs is at critical level. While once Tonga had one of the highest levels of health in the Pacific the dramatic rise of NCDs, particularly diabetes and cardiovascular disease, has meant life expectancy has fallen by several years since 2006.[6] NCDs now account for 73% of all deaths, at least a quarter of which are premature. Diabetes alone has doubled since 1973, and, with 15.1% of adults diabetic, Tonga now has the seventh highest prevalence globally.

Obesity is the leading risk factor for disease in Tonga.[7] The average adult BMI sits in the obese category at 31.7 kg/m^2 and, with 84% of the adult population classified as overweight and 57% as obese,[8] Tonga is the fifth most obese country in the world.[9] In children, 17% of under-5 year olds and 60% of adolescents are overweight or obese.[10]

While genetic factors have contributed to this rise of NCDs, behavioural risk factors are evident throughout Tonga. Over 90% of adults are not consuming the recommended five servings of fruit and vegetables a day, and 33.5% show low levels of physical activity (particularly women at 53.7%).[12] Each year the average Tongan consumes 31 L of soft drinks (not including juice) a year, the equivalent of 3.3 kg of sugar (approximately two teaspoons of sugar per day).[11]

Food and feasing are integral parts of Tongan culture, as health advocate Rev Dr Ma'afu Palu explains, 'Good food, in a Tongan sense, is lots of food.'[12] As a result, larger body size is often seen as a symbol of wealth and status. A dietary survey found the average daily calorie intake is between 2530 and 2900 calories,[13]well above the 2000 calories per day recommendation. Of this, half the calories came from imported foods—namely meat, canned foods, butter, flour, sugar, and noodles. These imported foods provide very few essential micronutrients (calcium, iron, and vitamins A and C) and are often high in unhealthy fats, salt, and sugar, exacerbating the risk of NCDs. One food that has gained a lot of attention from the media and health professionals is 'sipi'—mutton flaps, which are cheap, fatty cuts of meat imported from Australia and New Zealand which contain over 40 g of fat per 100 g. Health Planning Officer Sunia Soakai says, 'There's this whole generation in Tonga that was brought up on mutton flaps. It's not unusual for Tongans to eat 1 kg of mutton flaps in one sitting.' As Papiloa Bloomfield Foliaki, a retired Tongan nurse explains, 'Something Western, something modern, people think is better. People associated Tongan style of homes with poverty. Just like with our food.' As a result, growing reliance on imported foods has come at the expense of local agriculture, which has seen a 14.7% reduction since 2006.

How was this particular approach selected?

Recognizing the burden of NCDs was impeding Tonga's economic and social development, NCD prevention and control objectives were incorporated into the National Strategic Development Framework (NSDF).[17] The high level of political commitment contributed to major achievements, although early success was limited as interventions and programmes were often restricted to the health sector and faced implementation issues that minimized impact. For example, when the government raised excise tax on cigarettes, failure to collaborate with the agriculture sector resulted in increased local tobacco production, hindering positive impacts on smoking outcomes.[10]

A 2010 analysis identified that 60 to 80 separate policy problems undermined a healthy food environment in Tonga. These policies impacted food price, marketing, agriculture, fisheries, trade, and education. Identifying the broad range of health determinants—from agriculture and education to trade and law enforcement—highlighted that the responsibility to address NCDs lay beyond the health sector alone.[18] To create sustainable and holistic changes would require coordinated, multisector action from all divisions of the government and community to not only control NCDs in clinical settings, but to reshape public policy to create healthy environments which work to address behavioural risk factors and prevent NCDs.

To strengthen national NCD action, the Tonga Commitment to Promote Healthy Lifestyles and Supportive Environment was declared in 2003.[19] As an outcome of this commitment, Tonga became the first Pacific island country to develop a comprehensive National Strategy to Prevent and Control NCDs,[20] governed by the National NCD Committee (NNCDC). The NNCDC is comprised of multisector stakeholders who represent a collection of major sectors of the Tongan community and government; including government ministries, church leaders, and civil societies.

In 2007 the NNCDC's work led to the signing of the Health Promotion Foundation Act, which laid the foundation for the establishment of the Tonga Health Promotion

Foundation (also known as TongaHealth).[21] TongaHealth functions as an independent body acting as a link between the community, non-governmental organizations (NGOs), and the government to implement evidence-based approaches to promote healthy living and help prevent and control non-communicable diseases.

TongaHealth has been instrumental in developing and implementing the National Strategy to Prevent and Control NCDs.[22] As a constantly evolving and diversifying organization, TongaHealth's success has seen it expand beyond the traditional roles of a health promotion organization. In 2014, TongaHealth was appointed as the NCD secretariat in charge of designing and implementing the national NCD strategy, under direction from the NNCDC, focusing on strengthening and delivering multisector action.[23] TongaHealth seeks to strengthen and harmonize donor funds to ensure health promotion funding is coordinated against delivery of the national NCD Strategy.

Figure 13.3 outlines the architecture of the national NCD strategy, highlighting the multisector nature of the NNCDC, TongaHealth's role as secretariat, and influential national and international priorities.[15]

What are the main aims/objectives/targets?

TongaHealth consists of a core staff of nine, governed by the TongaHealth Board. The board is made up of multisector representatives appointed by the Minister of Health. TongaHealth's vision is for a healthy Tonga where everyone is responsible for promoting health and everyone shares in the benefits of a healthy population. The four priorities for programme delivery are:

- Healthy eating
- Physical activity
- Tobacco control
- Reduction of harm from alcohol misuse.

They pursue this vision via:

- Coordinating, planning and implementing the national NCD strategy;
- Funding activities, through competitive grants schemes and sponsorships, which aim to increase the capacity of organizations, communities, and individuals to improve health. NGOs, government institutions, and church and community organizations can apply for funding on a competitive basis, according to published eligibility criteria;
- Acting as a catalyst or advocate for the development of health-promoting policies, programmes, and environments, based on sound evidence;
- Designing and conducting locally relevant social marketing campaigns, in partnership with other health promotion organizations, to communicate healthy messages for behaviour change to the whole population through TV, radio, print media and other activities;

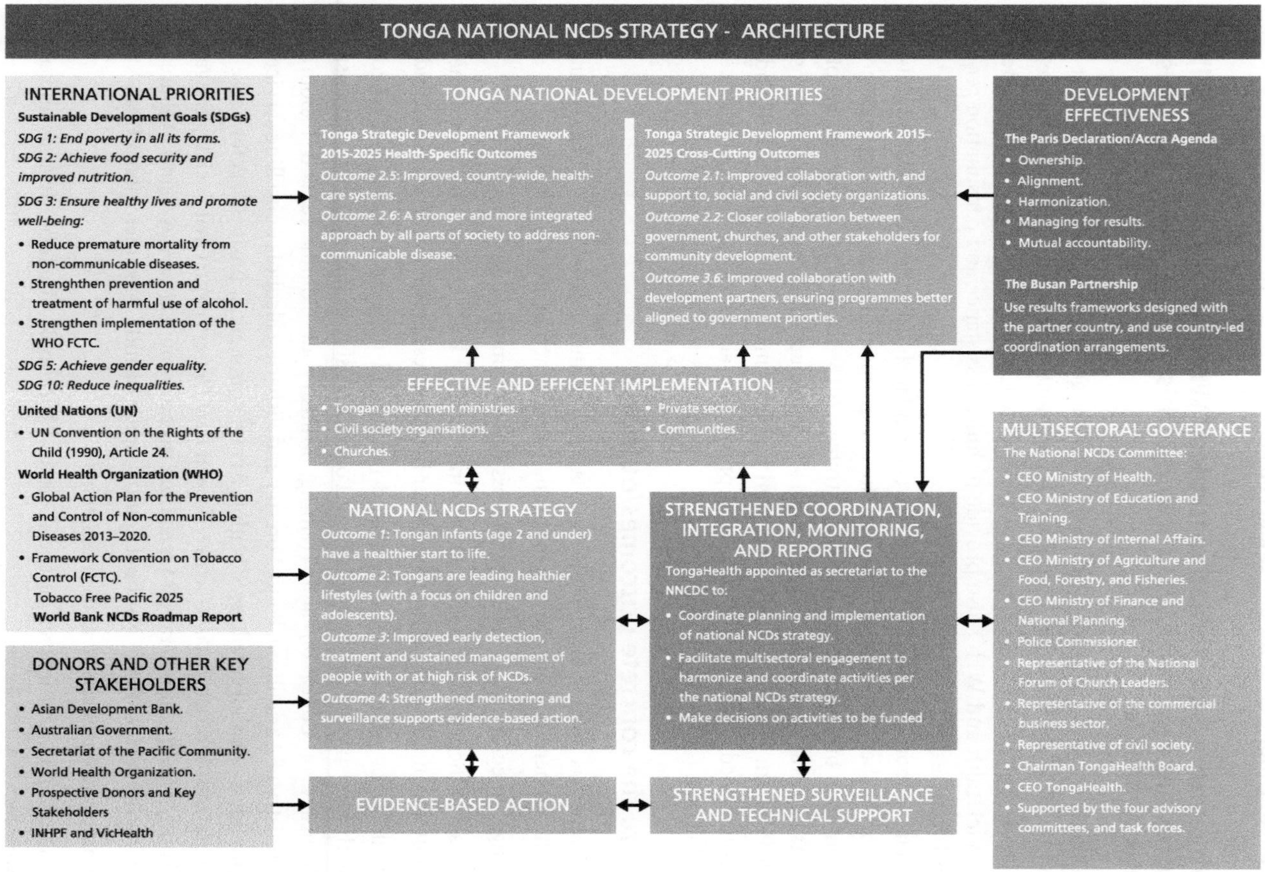

Figure 13.3 The architecture of Tonga's national NCDs strategy.

Reproduced with permission from **Tonga Health Promotion Foundation**. *Hala Fononga: Path to Good Health*, http://media.wix.com/ugd/5ce0eb_cf16fa42674049329e737e0236e804f3.pdf, accessed 10 Aug. 2016. Copyright © 2016 Tonga Health Promotion Foundation (TongaHealth). All Rights Reserved.

- Focusing delivery in key settings and population groups and remote areas where inequalities exist; and
- Facilitating multisector initiatives and consultation.

How/by whom is the initiative funded? What other (non-financial) resources are required? Why/how did this money/these resources become available?

TongaHealth receives its funding from the Tongan government, development partners, particularly through the Australian Department of Foreign Affairs and Trade, Asian Development Bank, Secretariat of the Pacific Community, WHO, and private donors. VicHealth and WHO also provide technical assistance and consultation services to TongaHealth.[23,15]

Financial support from the Australian Government includes a five-year AUS$2.1 million agreement, between TongaHealth and the Government of Australia to support the implementation of Tonga's National NCD Strategy 2015–2020. This support is part of Australia's bilateral support to Tonga's health sector through the Tonga Health Systems Support Program Phase 2 (THSSP 2). Based on performance against the NSDP, and the ongoing need, funding towards NCD prevention activities has increased since phase 1 in 2009.

What are the concrete outcomes/outputs?

TongaHealth has consolidated multisectorial action and collaboration throughout Tonga. The numerous achievements of this nationwide action are listed below:

- Stronger integrated approaches to address non-communicable diseases:[15]
  - Establishment of the Health Promoting Church Partnership, which uses the churches' influential position to deliver healthy messages and interventions; and
  - Multisector partnerships with shared health and policy outcomes established with Ministry of Health; Ministry of Police; Ministry of Revenue and Customs; Ministry of Education and Training; Ministry of Commerce and Labour; Ministry of Agriculture, Food, Forestry and Fisheries; alcohol counselling service providers; alcohol retailers; Salvation Army; commercial business sector representatives; Women's Crisis Centre; Crown Law Department; Civil Society; Tonga Family Health Association; Mai e Nima programme; Latter Day Saints Welfare; Ports Authority; Tonga National Youth Congress; and Consumer Affairs Unit.
- Community engagement and awareness:[22]
  - The creation and upkeep of social media (Facebook, YouTube) forums and a website;
  - Periodic health promotion radio programmes, TV and radio spots, newspaper articles, billboards, social and print media, and radio; and

- 'Tonga Mo'ui Lelei', a 30-minute television show which promotes the multisectoral partnerships.

◆ Fiscal measures:[14]

- Establishment of the TongaHealth promotion fund for sourcing and distributing funding to community-run NCD programmes and activities;
- Embarked on a process of incrementally raising excise rates so that they will reach 60% of the final price of cigarettes;
- Excise tax of TOP $0.50 per litre imposed on carbonated drinks;
- Import duty for healthy food including fish removed to promote healthy living; and
- Import duty for sports equipment and footwear removed to encourage participation of the public in sports and other physical activities.

Promoting healthy behaviours and reducing NCD risk factors

◆ Healthy eating:

- Supported *Mai e Nima* (Give me Five)—a collaborative effort between the Ministry of Education and TongaHealth involving a Healthy Eating Teaching Resource kit which promotes fruits and vegetables and is used in all primary schools throughout the kingdom; and
- 1,856 households have participated in TongaHealth's Community Gardening Programme since 2009. Families are provided with seedlings and gardening equipment to grow vegetables and eight different fruit trees in their home gardens.

◆ Tobacco:

- In 2014, Tonga received a 'World No Tobacco Day Award' for its tobacco tax measures;[15]
- Funded the placement of over 2,000 non-smoking signs in public places such as churches, markets, community halls, hospitals, restaurants, and bars; and
- Authorized officers monitor non-compliance by businesses and individuals and enforce fines according to the Tobacco Control Act 2000.

◆ Physical activity:

- Sponsored three Community Champions (and five assistants) to deliver regular fitness classes within villages. Over 550 individuals from churches, workplaces, and villages participated in these classes in 2012;[22]
- Provided over 61 grants and sponsorships within villages, churches, schools, and workplaces to purchase their own sports equipment for physical activity events, reaching 55,779 individuals;

- Ministries of Education, Internal Affairs, and Health work collaboratively to raise demand for sport in school children and make public spaces available for exercising; and
- In 2013, Tonga was awarded the WHO 'Healthy Islands' in recognition for the 'Kau Mai Tonga' women's physical activity programme.

◆ Alcohol consumption:
- Work alongside Tonga police to raise awareness of the dangers of binge drinking and drunk driving, as well as enforcing liquor licensing laws.

◆ Strengthen the collection, collation, and timely reporting of NCD data
- Incorporation of NCDs into the Millennium Development Goals has led to the substantial improvement in the collection of indicators such as death rates, incidence, and/or prevalence of diabetes, CVD, hypertension, overweight, and obesity; and
- A robust Monitoring and Evaluation Framework has been developed to monitor and report on corporate output as well as progress of health promotion interventions.

Health outcomes

In 2014 Tonga was the first Pacific Island to publish its second NCDs STEPS report. Shown in Table 13.2, results revealed that between 2004 and 2012 Tonga reported significant improvements in reducing physical inactivity (with an apparent reduction in physical inactivity by 20%), increasing adequate fruit/vegetable intake by 19%, and reducing alcohol consumption and marginally reducing smoking.[24] Promisingly, the

Table 13.2 Tonga STEPS survey results from 2004 and 2012

NCD Indicators for 25–64 years	STEPS Survey 2004 results (%)	STEPS Survey 2012 results (%)	Difference
Low physical activity (<600 MET minutes per week)	43.9	23.7	Reduced by 20.2%
Fruit and vegetable consumption (less than 5 servings per day)	92.2	73.1	Reduced by 19.1%
Alcohol consumption (in past 12 months)	8.9	5.7	Reduced by 3.2%
Smoke any tobacco product (such as cigarettes, cigars, or rolled tobacco)	29.8	29.3	Reduced by 0.5%
Overweight	92.1	90.7	Reduced by 1.4%
Obese	68.7	67.6	Reduced by 1.1%

Source: data from WHO Western Pacific Region. *Kingdom of Tonga NCD Risk Factors—STEPS Report*, http://www.who.int/chp/steps/2004_TongaSTEPSReport.pdf, accessed 01 Nov. 2016, Copyright © 2012 WHO.

results suggest these improvements in behavioural risk factors are influencing levels of overweight and obesity with a 1.4% and 1% reduction, respectively.

Conclusions

Though faced with a critical burden of NCDs and a long road ahead, Tonga has laid the foundations for creating health-promoting environments to stem the rise of NCD morbidity and mortality. The establishment of TongaHealth has strengthened multisector action to activate all areas of the government and community to work in collaboration towards sustainable changes and long-lasting impact on the health status of Tonga. Through its lessons and successes, it serves as a role model to other Pacific islands to progress their own multisector NCD strategies.

Acknowledgements

This chapter is based on presentations by Dr Shanti Mendis, Dr Xuefeng Zhong, Prachi Bhatnagar, and Dr Aaron Reeves, with case study information provided by Jessica Pullar and Dr Temo Waqanivalu.

References

1. **World Health Organization**. *Health in All Policies (HiAP) Framework for Country Action.* Geneva: World Health Organization, 2014.
2. *Adelaide statement on health in all policies: moving towards a shared governance for health and well-being.* WHO, Government of South Australia, Adelaide, 2010.
3. **Republic of Palau**, Executive Order No 295, 4 May 2011.
4. **Secretariat of the Pacific community**. Pacific in an crisis, leaders declare (9 September 2011). Available at: http://www.spc.int/hpl/index.php?option=com_content&task=view&id=124
5. See **World Health Organization**. *Noncommunicable Diseases and Mental Health: Tools for Developing, Implementing and Monitoring the National Multisectoral Action Plan for NCD Prevention and Control.* Geneva: World Health Organization, 2016. Available at: http://www.who.int/nmh/action-plan-tools/en/ . Accessed 20 July 2016.
6. **World Bank**. *The economic costs of non-communicable diseases in the Pacific Islands—A rapid stocktake of the situation in Samoa, Tonga and Vanuatu.* 2013. Available at: http://www.worldbank.org/content/dam/Worldbank/document/the-economic-costs-of-noncommunicable-diseases-in-the-pacific-islands.pdf
7. **Institute for Health Metrics and Evaluation**. *The Global Burden of Disease Profile: Tonga.* 2010. Available at: http://www.healthdata.org/sites/default/files/files/country_profiles/GBD/ihme_gbd_country_report_tonga.pdf
8. **Ministry of Health Kingdom of Tonga** and **WHO Western Pacific Region**. *Kingdom of Tonga NCD Risk Factors STEPS Report [Internet].* Manila (PHL): World Health Organization, 2012 [cited 2014 Apr 10]. Available from: http://www.who.int/chp/steps/reports/en/
9. **Ng M, Fleming T, Robinson M, Thomson B, Graetz N, Margono C**, et al. Global, regional, and national prevalence of overweight and obesity in children and adults during 1980–2013: a systematic analysis for the Global Burden of Disease Study 2013. *Lancet* 2014; **384**(9945):766–78.

10. **Kessaram T, McKenzie J, Girin N, Merilles OE Jr, Pullar J, Roth A**, et al. Overweight, obesity, physical activity and sugar-sweetened beverage consumption in adolescents of Pacific islands: results from the Global School-Based Student Health Survey and the Youth Risk Behavior Surveillance System. *BMC Obesity* 2015; **2**:34.

11. **Pak N, McDonald A M, McKenzie J, Tukuitonga C.** Soft drink consumption in Pacific island countries and territories: a review of trade data. *Pacific Health Dialogue* 2014; **20**(1):59–66.

12. **Watson K, Treanor S.** How mutton flaps are killing Tonga. *BBC News Magazine* 2016. Available at: http://www.bbc.co.uk/news/magazine-35346493

13. **Konishi S, Watanabe C, Umezaki M, Ohtsuka R.** Energy and nutrient intake of Tongan adults estimated by 24-hour recall: the importance of local food items. *Ecology of Food and Nutrition* 2011; **50**(4):368–74.

14. **Chinese Center for Disease Control and Prevention.** *China national plan for NCD prevention and treatment (2012–2015).* 25 July 2015. Available at: http://www.chinacdc.cn/en/ne/201207/t20120725_64430.html

15. **Ministry of Healthcare and Nutrition, Sri Lanka.** *The National Policy & Strategic Framework for Prevention and Control of Chronic Non-Communicable Diseases.* 2009.

16. **Parra D, Gomez L, Pratt M, Sarmiento OL, Mosquera J, Triche E.** Policy and built environment changes in Bogotá and their importance in health promotion. *Indoor and Built Environment* 2007; **16**:344–8.

17. **Government of Tonga.** *Tonga Strategic Development Framework 2015-2025.* Ministry of Finance and National Planning, 2014. Availabe at: http://www.adb.org/sites/default/files/linked-documents/cobp-ton-2016-2018-ld-05.pdf

18. **Snowdon W, Lawrence M, Schultz J, Vivili P, Swinburn B.** Evidence-informed process to identify policies that will promote a healthy food environment in the Pacific Islands. *Public Health Nutrition* 2010; **13**(6):886–92.

19. **WHO Regional Office for the Western Pacific.** *Tonga Commitment to Promote Healthy Lifestyles and Supportive Environment.* 2003. Available at: http://www.wpro.who.int/publications/PUB_9290610603/en/

20. **Ministry of Health, Tonga.** *Tonga National Strategy to Prevent and Control Non Communicable Diseases (2010–2015).* 2010. Available at: https://www.mindbank.info/item/1168

21. **Tonga Health.** History of Tonga health. 2016. Webpage, available at: http://www.tongahealth.org/#!about_us/csgz

22. **WHO Regional Office for the Western Pacific.** The Kingdom of Tonga health system review. *Health Systems in Transition* 2015; **5**(6). Available at: http://www.wpro.who.int/asia_pacific_observatory/hits/series/tonga_health_systems_review.pdf?ua=1

23. **Ministry of Health, Tonga.** *Tonga National Strategy to Prevent and Control Non-Communicable Diseases (2015–2020).* 2015. Available at: http://media.wix.com/ugd/5ce0eb_cf16fa42674049329e737e0236e804f3.pdf

24. **TUFI Policy and Strategic Management Consultancy Services.** *Tonga Millennium Development Goals Final Report.* 2015. Available at: http://www.finance.gov.to/sites/default/files/Tonga%203rd%20MDG%20Report%20FINAL%20COPY%20(003).pdf

Further Reading

On multisectoral action:

Adelaide statement on health in all policies: moving towards a shared governance for health and well-being. WHO, Government of South Australia, Adelaide, 2010.

Part V

Monitoring progress

Chapter 14

Evaluation and monitoring

14.1 Defining evaluation and monitoring

Despite our deepening understanding of non-communicable disease (NCD) control and prevention, there is no single blueprint for NCD policies or programmes. A complex set of issues requires sophisticated and complex solutions, and an element of learning from experience (trial and error) is also important. This is why evaluation and monitoring are absolutely essential.

Monitoring and evaluation are separate, but related, activities (Box 14.1). Crucially, monitoring is an ongoing review process, described by the World Health Organization (WHO) as 'keeping track of events'.[1] Evaluation also involves making a judgement about whether, or to what degree, an initiative has been successful. Evaluation differs from research into the effectiveness of interventions in that it takes place in a real-life situation. Research into effectiveness, in contrast, is generally conducted under conditions which are controlled.

14.2 Evaluation

There are numerous reasons for evaluating a programme. One purpose is to identify whether the programme's aims and objectives have been achieved. Another reason may be to find out what went well and what could be improved and to use this information to inform the development of the programme. Finally, evaluation may provide valuable feedback for stakeholders, funders, supporters, and media.

In fact, the precise purpose and focus of any evaluation will depend on the values of those who design the evaluation exercise. It is important to recognize that all the various groups involved in a programme—service users, participants, funders, service providers, staff—may have different ideas about what is important to measure and evaluate. This will depend on how people define success, and perceptions of strengths and weaknesses in the programme. Success for programme participants, for example, might be related to how they feel, whereas success for policy-makers may relate to the cost savings achieved or politicians may be interested in media coverage of the programme. The first task in any evaluation, therefore, should be to bring all stakeholders together and agree on what to evaluate and how to focus the evaluation.

Box 14.1 Defining monitoring, evaluation, and research

Monitoring—the process of appraising and assessing work activities through performance monitoring.

Evaluation—a formal and systematic activity where assessment is linked to original intentions and the findings are fed back into the planning process.

Research into the effectiveness of interventions—a formal and systematic activity where the intervention and method of assessment are constructed by researchers with the intention of making the findings generalizable to other contexts.

The complexity of public health issues—and the sometimes-distant relationships between public health interventions and actual health outcomes—suggests a need for sophisticated evaluation. This means combining different methods and using a variety of data and sources of information. It may involve using both qualitative and quantitative research methods and a combination of subjective and objective measures.

14.3 Types of evaluation

There are three main types of evaluation.

14.3.1 Formative evaluation

Formative evaluation is used to help develop a programme and its implementation. A good example would be to 'pilot' materials such as questionnaires or educational leaflets with a small sample of the target audience and making refinements based on their feedback. It may also involve testing methods to be used, e.g. cognitive behavioural therapy interviews or provision of gym passes and refining delivery and implementation methods. Formative evaluation can be used to reduce the potential for project messages to be misunderstood or executed inappropriately, to check that the target group understands the language and images used, and to anticipate potential unforeseen consequences. In this way, it can act as an early warning system.

The steps involved in formative evaluation include finding out the target group's needs and concerns, helping to establish and clarify aims and objectives, establishing knowledge or attitude baselines and also identifying barriers to implementation. Formative evaluation can be particularly useful in clarifying whether the chosen methods are appropriate for the task and whether the development process is flexible enough. It can also help to establish realistic timescales.

Table 14.1 Advantages and disadvantages of process evaluation

Process evaluation can ...	However, it may also ...
show if the project has done what it set out to do	show the project does not work
show what worked well	use resources which could be used for implementation
show what did not work	be time consuming
improve the intervention through learning	be used to whitewash project results
demonstrate progress to stakeholders	be used to torpedo projects.
inform practice.	

14.3.2 **Process evaluation**

Process evaluation aims to explain how and why intended outcomes of a project were (or were not) achieved. It does this by describing what happens when a programme is implemented. Process evaluation helps to understand why and how interventions work or fail, and helps to avoid wrongly attributing success or failure to particular elements of project design. Process evaluation focuses on the actual programme activities, contact between the project and target group, relationships with key partners, and the environmental context in which the activity takes place. Process evaluation needs to be built in from the start of a project and should be carried out in partnership with all parties involved (Table 14.1).

14.3.3 **Outcome evaluation**

Outcome evaluation focuses on the various impacts of a project over time. In other words, does the intervention actually work? Outcome evaluations can be quantitative (assessing whether there is a relationship between the intervention and outcomes) and/or qualitative (seeking to explain why there is such a relationship). In fact, evaluations should ideally combine both quantitative and qualitative elements. They should also include a variety of outcome variables.

Outcome evaluation may often appear to be the most obvious choice, and is often the favoured option of funders and policy-makers. It is important to recall, however, that the nature and complexity of public health problems and interventions, along with measurement challenges, may mean that the size of the effect which one can expect to observe in any evaluation is modest. If the evaluation focuses solely on outcome, there is a risk that little will have been learned about whether, how, or why the intervention did or did not work. For this reason, it is important to consider evaluating process outcomes to be able to learn from experience and apply lessons to improve the intervention. Figure 14.1 illustrates the six stages of research and evaluation for public health programmes to illustrate how the three different types of evaluation fit into the process.

14.4 **Formulating an evaluation plan**

Like any other project, evaluation requires careful planning and must be tailored to the specific circumstances. The plan should include details of evaluation questions, which

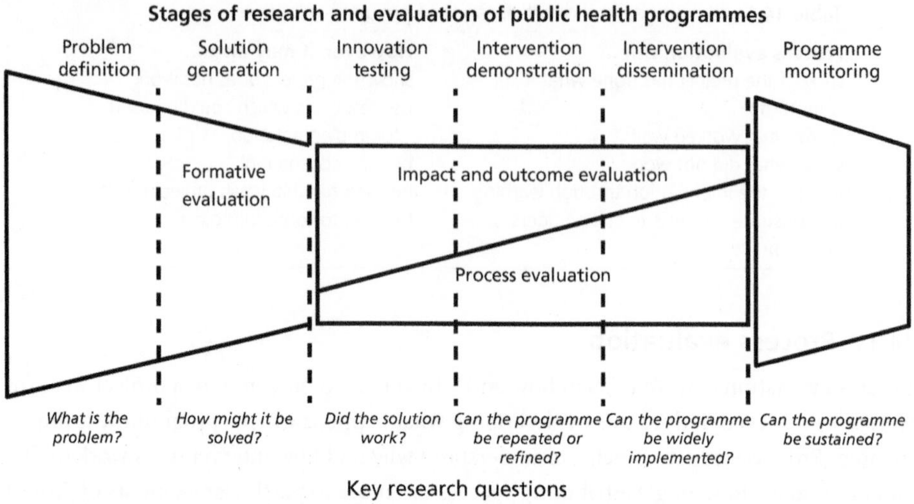

Figure 14.1 Stages of evaluation in public health programmes.
Reproduced with permission from **Nutbeam D** and **Bauman AE**. *Evaluation in a Nutshell: A Practical Guide to the Evaluation of Health Promotion Programs*. McGraw-Hill Education, Australia, Copyright © 2006 McGraw-Hill Education, Australia.

should be in keeping with the aims of the project. It should also include the methods to be used to collect information, what information will be collected, and how these will be analysed. Finally, it should be clear what to do with the results.

In addition to a plan, every evaluation needs four other essential elements: funds, time, people, and tools. Drawing up an evaluation plan will enable assessment of exactly what is needed (Box 14.2).

14.5 **Choosing reliable and valid measures**

At some point in any evaluation there will be a need to measure something—whether that is an action undertaken as part of the programme, a desired outcome, or another element of the programme. Once the factors to be measured have been identified, selection of feasible, appropriate, accurate (valid), consistent (reliable), and sensitive (to change) measures is required. Box 14.3 sets out some of the issues to consider in choosing measures.

The *validity* of any instrument reflects how well it actually measures what it is supposed to measure. There are various different aspects of validity—face, construct, content, convergent, concurrent, and criterion. Tools will often already exist with these dimensions tested and established; these should be considered for appropriateness and feasibility in programme design. Sometimes it will be necessary to attempt to measure something new, or more likely in a previously untried setting (or language). In these cases, time and resources need to be allocated to establishing the validity of the measure in this new context.

As well as being valid, the chosen tool or instrument needs to be consistent and produce repeatable results. *Reliability* reflects how well an instrument gives the same measurement

Box 14.2 Stages in formulating an evaluation plan

Define the evaluation question/s

What is to be evaluated? What are its aims? Whom is it aimed at? Where is it taking place? What is its timescale?

Choose indicators

Select measures which are valid, reliable and sensitive.

Select appropriate methods

How will information be collected? How will the information be assessed (analysis)? What will be done with the results? Plan for who does what, by when, and how.

Budget

WHO recommends that at least 10% of the total financial resources of an initiative should be allocated to evaluation.[2] Remember to cost for planning, meetings, preparation and printing of materials, data collection, participants' travel expenses, data entry or transcription, data analysis, report writing, training of those involved, management time, value-added (or sales) tax, and overheads.

each time it is used in the same circumstances. It is also important that an instrument gives consistent results when used by different people (have good inter-rater reliability).

The stability of the behaviour will also influence reliability. It is important to consider whether the measure of interest (e.g. health behaviour) is likely to change day to day, week to week, or season to season regardless of the intervention/programme. Once again, it is important to consult the literature and consider how reliability might influence the number of repeated measurements that are needed, the sample size, or the ability to detect change.

There are some concepts that it is particularly important to take into account when designing an evaluation for NCD prevention:

The Hawthorne effect means that participants may change what they do (or what they say they do) because they are being studied. This is particularly relevant to self-reported health-related behaviour. It is important to consider carefully whether to use subjective or objective measures.

The ceiling effect describes where participants start with a relatively high score for a particular variable. As a result, a programme may show a more limited effect than it would on a population with a lower baseline. It may make sense to screen out participants who score highly or to adjust the scale. Interventions to increase physical activity, for example, may want to screen out participants who are already very active even though these individuals would be enthusiastic and willing participants.

Box 14.3 Checklist of issues to consider in choosing measures

Feasibility

Consider cost, equipment required and data coding, storage, and analysis requirements.

Timeframe

Include considerations of timeframe in definitions. This is particularly important for health-related behaviours. If, for example, the aim is to measure participants' physical activity, what period is of interest? Yesterday? The previous seven days? The last 12 months? Is it likely that the construct to be measured will change in the timeframe of the programme? Outcomes such as fitness or body mass index (BMI) might change at different rates to smoking or alcohol consumption.

Participant burden

How much effort does it require participants to put in? Participants need clear and honest explanations of what is involved. It is important to consider the intrusiveness of the measurement proposed.

Ethics

It is important to use instruments that are appropriate to the cultural setting, respecting differences in culture, customs, religious beliefs, etc. The process should be honest and transparent and pay careful attention to confidentiality considerations (it should not be possible to trace sensitive information back to its source).

Validity

Does the instrument really measure what it is supposed to measure according to the evaluation design? Consult the relevant measurement literature or seek expert advice.

Reliability

Are measurements consistent and repeatable? Some behaviours are not stable; for example, exercise levels might change from day to day. Consider how many measurements at baseline and follow-up(s) are needed to characterize normal patterns of behaviour. Sometimes a physiological measurement (such as cardiovascular fitness) might be more stable than a related health behaviour (exercise).

Learning from others

What can be learned from how others measure these variables? Where possible, and appropriate, use harmonized instruments for comparability.

Case study: Evaluating Mexico's tax on sugar-sweetened drinks

When Mexico announced in 2013 that an excise tax would be levied on sugary drinks, policy-makers and health advocates from around the world were keen to observe the impact of the new tax. They were also eager to understand how Mexican policy-makers had succeeded in implementing such a controversial measure—similar to those that had encountered fierce opposition in other jurisdictions. As a result, the Mexican experience has been evaluated in a number of different ways.

As part of efforts to tackle one of the world's highest obesity rates, the Mexican government introduced an excise tax on sugar-sweetened beverages in an attempt to reduce demand for sugary drinks. The 1 peso per litre tax on non-dairy and non-alcoholic beverages with added sugars—announced in October 2013 as part of the National Strategy for the Prevention and Control of Overweight, Obesity and Diabetes—came into effect on 1 January 2014. The amount represented a price increase of around 10% and research suggests that all of this was passed on to Mexican consumers. Drinks sweetened with artificial sweeteners, sparkling mineral water, plain water, juices with no added sugars, and milk with no added sugars are exempt. At the same time, the government launched a mass-media information campaign to promote healthy diets and implemented some other national measures.

Researchers from the Instituto Nacional de Salud Publica in Mexico and the University of North Carolina at Chapel Hill conducted an outcome evaluation that examined the effect on purchases of taxed and untaxed beverages.[3] They conducted an observational study using scanned and recorded food purchase data on beverage purchases from a representative group of 6,253 households involved in Nielsen Mexico's Consumer Panel Services from January 2012 to December 2014. The authors used a difference-in-difference fixed effects model that adjusts for macroeconomic variables and pre-existing trends. This is particularly important because sugar-sweetened beverage intakes were already falling before the tax was introduced. The study compared, therefore, the volumes of taxed and untaxed beverages purchased in 2014, after the tax had been introduced, with the estimated volumes that would have been bought if the tax had not been introduced based on pre-tax trends (this is referred to as 'the counterfactual').

During the first year of the tax, the average volume of taxed beverages purchased monthly was 6% lower in 2014 than would have been expected without the tax and the reductions accelerated, reaching a 12% decline by December 2014 (Figure 14.2). There were lower purchases of taxed beverages in all three socioeconomic groups, but the reductions were higher among low socioeconomic status households (average 9% decline during 2014, with a 17% decrease by December 2014). People bought more untaxed beverages than would have been expected without the tax (4% higher than the counterfactual), mainly due to an increase in bottled plain water purchases.

The effective level of the tax—at 10%—is only half of the 20% that is often recommended as necessary to have enough impact on consumption to affect health outcomes.

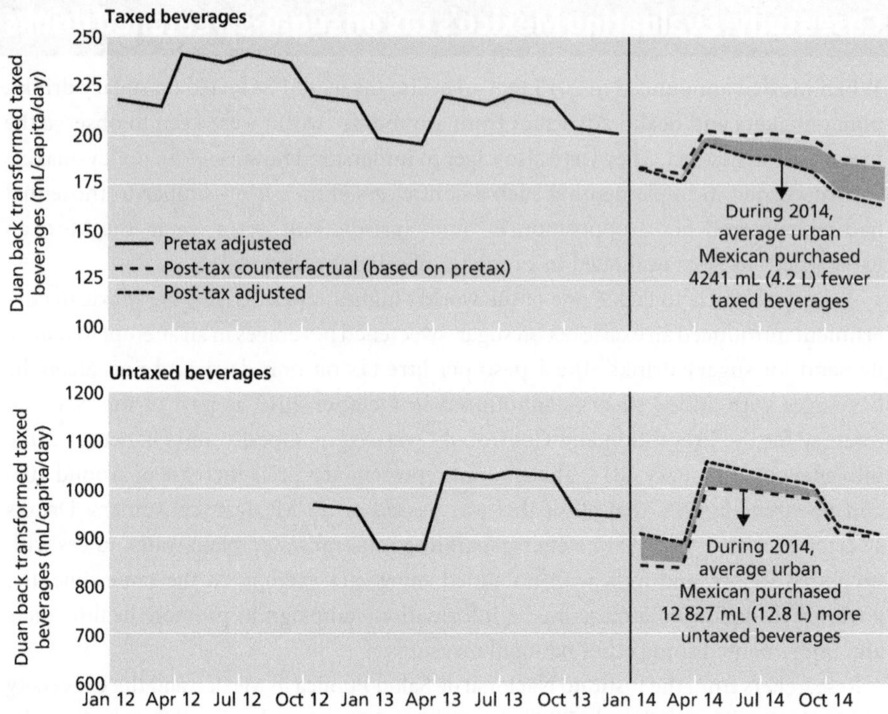

Figure 14.2 Monthly predicted purchases of taxed and untaxed beverages between January 2012 and end of 2014. Note: The figures compare the estimated purchases if pre-tax trends had continued without imposition of the tax (the 'counterfactual', shown in large-dash line) with post-tax purchases (in small-dash line).

These results suggest that even a relatively small tax can make a difference to demand for sugar-sweetened drinks. Projections based on these results suggest that there will be a positive impact on the reduction of overweight, obesity, and diabetes.[4]

Some limitations of this evaluation include the fact that causality cannot be established because there may have been other changes at the same time as the tax was introduced, incomplete data on dairy beverages prior to October 2012, and the data are based on people living in cities with more than 50,000 residents so do not represent the population living in small towns and rural areas. The evaluation does not really explore the impact of possible industry tactics in response to the tax—further work is needed to monitor industry marketing and promotions, and their impact on consumption. Long-term evaluation should continue to monitor purchase trends, explore substitution effects, and understand the impact on diets, particularly among those who consume the largest quantities of sugary soft drinks.

The impact of the tax has also been measured by monitoring the collection of revenue as a result of the excise tax. Between January and December 2014, collection of duties led to revenues of MXN 124,016,000 (US$9,152,472), representing a 51.1% increase on the previous year, as a result of the expansion of the tax to sugar-sweetened beverages and energy-dense foods (a tax on energy-dense foods was introduced at the same time as the sugar-sweetened beverage tax).

An evaluation by Johns Hopkins Bloomberg School of Public Health attempted to identify lessons for policy-makers or other stakeholders that want to advocate for a similar tax by examining the tactics employed in Mexico by proponents and opponents of the measure in the run-up to the law's approval in October 2013.[5] Qualitative data were collected from 20 interviews with purposively sampled key informants and a review of documents.

The case study concluded that a strong and effective advocacy strategy was at the core of the successful campaign, and that this was complemented by strong science and informed by the political and social context. This campaign was thus able to fend off industry lobbying and media attacks. The author identified three important lessons for health policy advocates:

- Engage organizations with a strong background in media advocacy and strategic campaign development and who are respected and recognized as legitimate defendants of the public's interest.
- Develop a keen understanding of the scientific literature with a focus on how the evidence can inform the selection and defence of policy measures and development of campaign messages.
- Understand the political context, and windows of opportunity, to influence policy change.

A report on the tax by the Pan American Health Organization/WHO Regional Office for the Americas noted that the government had also launched other initiatives—including a mass media campaign on healthy eating—and that, therefore, the tax may not have been the only factor responsible for the reduction in demand.[5] Another element that may have had an effect, and may continue to do so, is civil society's advocacy for provision of drinking water in schools and public spaces, leading to a new legal duty on schools to have sufficient fountains to guarantee a constant supply of drinking water. The new decree also requires earmarking of the equivalent of the federal revenue raised by the tax for programmes to combat malnutrition, treat and prevent obesity, and improve access to drinking water in rural areas, schools, and public spaces.

Source: data from **Colchero MA**, **Popkin BM**, **Rivera JA**, and **Ng SW**. Beverage purchases from stores in Mexico under the excise tax on sugar sweetened beverages: observational study. *British Medical Journal*, Volume 352, Article h6704, Copyright © 2016 BMJ Publishing Group Ltd.; **Donaldson E**. *Advocating for Sugar-Sweetened Beverage Taxation: A Case Study of Mexico*. Baltimore, MD: Johns Hopkins Bloomberg School of Public Health, Copyright © 2015 Johns Hopkins Bloomberg School of Public Health, http://www.jhsph.edu/departments/health-behavior-and-society/_pdf/Advocating_For_Sugar_Sweetened_Beverage_Taxation.pdf, accessed 10 Aug. 2016; **PAHO/WHO**. *Taxes on Sugar-Sweetened Beverages as a Public Health Strategy: The Experience of Mexico*. PAHO/WHO Regional Office for the Americas, Copyright © 2015 Pan American Health Organization, https://ncdalliance.org/sites/default/files/resource_files/9789275118719_eng.pdf, accessed 10 Aug. 2016.

Case study: Evaluating the Active Teen Leaders Avoiding Screen Time (ATLAS) initiative to prevent adolescent obesity in New South Wales, Australia

Adolescent obesity represents great public health concern, associated with a broad range of negative health outcomes. The development of obesity is driven by complex, interrelating factors, and any intervention to prevent obesity must be multicomponent, operating at multilevels to tackle the complexity of this health issue.

The age period of adolescence offers a unique opportunity to intervene for obesity, as it is during this time that key independent lifestyle behaviours are developed. School settings have been identified as ideal environments to deliver such interventions due to the opportunity to target large groups of young people, and educational institutions often hold the resources to implement intervention initiatives. Recent trials for such interventions indicate preliminary success. Recommendations for future interventions are to examine and evaluate interventions for those at increased risk for obesity, such as youth from low-income communities, and to explore gender-specific health behaviour programmes.

In response to the above recommendations, the Active Teen Leaders Avoiding Screen-time (ATLAS) programme was developed with the aim of preventing obesity among Australian secondary school adolescent males living in low-income communities.[6] The programme was based on successes observed in the pilot trial, the Physical Activity Leaders programme, which demonstrated feasibility and efficacy to reduce healthy weight loss among adolescent males from disadvantaged secondary schools.

The ATLAS intervention was a cluster randomized controlled trial, operating in 14 coeducational, public secondary schools in New South Wales, Australia. The 8-month intervention targeted adolescent males in Year 8 (second year of secondary school), aged 12–14 years. Eligible study participants were those who failed to meet international recommendations for physical activity and screen-time, and were therefore considered at risk for obesity. Study participants were randomized at the school level to either ATLAS intervention or wait list control group. Baseline measures occurred in November–December 2012 and were repeated post-programme (July–September 2013), and 18 months post baseline (April–June 2014).

The ATLAS programme aimed to prevent obesity through targeting health behaviours in physical activity, screen-time, and sugar-sweetened beverage consumption. The programme was informed by self-determination theory and social cognitive theory in that the psychological needs of adolescents were targeted in addition to the provision of opportunities, to motivate and support the engagement in health behaviours.

The control group maintained usual practice, including regularly scheduled school sports and physical education lessons, for the duration of the intervention. The control group would receive an equipment pack and a condensed version of the programme after the 18-month assessment.

Evaluation

Formative evaluation occurred during the pilot trial, the Physical Activity Leaders programme that ran from June to December 2009. Outcome evaluation for ATLAS occurred at baseline (November 2012), post-intervention (July 2013), and 18-month post baseline (April 2014). Assessors were blind to school allocation at baseline, but not at post-intervention. Primary outcome measures were objectively measured height, weight, and waist circumference. Secondary measures were body fat percentage, a range of physical activity indicators (accelerometer data, muscular fitness, resistance training skill competency), recreational screen-time, sugar-sweetened beverage consumption, physical self-concept, well-being, video gaming, aggression, and sleepiness. Primary and secondary measures were taken at baseline, post-programme, and 18-months post baseline. The purpose of repeating outcome measures 18-months post baseline was to monitor potential ongoing impact beyond the intervention period, and to determine the sustainability of the programme.

Hypothesized cognitive mediators (motivation, locus of control, self-perceived competence, etc.) were assessed at baseline and at 6-months post baseline, prior to post-programme assessment. This was due to the expectation that for true mediation to occur, the change in cognition should precede behaviour change.

A range of process data was collected during the intervention period. Process measures included student attendance at sport sessions; student leadership accreditation; teacher satisfaction with professional learning workshops; parental involvement; participant satisfaction with intervention initiatives; and intervention fidelity (based on sport observation sessions). A checklist was completed by observing researchers during sport sessions (two per school), to determine whether the session adhered to assigned structure and the degree to which the session demonstrated predetermined teaching principals that supported students' psychological needs. Teachers had previously participated in workshops and were familiarized with such principles. Feedback was provided to teachers at the conclusion of the sport session, including strengths and possibilities for improvement. A limitation of the ATLAS programme was lack of economic evaluation and this precluded determining the cost-effectiveness of the programme.

Impact/effectiveness

The evaluation found that although there were no significant intervention effects for body composition (body mass index, waist circumference, percentage of body fat), there were significant behavioural findings. There was a significant decrease in screen-time and consumption of sugar-sweetened beverages among the intervention group compared to control. Significant intervention effects were also found in improved muscular fitness and resistance training skills. A small but statistically significant improvement in psychological well-being was found in intervention compared to comparison group.

Process evaluation data reported that no adverse effects or injuries occurred during the intervention-specific activities. Process data also revealed that two-thirds of adolescent males attended a satisfactory number of sport sessions, although participation at lunchtime sessions was low. Adolescent males reported lower satisfaction with lunchtime activities. Compliance with the sport session structure was moderate in the initial phases of the intervention, but was reported to improve substantially. Moderate usage was reported for the smart phone application, and all teachers agreed or strongly agreed that students benefited from the programme.

The ATLAS programme was a multicomponent, school-based intervention using a broad range of intervention initiatives to promote health behaviours among disadvantaged, male adolescents. Post-intervention findings indicated improvements in key weight-related behaviours and psychological well-being among the intervention group. Further planned follow-up evaluation at 18 months (yet to be reported) will reveal the longer term effectiveness and sustainability of the ATLAS programme. Early successes indicate potential for targeted obesity prevention interventions for specific groups, incorporating a broad range of weight, psychological, and behavioural initiatives.

Case study: Integrating Nutrition Promotion and Rural Development (INPARD) in Sri Lanka

Sri Lanka is a lower-middle income country experiencing rapid development and a double burden of under- and overnutrition. According to the WHO, NCDs are estimated to account for 75% of total deaths, and the probability of dying between ages 30 and 70 years from the four main NCDs is 18%.[7] In addition to their major human and social costs, NCDs place a major challenge on development[8] and there is increased recognition of the need for multisectoral action to address NCDs.[9]

The Integrating Nutrition Promotion and Rural Development (INPARD) project seeks to examine the feasibility of linking multiple sectors together to implement a community-led NCD prevention intervention. Specifically, it focuses on linking rural development with nutrition promotion. It involves a wide range of sectors and stakeholders from rural development, education, agriculture, and nutrition, amongst others.

Sri Lanka's national District Nutrition Action Plan (DNAP) recommends that health and non-health sectors work together to improve nutrition, and the WHO office for Sri Lanka prioritizes addressing the social determinants of health through multiectoral and multistakeholder coordination. It also emphasizes the value of research and generating evidence-based projects. INPARD is designed to generate evidence which may be used to inform future efforts to link development with multisectoral NCD prevention interventions.

INPARD's main objectives are as follows:

- Evaluate the feasibility of integrating nutrition promotion with rural development to improve nutrition outcomes.
- Identify pathways to promote nutrition with multiple stakeholders.
- Provide evidence on ways to operationalize multisectoral approaches to NCD prevention.
- Evaluate and compare nutrition-related health outcomes between INPARD and control groups.

The INPARD intervention involved a range of community-led activities that were implemented within villages and schools to promote nutrition. INPARD developed a curriculum to provide training for stakeholders involved in designing and implementing nutrition-promotion interventions. INPARD involved coordinating representatives from government offices (development, health, public health, administrators, education, and agriculture) and a local coordinator (called the 'Village Development Officer').

INPARD developed training materials on linking rural development and nutrition, health promotion through rural development, and multisectoral collaboration. In addition to providing training to multisectoral stakeholders, it hosted a range of workshops and activities within villages and schools to promote nutrition and provided feedback on improving intersectoral coordination. After delivering training to the group of stakeholders, the team conducted a needs assessment within schools and villages, developed an action plan, and identified the mechanisms to deliver a nutrition-promotion intervention.

INPARD was responsible for coordinating this process. It worked with the teams to ensure that the officers from the various departments were able to meet on the same day and arranged a common meeting place for fortnightly meetings. Additionally, INPARD appointed one officer who was responsible for coordinating meetings and taking minutes.

This process led to a number of interventions. For example, one village identified the problem of low levels of dietary protein. The stakeholders identified a possible solution to introduce yoghurt to the market. They identified barriers to this process, which included a lack of financial assistance to initiate the business, a lack of demand for the product, misconceptions, and a lack of technical knowledge. The multisectoral team then came up with solutions in their respective sectors. For example, agriculture officers provided technical knowledge, public health instructors helped link yogurt producers to suppliers and to complete business registrations, and development officers provided financial support and loans. As a result of this community-led effort, yogurt was made available in school canteens for half its usual price (dropping from 30 rupees per serving to 15 rupees). Additionally, it generated a source of employment for local community members.

The INPARD intervention was delivered in more than 100 villages in Ampara (n = 57 villages) and Moneragala (n = 55 villages) and covered a population of nearly 130,000 people living within these rural areas. INPARD has the potential to have a wider impact, and reach more direct beneficiaries, if it is rolled out internationally.

In addition to these direct beneficiaries, others may benefit indirectly from the initiative. These could include governmental and non-governmental organizations (local and international) and researchers concerned with nutrition, sustainable development and NCD prevention, and Sri Lankan stakeholders and sectors collaborating within the INPARD network.

The project, funded by the South Asia Food and Nutrition Security Initiative, involved stakeholders from organizations including the World Bank, Sri Lanka Ministry of Economic Development, University of Colombo, University of Oxford, and Australian National University. Community members from the rural districts of Ampara and Moneragala played a key role in the intervention and evaluation. Community members from Kurunegala played a key role in the evaluation of the INPARD project.

Outcomes include baseline and post-intervention data from intervention and control districts. These include health-related measures from adults and children (nutrition, anthropometrics, physical activity, and other health behaviours). Table 14.2 shows the INPARD outcome indicators and the tools which were used to collect the data.

To evaluate the INPARD intervention, the study followed a longitudinal quasi-experimental design. Data were collected at baseline (before the INPARD intervention) and one year following the intervention. The INPARD intervention was implemented within selected villages (n = 112) and schools (n = 20) within two districts (Ampara and Moneragala). Outcomes from these intervention districts will be compared to outcomes from controls in non-INPARD villages located within Ampara, Moneragala, and Kurunegala. In total, INPARD collected data from more than 4,000 individuals living within three districts, 50 villages, and 49 schools.

To evaluate the effect of the intervention (ongoing at the time of writing), baseline measures are compared to post-intervention measures, requiring a multilevel analytical approach to account for the clustered nature of the data (individuals within villages, children within schools).

In addition to the specific outcomes (Table 14.2), project outputs include a range of data collection tools, training materials on nutrition, health promotion and intersectoral collaboration, research symposiums, and peer-reviewed publications.

INPARD has received high-level recognition as an example of implementing multisectoral NCD prevention interventions within a low- to middle-income country (LMIC). INPARD was featured as a case study in a report of the first dialogue convened by the WHO Global Coordination Mechanism on NCDs in April 2015.[10]

Table 14.2 INPARD outcome indicators and data sources

Age group/ level and outcome	Outcome indicator	Data source
Children 12-18 years of age		
Diet	Proportion of children meeting SL food-based standards	WHO Global School-Based Health Survey (GSHS) and Food Frequency Questionnaire (FFQ)
Anthropometric	Proportion of children classified as under-weight, healthy weight, overweight, and obese	Anthropometric measurements taken by trained researchers following standard protocol
Physical activity	Proportion meeting recommendations of 150 min/week	GSHS
Other health behaviours	Proportion of children who are current smokers and consume alcohol (current/ever consumed)—(WHO definitions)	GSHS
Children 5-12 years of age (Note: Children's outcomes will be segregated by sex)		
Diet	Proportion of children meeting SL food-based standards	24 hour dietary recall (parent-report)
Anthropometric	Proportion of children classified as under-weight, healthy weight, overweight, and obese	Anthropometric measurements taken by trained researchers following standard protocol
Children 1–5 years of age		
Diet	Proportion of children meeting SL food-based standards	24-hour dietary recall (parent report)
Anthropometric	Proportion of children classified into different Child Health Development Record categories by measuring weight against age (e.g. extremely low, low, risk of low, normal, and overweight) and height against age (short, at risk, normal)	Anthropometric measurements taken by trained researchers following standard protocol and values recorded in the CHDR
Adults (Note: Adult's outcomes will be segregated by sex and 10 year age groups)		
Diet	Proportion of adults meeting SL food-based standards	WHO STEPwise Approach to Chronic disease Risk Factor Surveillance (STEPS) and FFQ
Anthropometric	Proportion of adults classified as underweight, healthy weight, overweight, and obese	Anthropometric measurements taken by trained researchers following standard protocol
Physical Activity	Proportion of adults meeting recommendations of 150 min/week	STEPS
Smoking	Proportion of current smokers (WHO definition)	STEPS
Alcohol	Proportion of adults who consume alcohol (current/ever)	STEPS

Age group/ level and outcome	Outcome indicator	Data source
Area level measures		
School	Nutrition friendliness of the school (score based on WHO Nutrition-Friendly Schools Initiative criteria)	NFSI Assessment Tool
Village	Food availability and access (price and the presence of food items available for purchase in village)	Food availability and price data collected by researchers

14.5.1 Monitoring: model for a three-dimensional framework

While evaluation is essential to be able to judge whether, and why, an intervention has been successful or unsuccessful, ongoing monitoring is important to keep track of the situation over the longer term.

Monitoring efforts have tended to focus on disease end points, with some inclusion of risk factors such as smoking and obesity. The ideal monitoring approach would be much more comprehensive—taking account of upstream determinants of health, such as socioeconomic factors. In addition to monitoring this broader range of outcomes, this approach would also monitor actions and interventions undertaken.

Regardless of whether a broad or relatively narrow range of indicators is monitored, it is important to be able to conduct meaningful analysis of the data. This means being able to track changes over time. It is also important to collect enough data to be able to disaggregate by, for example, sex and socioeconomic status.

Figure 14.3 illustrates one possible model for NCD monitoring, which takes into account disease and upstream outcomes, as well as process indicators (actions).

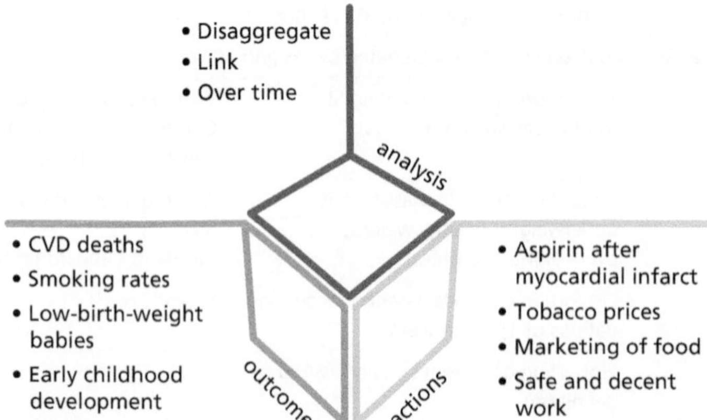

Figure 14.3 Example of a three-dimensional model for an NCD monitoring framework.

In reality, even wealthier countries currently struggle to gather enough data to be able to implement such a comprehensive approach to monitoring. National reporting of comparable and standardized health data is often lacking, even in wealthier regions. Even when it comes to reporting death rates, comparable and standardized reporting is not guaranteed. The problems are even more pronounced in relation to monitoring NCD risk factors. Furthermore, data collection that is sufficiently comprehensive to enable disaggregated analysis by, for example, population groups is even rarer.

14.6 The global NCD monitoring framework

A global monitoring framework has been developed to monitor progress on the Global NCD Action Plan. This monitoring framework, approved by the World Health Assembly in 2013, set out nine voluntary targets (see Chapter 5) and 25 outcome indicators to monitor the development of interventions, risk factors, and the overall burden. In some cases, countries will select the indicators as appropriate to the national context (e.g. for harmful use of alcohol, prevalence of overweight, and obesity) (Table 14.3).

In addition, to the outcome indicators, some time-bound commitments have been defined and, in relation to these time-bound commitments, some progress indicators

Table 14.3 Monitoring global progress: outcome indicators

Outcome indicators	
Mortality and morbidity	Unconditional probability of dying between 30 and 70 from CVD, cancer, diabetes, or chronic respiratory disease
	Cancer incidence, by type of cancer, per 100,000 population
Behavioural risk factors	Total (recorded and unrecorded) alcohol per capita (aged 15+ years old) consumption within a calendar year in litres of pure alcohol, as appropriate, within the national context
	Age-standardized prevalence of heavy episodic drinking among adolescents and adults, as appropriate, within the national context
	Alcohol-related morbidity and mortality among adolescents and adults, as appropriate, within the national context
	Prevalence of insufficiently physically active adolescents, defined as less than 60 minutes of moderate to vigorous intensity activity daily
	Age-standardized prevalence of insufficiently physically active persons aged 18+ years (defined as less than 150 minutes of moderate to intensity activity per week or equivalent)
	Age-standardized mean population intake of salt per day in grams in persons aged 18+ years
	Prevalence of current tobacco use among adolescents
	Age-standardized prevalence of current tobacco use among persons aged 18+ years
	Age-standardized prevalence of raised blood pressure among persons aged 18+ years (defined as systolic blood pressure ≥ 140 mmHg and/or diastolic blood pressure ≥ 90 mmHg) and mean systolic blood pressure

Outcome indicators	
Biological risk factors	Age-standardized prevalence of raised blood glucose/diabetes among persons aged 18+ years (defined as fasting plasma glucose concentration ≥ 7.0 mmol/L (126 mg/dL) or on medication for raised blood glucose)
	Prevalence of overweight and obesity in persons aged 18+ years (BMI ≥ 25 kg/m^2 for overweight and BMI ≥ 30 kg/m^2 for obesity)
	Age-standardized mean proportion of total energy intake from saturated fatty acids in persons aged 18+ years
	Age-standardized prevalence of persons (aged 18+ years) consuming less than five total servings (400 g) of fruit and vegetables per day
	Age-standardized prevalence of raised total cholesterol among persons aged 18+ years (total cholesterol ≥ 5.0 mmol/L or 190 mg/dL); and mean total cholesterol concentration
National systems response	Proportion of eligible persons (aged 40+ with a 10-year cardiovascular risk ≥ 30%, including those with existing CVD) receiving drug therapy and counselling (including glycaemic control) to prevent heart attack and strokes
	Availability and affordability of quality, safe, and efficacious essential non-communicable disease medicines, including generics, and basic technologies in both public and private facilities
	Access to palliative care assessed by morphine-equivalent consumption of strong opioid analgesics (excluding methadone) per death from cancer
	Adoption of national policies that limit saturated fatty acids and virtually eliminate partially hydrogenated vegetable oils in the food supply, as appropriate, within the national context and national programmes
	Availability, as appropriate, if cost-effective and affordable, of vaccines against human papillomavirus, according to national programmes and policies
	Policies to reduce the impact on children of marketing of foods and non-alcoholic beverages high in saturated fats, trans fatty acids, free sugars or salt
	Vaccination coverage against hepatitis B virus monitored by number of third doses of hep-B vaccine administered to infants
	Proportion of women, 30–49, screened for cervical cancer at least once, or more often, and for lower or higher age groups according to national programmes or policies

were developed, as a basis for reporting back on progress to the UN General Assembly. Table 14.4 shows the time-bound commitments for 2015 and 2016, along with the ten progress indicators linked to these commitments.

Progress against those indicators was reported in the *NCD Progress Monitor 2015*.[11] This provides a global snapshot of achievements and challenges for countries taking action towards the voluntary NCD targets and the time-bound commitments (Table 14.5).

Table 14.4 Monitoring global progress: time-bound commitments and linked progress indicators

Time-bound commitment	10 progress indicators
By 2015, consider setting national targets for 2025 and process indicators based on national situations, taking into account the nine voluntary global targets for NCD, building on guidance provided by the World Health Organization, to focus on efforts to address the impacts of non-communicable diseases and to assess the progress made in the prevention and control of NCDs and their risk factors and determinants.	1. Member state has set time-bound national targets and indicators based on WHO guidance. 2. Member state has a functioning system for generating reliable cause-specific mortality data on a routine basis. 3. Member state has a STEPS survey or a comprehensive health examination survey every 5 years.
By 2015, consider developing or strengthening national multisectoral policies and plans to achieve the national targets by 2025, taking into account the WHO Global NCD Action Plan 2013–2020.	4. Member state has an operational multisectoral national strategy/action plan that integrates the major NCDs and their shared risk factors.
By 2016, as appropriate, reduce risk factors for NCDs and underlying social determinants through the implementation of interventions and policy options to create health-promoting environments, building on guidance set out in Appendix 3 to the WHO *Global NCD Action Plan 2013–2020*.	5. Member state has implemented the following four demand-reduction measures of the WHO *Framework Convention on Tobacco Control* (FCTC) at the highest level of achievement: a. Reduce affordability of tobacco products by increasing tobacco excise taxes. b. Create by law completely smoke-free environments in all indoor workplaces, public places, and public transport. c. Warn people of the dangers of tobacco and tobacco smoke through effective health warnings and mass media campaigns. d. Ban all forms of tobacco advertising, promotion, and sponsorship. 6. Member state has implemented, as appropriate according to national circumstances, the following three measures to reduce the harmful use of alcohol as per the WHO Global Strategy to Reduce the Harmful Use of Alcohol: a. Regulations over commercial and public availability of alcohol. b. Comprehensive restrictions or bans on alcohol advertising and promotions. c. Pricing policies such as excise tax increases on alcoholic beverages. 7. Member state has implemented the following four measures to reduce unhealthy diets: a. Adopted national policies to reduce population salt/sodium consumption. b. Adopted national policies that limit saturated fatty acids and virtually eliminate industrially-produced trans fatty acids in the food supply. c. WHO set of recommendations on marketing of foods and non-alcoholic beverages to children. d. Legislation /regulations fully implementing the International Code of Marketing of Breast-milk Substitutes. 8. Member state has implemented at least one recent national public awareness programme on diet and/ or physical activity.

(*continued*)

Table 14.4 Continued

Time-bound commitment	10 progress indicators
By 2016, as appropriate, strengthen and orient health systems to address the prevention and control of NCDs and the underlying social determinants through people-centred primary health care and universal health coverage throughout the life cycle, building on guidance set out in Appendix 3 to the WHO *Global NCD Action Plan 2013–2020*.	9. Member state has evidence-based national guidelines/protocols/standards for the management of major NCDs through a primary care approach, recognized/approved by government or competent authorities. 10. Member state has provision of drug therapy, including glycaemic control, and counselling for eligible persons at high risk to prevent heart attacks and strokes, with emphasis on the primary care level.

Table 14.5 Progress on implementation of the Global NCD Action Plan

Indicator	Fully met	Partially met	Not met
1. National NCD targets and indicators	59	29	69
2. Mortality data	70	51	73
3. Risk factor surveys	55	99	20
4. National NCD policy/strategy/action plan	64	23	86
5.a. Tobacco taxation	3	65	117
5.b. Tobacco smoke-free policies	48	76	70
5.c. Tobacco health warnings	42	93	59
5.d. Tobacco advertising bans	29	106	59
6.a. Alcohol availability regulations	30	146	3
6.b. Alcohol advertising and promotion bans	38	84	57
6.c. Alcohol pricing polices	42	98	37
7.a. Salt/sodium policies	62		98
7.b. Saturated fatty acids and trans-fats policies	40		118
7.c. Marketing to children restrictions	42		118
7.d. Marketing of breast-milk substitutes restrictions	72		60
8. Public awareness on diet and/or physical activity	119		41
9. Guidelines for the management of major NCDs	50	47	48
10. Drug therapy/counselling for high-risk persons	28	11	92

Reproduced with permission from **Bettcher D**. *Transforming the World: Promoting Healthy Lifestyles and NCDs Control* [presentation given at UN Sustainable Development Summit 2015, New York], http://www.who.int/nmh/publications/UN-Summit-Dir-PND-NCD-Progress-Monitor-2015.pdf?ua=1, accessed 10 Aug. 2016, Copyright © World Health Organization.

Acknowledgements

This chapter is largely drawn from the presentations by Dr Charlie Foster, Dr Paul Kelly, and Dr Gauden Galea, with case study material provided by Erin Hoare, Julianne Williams, and Dr Kremlin Wickramasinghe.

References

1. **World Health Organization.** Health impact assessment (HIA): Glossary of terms used, F–P. Available at: http://www.who.int/hia/about/glos/en/index1.html
2. **WHO Europe.** *Health Promotion Evaluation: Recommendations to Policy-Makers.* Report of the WHO European Working Group on Health Promotion Evaluation (E60706). Copenhagen: World Health Organization, 1998
3. **Colchero MA, Popkin BM, Rivera JA, Ng SW.** Beverage purchases from stores in Mexico under the excise tax on sugar sweetened beverages: observational study. *BMJ* 2016; **352**:h6704 http://dx.doi.org/10.1136/bmj.h6704
4. **Pan American Health Organization.** *Taxes on Sugar-Sweetened Beverages as a Public Health Strategy: The Experience of Mexico.* PAHO/WHO Regional Office for the Americas.
5. **Donaldson, E.** *Advocating for Sugar-Sweetened Beverage Taxation: A Case Study of Mexico.* Johns Hopkins Bloomberg School of Public Health.
6. **Smith JJ, Morgan PJ, Plotnikoff RC, Dally KA, Salmon J, Okely AD,** et al. Rationale and study protocol for the 'Active Teen Leaders Avoiding Screen-time' (ATLAS) group randomized controlled trial: an obesity prevention intervention for adolescent boys from schools in low-income communities. *Contemporary Clinical Trials* 2014; **37**(1):106–19.
7. **World Health Organization.** Country profiles, Sri Lanka. Available at: http://www.who.int/nmh/countries/lka_en.pdf?ua=1
8. **United Nations General Assembly.** Outcome document of the high-level meeting of the General Assembly on the comprehensive review and assessment of the progress achieved in the prevention and control of non-communicable diseases (A/RES/68/300). United Nations, 2014. Available at: http://www.who.int/entity/nmh/events/2014/a-res-68-300.pdf?ua=1.
9. **World Health Organization.** *Global Action Plan for the Prevention and Control of Noncommunicable Diseases, 2013-2020.* Geneva: World Health Organization, 2013.
10. **World Health Organization.** *Report of the First Dialogue Convened by the World Health Organization Global Coordination Mechanism on Noncommunicable Diseases.* Geneva: World Health Organization, 2015. Available at: http://www.who.int/global-coordination-mechanism/final_meeting_report_dialogue_ncd_development_april15_en.pdf?ua=1
11. **World Health Organization.** *Noncommunicable Diseases Progress Monitor 2015.* Geneva: World Health Organization, 2015.

Further Reading

Nutbeam D, Bauman A. *Evaluation in a Nutshell—A Practical Guide to the Evaluation of Health Promotion Programs.* Sydney: McGraw-Hill, 2006.

Rootman I, Goodstadt M, Hyndman B, McQueen DV, Potvin L, Springett J, Ziglio E. *Evaluation in Health Promotion—Principles and Perspectives.* WHO Regional Publications European Series, No. 92. World Health Organization: Copenhagen, 1992.

Chapter 15

Revisiting the stages of the policy cycle

15.1 The policy cycle for the prevention of NCDs

This book is structured around the policy cycle shown in Chapter 1 and repeated as Figure 15.1. It is suggested throughout this document that using the policy cycle is a good way of thinking about the steps necessary for effective non-communicable disease (NCD) prevention. The version of the policy cycle illustrated in Figure 15.1 is the simplest way of conceiving of the policy cycle; other, more complicated, ways can also be found.

To recap: the stages of the policy cycle are (1) problem definition; (2) solution generation; (3) resource mobilization and implementation; and (4) evaluation.

15.1.1 Problem definition

- See **Chapters 2–7**

In the case of NCD prevention this involves establishing both the nature and the extent of the problem of NCDs in a particular situation. But it also involves coming to an understanding of the causes of the problem (i.e. the risk factors for NCDs) and also of the causes of those causes (i.e. the wider determinants of health). This understanding needs to have a general dimension—i.e. with reference to the literature available—but also a more specific dimension, i.e. with reference to the particular context for which the NCD prevention is planned.

15.1.2 Solution generation

- **See Chapters 8–10**

This involves a general assessment of the evidence for the potential costs and benefits of particular interventions aimed at preventing NCDs but again with specific reference to the particular context for which NCD prevention is planned. It involves a consideration of the potential barriers to, and facilitators of, different solutions. Solutions may have a low cost–benefit ratio (be cost-effective) but still have too small a benefit to have much impact or be too costly to carry out on a wide scale if, for example, the problem is widespread. Solutions may have either detrimental or beneficial effects on health inequalities.

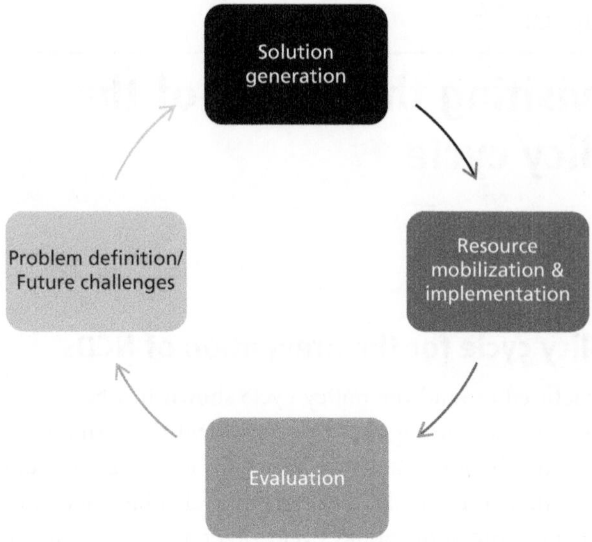

Figure 15.1 The policy cycle.

Some solutions may be controversial because they involve measures which affect personal autonomy and choice so a consideration of the ethical and political dimensions of different solutions will be necessary. Because many solutions are generally possible, solution generation involves a prioritization of possible actions—bearing in mind that it is likely that many will be needed. Finally, solution generation involves the development of a plan.

15.1.3 Resource mobilization and implementation

◆ **See Chapters 11–13**

The resources needed to implement interventions designed to prevent NCDs can be divided into money and people. Money is often needed for the material aspect of interventions: the infrastructure, equipment, salaries, etc. Interventions invariably involve people—to plan for and carry out the interventions—and these people will require training to enhance their knowledge and skills, but also leading, motivating, connecting with others, etc. One aspect of mobilizing human resources is building capacity. Implementation can be simple or challenging, depending on the nature of the intervention and, again, context.

15.1.4 Evaluation

◆ **See Chapter 14**

Evaluations can be specifically designed to assess whether the interventions for preventing NCDs, once implemented, meet their aims and objectives or to generate evidence that is generalizable to other situations. A good way of viewing evaluation is to see it as the attempt to ask a series of questions: what were the costs of the interventions and what were their benefits (both intended and unintended)? What worked for whom and in what circumstances? How were any costs accrued and any benefits achieved?

It is clearly the case that NCD prevention—as actually practiced—does not always follow the stages of the policy cycle in a strict sequence. For instance, evaluation ideally needs to be built into an NCD prevention programme from the outset and should begin prior to the implementation stage if at all possible.

The cycle as portrayed suggests that all four stages need to be completed before redefining the problem and starting again. This is clearly not the case. For example, when generating solutions, it might turn out that the problem needs further definition before any implementation takes place. There is no need to wait for a full evaluation of the effectiveness of a possible action if it has already been discovered that it is not addressing an important need.

Hindsight, is as they say, a wonderful thing! And issues uncovered in later stages of the cycle, had they been known about previously, might have influenced decision-making at earlier stages. For instance, issues uncovered during the implementation stage are likely to be highly relevant to solution generation.

However, having followed all the steps in the policy cycle, it is very probable that preventive interventions—either in part or in whole—will need revising, either because they have worked or because they have failed, or more likely worked up to a point. It will be necessary, in other words, to start again and to revisit each stage of the policy cycle in the light of the experiences of all involved and the results of any monitoring and evaluation that have taken place .

In revisiting these steps, it will be necessary to ask some new questions about the problem and the solution before proceeding to a new round of implementation.

Problem definition

- Has the problem changed in any way and if so how?
- If the problem has changed, was this a result of any interventions implemented or of factors beyond your control?
- What do the results of the evaluation tell you about the nature of the problem post implementation of the intervention(s)?

Solution generation

- Did the interventions work? What effect did they have on the problem and, if so, what worked for whom and in what circumstances?
- Is there evidence from elsewhere that has changed your views on the effectiveness of possible solutions?

In the development of NCD prevention programmes and projects it is clearly possible to see how interventions have been modified by reflection on these questions, and there are examples throughout the previous chapters. In Chapter 2, for example, the development of NCD targets, indicators, and an operational policy in Zambia is clearly informed by the answer to the question 'Has the problem changed in any way?' While the country continues to face a considerable disease burden from infectious disease and undernutrition, it is being forced to adapt to an emerging burden of chronic disease, including overweight, obesity, and diet-related NCDs. The case study on public health impacts of austerity, in Chapter 4, describes how both Greece and Iceland were faced with changing public health contexts as a result of economic crises. Similarly, the case studies in Chapter 6 on advocacy on nutrition labelling and salt reduction describe situations in which the political context for the interventions changed—in both cases, the need for a more independent regulatory regime in the UK to ensure safe and healthy food in the wake of the bovine spongiform encephalopathy (BSE) scandal helped shape an environment more receptive to advocacy on those issues. In Chapter 7, a case study describes how the US Behavioural Risk Factor Surveillance Survey was able to change understanding of the obesity problem—even if the problem itself had not changed—by uncovering the worrying prevalence of severe obesity (BMI > 40), and the important implications for health and other services from this changed understanding of the obesity epidemic.

The further examples in Box 15.1 and Box 15.2 illustrate how emerging evidence at different stages of the policy cycle had an impact on policy interventions.

When it comes to new rounds of resource mobilization, implementation and evaluation, it will be worthwhile reflecting upon what lessons might be learnt from previous rounds. For example, when considering a new round of interventions it will be worth asking, 'What were the issues the issues faced during resource mobilization last time and how could implementation be improved?', and 'Were the methods used during the evaluation last time adequate and if not how could they be improved?'

Box 15.1 Reducing exposure to second-hand smoke in the UK—How evidence and advocacy changed the approach

By 1998, the then UK government accepted that passive smoking was harmful and that there was a need to reduce exposure to second-hand smoke. The government was committed to dealing with the problem, but the 1998 White Paper proposed a market-led voluntary approach (the Public Places Charter) with an opt-out for the hospitality industry and an emphasis on ventilation as a solution.

By 2003, it was clear that this approach was ineffective—a 2003 report to the Department of Health found that only 43% of pubs complied with the charter, that one in three pubs was completely non-compliant, and that 56% of those premises that complied with the charter still allowed smoking throughout.

Campaigners in England, therefore, adopted a new approach which involved advocating for smoke-free legislation by building, over time, a coalition of organizations in order to exert pressure to lever political action.[1] This was achieved by promoting evidence-based arguments and generating media coverage in order to build positive public opinion. Important reports were published to set out the evidence for going smoke-free, medical and scientific experts expressed their concerns, and maximum publicity was obtained for new research publications on second-hand smoke. Research was produced to challenge some of the potential barriers presented to implementing smoke-free legislation—to show, for example, that an exemption for pubs that do not serve food could widen inequalities or to challenge the assertion that a ban on smoking in public places would harm children by leading to more smoking at home. Polling was conducted to assess public attitudes and also to foster debate—through an online/phone consultation—and raise awareness. A rise in the level of public support in England for smoke-free pubs and bars, reaching two-thirds by December 2005, was important for the campaign's success. Other important elements of the campaign included developing local action by working with local authorities, working with trade unions, employers, and lawyers, and, finally, developing support in parliament. Successful implementation of smoke-free legislation in other jurisdictions (e.g. Ireland) was also influential.

In 2005 the government published the Health Improvement and Protection Bill, which included the proposal to ban smoking in workplaces, but still included exemptions for pubs that did not serve food and private members clubs. The parliamentary health committee denounced the exemptions as 'unfair, unjust, inefficient and unworkable' and argued that bar workers also need protection. Parliamentary support was crucial in the end to securing a vote for comprehensive smoke-free legislation, including pubs that do not serve food. The legislation came into force in July 2007.

Source: data from **Arnott D**, **Dockrell M**, **Sandford A**, and **Willmore I**. Comprehensive smoke-free legislation in England: how advocacy won the day. *Tobacco Control*, Volume 16, Issue 6, pp. 423–428, Copyright © 2007 BMJ Publishing Group Ltd.

Box 15.2 Action to tackle smoking amongst Indigenous people in Australia

There had long been evidence to indicate high rates of Indigenous smoking in Australia. A 1994 survey of over 15,700 Indigenous Australians found that 49.7% of respondents over the age of 13 years smoked daily. A survey conducted a decade later (2004–5) similarly found that 50% of Indigenous Australians aged 18 years and over (n = 10,439) were current daily smokers.

Despite these data, there had been an absence of significant government investment specifically geared towards reducing Indigenous smoking rates prior to 2008. For instance, an expenditure analysis revealed that smoking was a focus in only 2 and 3% of Indigenous-specific alcohol and other drug intervention projects in 1999–2000 and 2006–7, respectively.

Research suggests that the increased political attention given to Indigenous smoking in the late 2000s was the product of a confluence of three factors:

(1) the publication of evidence showing that tobacco was the single largest contributor to the 'gap' between Indigenous and non-Indigenous health outcomes;

(2) the success of and advocacy campaign called 'Closing the Gap' which was led by Indigenous and civil society groups, and supported by the incoming Labour Government; and

(3) the appointment of a Health Minister committed to tobacco control, perhaps best evidenced in that government's decision to make Australia the first country in the world to introduce a law to mandate plain cigarette packaging.

The first of these elements—evidence that tobacco was the biggest contributor to excess mortality among Indigenous Australians—was cited as particularly important in raising the political prominence of Indigenous smoking. The study in question, by Vos and colleagues, used the burden of disease methodology, to examine the health gap between Indigenous and non-Indigenous Australians and found that the Indigenous health gap accounted for 59% of the total burden of disease for Indigenous Australians, thus pointing to enormous potential for health gain.[2] Analysis of the main risk factors contributing to the gap found that tobacco was the biggest single contributor, accountable for 17% of the health gap disability-adjusted life years (DALYs) in 2003.

On 20 March 2008 the Indigenous Tobacco Control Initiative was announced by then Prime Minister Kevin Rudd at an Indigenous Health Equality Summit. Through the Initiative, the Government committed AU$14.5 million over four years to:

- train Indigenous health staff in smoking cessation strategies;
- trial innovative community interventions, including culturally appropriate communication activities, in five or six pilot sites; and
- support Indigenous tobacco control research to 'help build the evidence base around what works'.

The Tackling Indigenous Smoking Measure formed part of the National Partnership Agreement on Closing the Gap in Indigenous Health Outcomes, signed in December 2008, and the government committed AU$100.61 million to reduce Indigenous smoking rates and the burden of tobacco-related disease through a number of measures including:

- establishing a national network of tobacco action coordinators;
- developing a national Indigenous tobacco action training programme for health workers and community educators;
- strategies to improve delivery of smoking cessation services, including nicotine replacement therapy;

- social marketing campaigns to reduce smoking-related harms among Aboriginal and Torres Strait Islander peoples; and
- enhancing a telephone advice service to provide culturally sensitive services.

This initiative proved challenging to implement but involved both commitment to expenditure on the part of the Government and enhancing capacity within the workforce—partly by recruiting Indigenous people to take part in implementing the programme amongst their peers and partly through additional training for them and others in smoking cessation.

Evaluation of interventions was built into the programme at an early stage so experience gained during the early phases of the programme was used to inform subsequent stages and a redesigned programme was introduced in 2015–16 with an emphasis on flexible approaches for regional tobacco control.

Sources: Vujcich D. *Where there is no evidence, and where evidence is not enough: an analysis of policy-making to reduce the prevalence of Australian indigenous smoking* (PhD Thesis), University of Oxford, UK, 2014, https://ora.ox.ac.uk/objects/uuid:f2d8fbe9-b506-4747-993a-0657cb1df7bf, accessed 10 Aug. 2016.

Vujcich D, Rayner M, Allender S, Fitzpatrick R. When there Is not enough evidence and when evidence is not enough:an Australian indigenous smoking policy sudy. *Frontiers in Public Health* 2016; 4:228.

15.2 **Conclusion**

The policy cycle should be seen as exactly that—a cycle, rather than a linear process with a defined start and finish. For effective policy-making new evidence, understanding, and reflection—whether as a result of interventions implemented or external factors—should feed into the cycle at different stages in order for policy to adapt and evolve.

The previous chapters have attempted to illustrate the many different elements that can feed into the policy cycle, and the various forms that these might take. These can range from the results of a specific evaluation of a particular intervention to a change in public opinion, and therefore political will, as a result of sustained advocacy. In addition to academic research on effectiveness, evidence from other countries' experience, modelling exercises to predict the potential impact of interventions, and analyses of cost-effectiveness can all usefully feed into the policy cycle.

NCDs are multifactorial conditions, with complex causal webs, and it is clear that there is no single, simple blueprint for their prevention. Such complex problems require a sophisticated mix of solutions, reflecting the specific context. The theoretical background, practical pointers, and country case studies described in the previous chapters, however, should help equip policy-makers, researchers, health advocates, and students with the knowledge and tools to contribute to reducing the burden of death and disability associated with NCDs.

Acknowledgements

This chapter is based on a presentation by Professor Mike Rayner and case study information provided by Daniel Vujcich.

References

1. **Arnott D, Dockrell M, Sandford A, Willmore I.** Comprehensive smoke-free legislation in England: how advocacy won the day. *Tobacco Control* 2007; **16**(6):423–8.
2. **Vos T, Barker B, Begg S, Stanley L, Lopez AD.** Burden of disease and injury in Aboriginal and Torres Strait Islander Peoples: the Indigenous health gap. *International Journal of Epidemiology* 2009; **38**(2):470–7.

Index

Tables are indicated by an italic *t*, boxes are indicated by an italic *b* and figures by an italic *f*, following the page number.